A COLOR HANDBOOK

Infectious Diseases
of the Dog and Cat

A COLOR HANDBOOK

Infectious Diseases of the Dog and Cat

Edited by

J SCOTT WEESE DVM DVSc DACVIM

Ontario Veterinary College
University of Guelph
Guelph, Ontario
Canada

MICHELLE EVASON BSc DVM DACVIM

Atlantic Veterinary College
University of Prince Edward Island
Charlottetown, Prince Edward Island
Canada

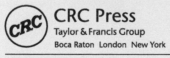

CRC Press
Taylor & Francis Group
Boca Raton London New York

CRC Press is an imprint of the
Taylor & Francis Group, an **informa** business

CRC Press
Taylor & Francis Group
6000 Broken Sound Parkway NW, Suite 300
Boca Raton, FL 33487-2742

First issued in paperback 2023

ISBN 13: 978-1-03-257010-5 (pbk)
ISBN 13: 978-1-4987-7551-9 (hbk)

DOI: 10.1201/9780429186646

Publisher's Note
The publisher has gone to great lengths to ensure the quality of this reprint but points out that some imperfections in the original copies may be apparent.

Visit the Taylor & Francis Web site at
http://www.taylorandfrancis.com

and the CRC Press Web site at
http://www.crcpress.com

To my parents, Paul and Lynda, for providing the foundation for my life and career. To Heather, Beth, Amy and Erin, for helping me keep priorities in perspective.

JSW

For the mammals in my universe (4 footed and 2), who encourage and support my taking on challenges … and to Amelie, Teghan and Jay, for never doubting my reasons to do so.

Thank you to my co-editor, for inviting me to play in the sandbox, despite knowing what would ensue.

ME

CONTENTS

The field of infectious diseases can be fascinating, daunting, frustrating and sometimes scary. All these make the area rewarding and challenging, descriptors that apply equally to the book writing process.

This book was written with the clinician in mind, and is an attempt to balance relevant background and guidance, and to optimize efficiency. As a handbook, it is meant to provide a pathway for clinicians through this complex field, by highlighting the most clinically relevant aspects of a wide range of diseases and granting them consideration for placement on dog and cat differential lists. Readers are referred to various other sources for depth of content (e.g. pathophysiology) beyond the scope (and page count) of this effort.

After considerable discussion, a system-based structure was used for organization, as opposed to a pathogen-based approach, i.e. viral, parasitic, bacterial, etc. As such, the book has been structured with chapters for major clinically affected systems (respiratory, gastrointestinal, genitourinary, neurological and skin), and includes a catch-all multisystem chapter for infectious diseases that refuse to be classified into single systems.

An additional adjective that can never be overlooked when discussing infectious diseases is "evolving". Infectious diseases continue to emerge and change, and our ability to understand, diagnose, treat and prevent disease changes in concert. This is another appealing and challenging nature of this dynamic field, and one that makes writing similarly challenging. Undoubtedly, information pertaining to diseases covered in this book will change. That is an inherent predicament of any constantly evolving field. We have attempted to ensure that all content is as accurate as possible at the time of writing, but are not under any illusions that some will change over time. However, we expect (and hope) that the material provided will assist clinicians with their understanding of, and ability to communicate about, infectious diseases of the dog and cat.

J Scott Weese
Michelle Evason

Darcy B Adin, DVM, DACVIM (Cardiology)
College of Veterinary Medicine
University of Florida
Gainesville, Florida, USA

**Julie Armstrong, DVM, MVSc, DACVIM
(Small Animal) (SAIM)**
True North Veterinary Diagnostics Inc.
Langley, British Columbia, Canada

**Vanessa Barrs, BVSc(Hons), PhD,
MVetClinStud, FANZCVS (Feline Medicine),
GradCertEd(Higher Ed)**
Sydney School of Veterinary Science and
 Marie Bashir Institute of Infectious Diseases
 and Biosecurity
University of Sydney
Sydney, New South Wales, Australia

Andrew S Bowman, MS, DVM, PhD, DACVPM
The Ohio State University
Columbus, Ohio, USA

Lisa Carioto, DVM, DVSc, DACVIM
Mobile Internal Medicine Referral Service
Montreal, Quebec, Canada

Kenneth Cockwill, BSc, DVM, DACVIM (SAIM)
Guardian Veterinary Centre
Edmonton, Alberta, Canada

Gary Conboy, DVM, PhD, DACVM
Atlantic Veterinary College
University of Prince Edward Island
Charlottetown, Prince Edward Island, Canada

Craig Datz, DVM, MS, DABVP, DACVN
Royal Canin USA
Columbia, Missouri, USA

Michelle Evason, BSc, DVM, DACVIM
Atlantic Veterinary College
University of Prince Edward Island
Charlottetown, Prince Edward Island, Canada

**M Casey Gaunt, DVM, MVetSc,
DACVIM (SAIM)**
Saskatoon, Saskatchewan, Canada

**Beth Hanselman, DVM, DVSc,
DACVIM (SAIM)**
Mississauga Oakville Veterinary Emergency
 Hospital
Oakville, Ontario, Canada

**Johanna Heseltine, DVM, MS, DACVIM
(SAIM)**
College of Veterinary Medicine and Biomedical
 Sciences
Texas A&M University
College Station, Texas, USA

**Roger A Hostutler, DVM, MS, DACVIM
(SAIM)**
MedVet Columbus
Columbus, Ohio, USA

Lee Jane Huffman, DVM, DAVDC
Head of Dentistry
Mississauga–Oakville Veterinary Emergency
 Hospital and Referral Services
Oakville, Ontario, Canada

Susan Kilborn, DVM, DVSc, DACVIM
Orleans Veterinary Hospital
Ottawa, Ontario, Canada
and
Antech Diagnostics
Fountain Valley, California, USA

Anette Loeffler, DrMedVet, PhD, DVD, DipECVD, MRCVS
Royal Veterinary College,
University of London
North Mymms, Hertfordshire, UK

Charlie Pye, BSc, DVM, DVSc, DACVD
Atlantic Veterinary College
University of Prince Edward Island
Charlottetown, Price Edward Island, Canada

Christine R Rutter, DVM, DACVECC
College of Veterinary Medicine & Biomedical Sciences
Texas A&M University
College Station, Texas, USA

Margie Scherk, DVM, DABVP (Feline)
catsINK
Vancouver, British Columbia, Canada

Robert G Sherding, DVM, DACVIM
The Ohio State University College of Veterinary
    Medicine
Columbus, Ohio, USA

Ameet Singh, DVM, DVSc, DACVS
Ontario Veterinary College
University of Guelph
Guelph, Ontario, Canada

Dennis Spann, DVM, DACVIM (SAIM)
Sacramento Area Veterinary Internal Medicine
Roseville, California, USA

John Speciale, DVM, DACVIM (Neurology)
Neurology Consultant
Rochester, New York, USA

Jason W Stull, VMD, MPVM, PhD, DACVPM
Atlantic Veterinary College,
University of Prince Edward Island
Charlottetown, Price Edward Island, Canada
and
College of Veterinary Medicine,
The Ohio State University
Columbus, Ohio, USA

Susan Taylor, DVM, DACVIM (SAIM)
Western College of Veterinary Medicine
University of Saskatchewan
Saskatoon, Saskatchewan, Canada

Jinelle A Webb, DVM, MSc, DVSc, DACVIM (SAIM)
Mississauga-Oakville Veterinary Emergency Hospital
Oakville, Ontario, Canada

J Scott Weese, DVM DVSc DACVIM
Ontario Veterinary College
University of Guelph
Guelph, Ontario, Canada

J Paul Woods, DVM, MS, DACVIM (IM, Oncology)
Ontario Veterinary College
University of Guelph
Guelph, Ontario, Canada

ABCB1	ATP-binding cassette subfamily B member 1 (gene)		EEEV	eastern equine encephalitis virus
AE	alveolar echinococcosis		ELISA	enzyme-linked immunosorbent assay
Ag	antigen		FA	fluorescent antibody (test)
A:G	albumin:globulin (ratio)		FCoV	feline coronavirus
AGID	agar gel immunodiffusion		FCV	feline calicivirus
AI	artificial insemination		FDP	fibrin degradation product
ALP	alkaline phosphatase		FECAVA	Federation of Companion Animal Veterinary Associations
ALT	alanine aminotransferase		FeLV	feline leukemia virus
AMB	amphotericin B		FeSV	feline sarcoma virus
APTT	activated partial thromboplastin time		FHV	feline herpesvirus
ARDS	acute respiratory distress syndrome		FIC	feline idiopathic cystitis
AST	aspartate transaminase		FISH	fluorescent *in situ* hybridization
BAL	bronchoalveolar lavage		FIV	feline immunodeficiency virus
BoNT	botulinum neurotoxin		FNA	fine-needle aspirate/aspiration
CAV-2	canine adenovirus type 2		FPV	feline panleukopenia virus
CBC	complete blood count		FURTD	feline upper respiratory tract disease
CDV	canine distemper virus		GABA	gamma-aminobutyric acid
CECoV	canine enteric coronavirus		GGT	gamma-glutamyl transferase
CFU	colony-forming units		GHLO	gastric *Helicobacter*-like organism
CHF	congestive heart failure		GI	gastrointestinal
CIRDC	canine infectious respiratory disease complex		GM	galactomannan (*Aspergillus*)
			GMS	Grocott's methenamine silver (stain)
CIV	canine influenza virus		GnRH	gonadotropin-releasing hormone
CK	creatine kinase		H	hemagglutinin (influenza virus)
CLG	canine leproid granuloma (syndrome)		H&E	hematoxylin and eosin
CME	canine monocytic ehrlichiosis		HIV	human immunodeficiency virus
CNS	central nervous system		IBD	inflammatory bowel disease
CPIV	canine parainfluenza virus		IFA	immunofluorescent assay
CPV	canine parvovirus		IFN	interferon
CSD	cat scratch disease		Ig	immunoglobulin
CSF	cerebrospinal fluid		IHC	immunohistochemical
CT	computed tomography		IM	intramuscular(ly)
CTVT	canine transmissible venereal tumor		IMHA	immune-mediated hemolytic anemia
DIA	disseminated invasive aspergillosis		IN	intranasal
DIC	disseminated intravascular coagulation		IRIS	International Renal Interest Society
DNA	deoxyribonucleic acid		ITP	immune-mediated thrombocytopenia
EDTA	ethylenediaminetetraacetic acid		ITZ	itraconazole

IV	intravenous(ly)	**PO**	orally (*per os*)
KCS	keratoconjunctivitis sicca	**PT**	prothrombin time
LMN	lower motor neuron	**PTT**	partial thromboplastin time
LPHS	leptospiral pulmonary hemorrhage syndrome	**PV**	papillomavirus
		q12h	every 12 hours (etc.)
LUTD	lower urinary tract disease	**RMSF**	Rocky Mountain spotted fever
MAC	*Mycobacterium avium-intracellulare* complex	**RNA**	ribonucleic acid
		rRNA	ribosomal ribonucleic acid
MALDI-TOF	matrix-assisted laser desorption/ionization–time of flight (mass spectrometry)	**RSAT**	rapid slide agglutination test
		RT-PCR	reverse transcriptase (or real-time) polymerase chain reaction
MAT	microscopic agglutination test	**SC**	subcutaneous(ly)
MDR1	multidrug resistance-1 (gene)	**Se**	(test) sensitivity
MIC	minimal inhibitory concentration	**SIRS**	systemic inflammatory response syndrome
MLV	modified live virus (vaccine)		
MODS	multiple organ dysfunction syndrome	**SN**	serum neutralizing (antibody)
MRI	magnetic resonance imaging	**SNA**	sinonasal aspergillosis
MRSA	meticillin-resistant *Staphylococcus aureus*	**SOA**	sino-orbital aspergillosis
		Sp	(test) specificity
MRSP	meticillin-resistant *Staphylococcus pseudintermedius*	**spp.**	species (plural)
		SSI	surgical site infection
N	neuraminidase (influenza virus)	**subspp.**	subspecies (plural)
NHPH	non-*Helicobacter pylori* helicobacter	**TAT**	tube agglutination test
NSAID	non-steroidal anti-inflammatory drug	**TLA**	transthoracic lung aspiration
		TTL	transtracheal lavage
NTM	non-tuberculous mycobacteria	**TTW**	transtracheal wash/aspiration
OU	in each eye (*oculus uterque*)	**UP:C**	urine protein:creatinine ratio
PAS	periodic acid–Schiff	**URT**	upper respiratory tract
PCR	polymerase chain reaction	**UTI**	urinary tract infection
PEP	post-exposure prophylaxis (rabies)	**VSD**	virulent systemic disease (feline calicivirus)
PFK	phosphofructokinase		
PG	prostaglandin	**WNV**	West Nile virus
PI	post-infection	**WSAVA**	World Small Animal Veterinary Association
PLN	protein-losing nephropathy		

CHAPTER 1

RESPIRATORY DISEASES

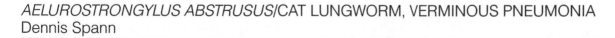

AELUROSTRONGYLUS ABSTRUSUS/CAT LUNGWORM, VERMINOUS PNEUMONIA
Dennis Spann

Definition
The metastrongyloid nematode *Aelurostrongylus abstrusus* causes lower airway disease in cats.[1] Infected cats cough secondary to inflammation from the parasite lodging in the terminal bronchioles and alveolar ducts.

Etiology and pathogenesis
Aelurostrongylus infestation occurs when a cat (definitive host) or dog consumes an intermediate (snail or slug) or paratenic host (frogs, lizards, birds, and rodents) with encysted larvae. The larvae travel through the lymphatics before entering the lung parenchyma and bronchioles. They penetrate the lung tissue deeply but extrude eggs into the bronchioles and alveolar ducts. The eggs then hatch into larvae, which travel up the mucociliary escalator and are swallowed; they exit via the gastrointestinal tract and pass into the environment (**Fig. 1.1**). Intermediate hosts, snails and slugs (**Fig. 1.2**), are penetrated by the L1 larvae, which then develop into L3 larvae. The intermediate host may be consumed by a paratenic host, in which the larvae encyst. Infection of the definitive host can occur via ingestion of the intermediate or paratenic host.[1, 2]

Geography
The parasite occurs worldwide.

Incidence and risk factors
The prevalence of larvae in feces has been estimated at 1.2% in indoor owned cats and up to 50% in free roaming cats in some areas.[1–3] Risk factors include hunting and increased time outdoors. Older cats may have higher prevalence due to cumulative hunting time.

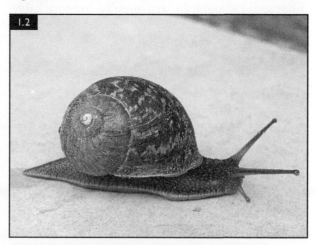

Fig. 1.1 L1 *Aelurostrongylus abstrusus* larvae from fecal float. (Courtesy of Drs Donato Traversa and Angela Di Cesare)

Fig. 1.2 *Cornu aspersum*, the garden snail, is a common intermediate host for *A. abstrusus*. (Courtesy of Rasbak, https://commons.wikimedia.org/wiki/File:Cornu_aspersum_(Segrijnslak).jpg)

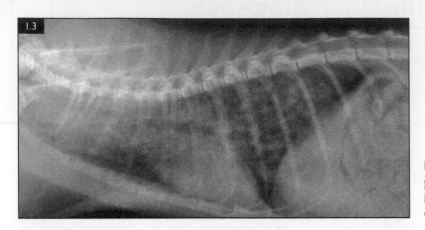

Fig. 1.3 Radiograph of a feline patient with a severe *A. abstrusus* infection. (Courtesy of Dr Maria Grazia Pennisi)

Clinical signs

Cats may be clinically normal if there is a low parasite burden. Disease is characterized by varying degrees of coughing, wheezing, respiratory distress, open-mouth breathing, abdominal effort and mucopurulent nasal discharge.[3] Debility and even death can occur in rare cases with severe infections or comorbidities.[3]

Diagnosis

Diagnosis is most often based on detection of larvae in feces via the Baermann technique. The larvae are approximately 360–400 µm in length and the tail ends in a kink with a dorsal subterminal spine (**Fig. 1.1**). Fecal floatation is less sensitive than Baermann testing, with zinc sulfate flotation having a higher yield than sucrose flotation. Thoracic radiographs are usually unremarkable, but a nodulointerstitial pattern can be present in severe cases (**Fig. 1.3**).

Therapy

Fenbendazole (50 mg/kg/day, PO, for 10–14 days), ivermectin (400 µg/kg, SC, twice at a 3-week interval) or an emodepside 2.1%/praziquantel 8.6% spot-on formulation can be used.[3, 4] Anti-inflammatory doses of a corticosteroid can be used in severe infections.

Prognosis/complications

Prognosis is fair with treatment. In rare instances, heavy infestations may cause tissue damage, pneumothorax or hydrothorax.

Prevention

Prevention of predation (hunting) is the main control measure.

BACTERIAL PNEUMONIA
J Scott Weese

Definition

Bacterial pneumonia is an infectious process occurring within lung parenchyma.

Etiology and pathogenesis

Disease occurs secondary to events such as progression of upper respiratory tract infection, aspiration, foreign body migration and hematogenous spread. The end result is a bacterial load within the lung parenchyma and airways beyond a level that inherent protective mechanisms and the immune system can manage. Factors such as the degree of bacterial burden, presence of debris (e.g. aspirated material), compromise of local immune defenses and systemic immunocompromise influence whether disease occurs, and its severity.

A range of bacteria can be involved, most commonly Enterobacteriaceae (e.g. *Escherichia coli*, *Enterobacter* spp., *Klebsiella* spp.), *Pasteurella* spp., *Bordetella bronchiseptica*, *Streptococcus* spp. and anaerobes.[5] *Mycoplasma* spp. are commonly identified but their role in disease is unclear, particularly in dogs.

Incidence and risk factors

The incidence is poorly described. It is a relatively common problem in dogs with megaesophagus, diseases that compromise laryngeal or pharyngeal function, or underlying pulmonary diseases (e.g. ciliary dyskinesia, bronchiectasis). Secondary pneumonia is uncommon following viral or bacterial upper respiratory tract infection but will develop in a small percentage of cases.

Clinical signs

It is important to differentiate upper respiratory tract infection from pneumonia. Dogs and cats with pneumonia typically have more severe signs. These indicate systemic disease and disease of the pulmonary parenchyma, and include fever, lethargy, decreased appetite, increased respiratory rate and effort, and auscultable crackles and wheezes. Signs of systemic inflammation may also be present.

Diagnosis

Clinical signs can be strongly suggestive of bacterial pneumonia, but radiographs are important for confirmation, to characterize the disease (and potential etiology) and to provide a baseline for monitoring response to treatment (**Figs. 1.4–1.6**). A lag between clinical signs and radiographic changes can occur, and initial radiographs may be normal or appear discordant with clinical severity.

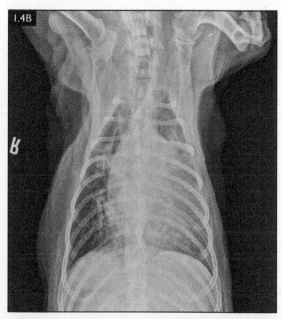

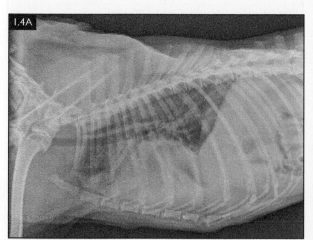

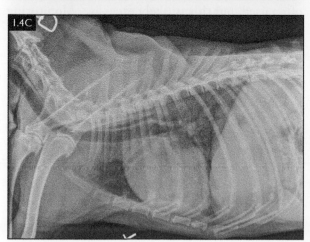

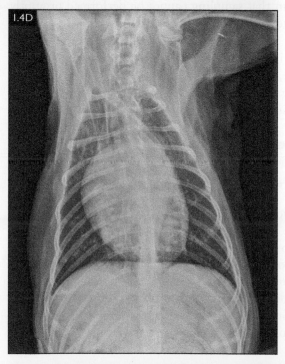

Fig. 1.4A–D Lateral and ventrodorsal radiographs of a dog with doxycycline-responsive pneumonia of unknown etiology before treatment (A, B) and six days later (C, D). Note the severe multilobar alveolar pattern that was present initially, most prominently in the left cranial lung lobe. (Courtesy of Atlantic Veterinary College)

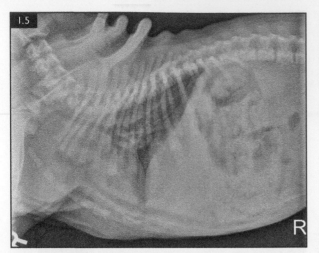

Fig. 1.5 Radiograph showing severe tracheal narrowing and concurrent bronchoalveolar pneumonia in a bulldog puppy with severe respiratory compromise. (Courtesy of Atlantic Veterinary College)

Table 1.1 **Antimicrobial dosing recommendations for bacterial pneumonia**	
DRUG	**DOSE**
Ampicillin	22–30 mg/kg IV IM q8h
Amoxicillin	22 mg/kg PO q8h
Clindamycin	Dogs: 10 mg/kg PO SC q12h Cats: 10–15 mg/kg PO SC q12h
Doxycycline	5 mg/kg PO q12h 10 mg/kg PO q24h
Enrofloxacin	Dogs: 10–20 mg/kg PO IM IV q24h Cats: 5 mg/kg PO IM IV q24h (avoid use in cats whenever possible)
Marbofloxacin	2.7–5.5 mg/kg PO q24h
Pradofloxacin	Tablets: 5 mg/kg PO q24h Oral suspension (cats): 7.5 mg/kg PO q24h

A CBC should be obtained as a baseline, to assess the degree of systemic response and provide a baseline for monitoring. A lower airway sample should ideally be collected for cytology and culture. The deeper the sample, the better, but transtracheal, endotracheal and bronchoalveolar lavage samples are all reasonable.[6] Samples are optimally collected before antimicrobials are administered, but treatment should not be delayed when patient stability or logistical factors mean that sampling cannot be performed promptly. Anaerobic culture should be considered in all cases and is particularly important when aspiration or a foreign body is suspected. In animals with severe disease, monitoring blood gases and oxygen saturation may be required to evaluate the need for (or response to) supplemental oxygen therapy.

Therapy

Antimicrobials should be administered promptly, along with supportive care. Doxycycline is a reasonable choice in patients with mild pneumonia but no evidence of sepsis (*Table 1.1*). With more advanced disease or evidence of systemic involvement, broader spectrum treatment is indicated, such as a fluoroquinolone in combination with either ampicillin or clindamycin. If *Streptococcus zooepidemicus* is the cause, either ampicillin or amoxicillin alone would be adequate.

Supportive treatment is indicated, based on severity of disease. Anti-inflammatories have been poorly

investigated in dogs and cats with pneumonia but should be considered. This could consist of NSAIDs, anti-inflammatory doses of corticosteroids (e.g. prednisone 0.5 mg/kg) or inhaled corticosteroids.

Duration of treatment is poorly understood. It has been recommended that treatment be reassessed after 10–14 days, to determine response and assist in deciding on the duration of antimicrobial therapy.[6] Four to six weeks of treatment is often used, but this is likely excessive. Monitoring CBC and radiographs can help to assess the response and antimicrobial treatment duration; however, infection likely resolves before radiographic resolution.

Prognosis/complications

Prognosis is highly dependent on the severity of infection and rapidity of progress by the time of treatment. In general, the prognosis is good. The prognosis is worse in animals with rapidly progressive disease (e.g. *S. zooepidemicus* hemorrhagic pneumonia), advanced age or comorbidities.

Prevention

Given that bacterial pneumonia is typically a secondary problem, preventing primary causes is important. This can include vaccination against upper respiratory tract pathogens and control of diseases that predispose to aspiration.

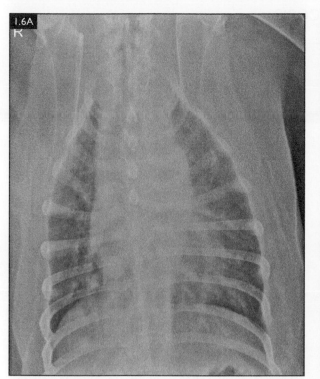

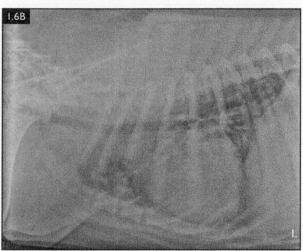

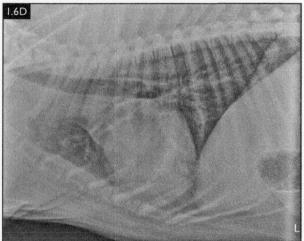

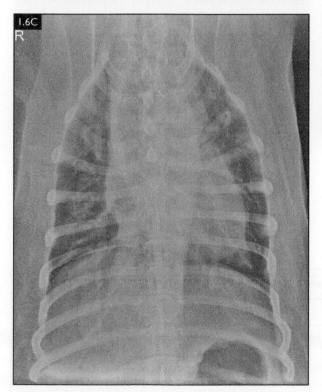

Fig. 1.6A–D Radiographs of a dog with suspected aspiration pneumonia. A diffuse alveolar pulmonary pattern, worse in the middle right lung lobe, is present initially (A, B), with substantial improvement 2 months later (C, D). (Courtesy of Atlantic Veterinary College)

BLASTOMYCES DERMATITIDIS/BLASTOMYCOSIS
M Casey Gaunt and Michelle Evason

Definition
Blastomycosis is a systemic fungal disease caused by the dimorphic fungus *Blastomyces dermatitidis*. It is most commonly diagnosed in dogs and humans, and is rare in cats.

Etiology and pathogenesis
Blastomyces dermatitidis is a dimorphic yeast that has two life phases, the infective mycelial form and the yeast form (*Table 1.2*).[7–9] Once within the animal, the mycelial phase transitions into the yeast form and pyogranulomatous inflammation occurs. Typically, *B. dermatitidis* replicates in the lungs and causes pulmonary disease. It may also travel through the blood to other tissues and organs and cause disseminated disease. Pyogranulomatous inflammation results at affected sites, most commonly the lungs, skin, eyes, bone and CNS.

Geography
Blastomyces dermatitidis has a relatively wide distribution in North America, including the Mississippi, Missouri and Ohio river valleys, the mid-Atlantic states, and southern Saskatchewan, Manitoba, Quebec and Ontario. High-risk areas tend to be focally identified within endemic regions. The disease has also been reported in Africa, India, Europe and Central America.

Incidence and risk factors
Dogs at greatest risk for developing blastomycosis are sexually intact, male, large breed dogs aged 1–5 years that live in endemic regions. Sporting dogs and hound breeds are predisposed, likely because of increased exposure to high-risk areas during hunting.[10] Living near a river or lake and access to recently excavated sites has been demonstrated to increase the risk of infection. Most cases of blastomycosis are diagnosed in late summer or early fall, though regional differences in seasonality occur.

Cats are rarely diagnosed with blastomycosis; however, clinical disease has been noted in indoor cats,[11] presumably through exposure to airborne *B. dermatitidis* spores.

Clinical signs
Clinical findings in dogs with blastomycosis are variable and commonly non-specific, e.g. anorexia, weight loss, lethargy and fever. Respiratory signs (exercise intolerance, cough, tachypnea, cyanosis or distress) reflect the lung lesions that occur in 65–85% of cases. Lymph node enlargement is common in dogs but not cats.[12, 13] Ocular lesions may be identified in 20–50% of cases (**Fig. 1.7**), with endophthalmitis as the most common abnormality.

The prostate, kidneys, testes, joints, nasal passages and brain are less frequently affected. CNS infections are identified in only 3–6% of cases,[12, 14] and findings may include depressed mentation, lethargy, neck pain, circling, cranial nerve deficits, head pressing, seizures, hypermetria, ataxia and tetraparesis.[10, 15, 16]

	MYCELIAL (MOLD)	YEAST
Location	Environment, mainly sandy, acidic soils near bodies of water	Tissues
Morphology	Thread-like, with production of conidia (spores)	Budding yeast
Infective	Yes, through inhalation, inoculation or wound contamination	Only through inoculation (e.g. needlestick from fine needle aspirate)
Disease causing	No	Yes

Table 1.2 **Comparison of the forms of *Blastomyces dermatitidis***

Dermatologic signs occur in 20–50% of infected dogs. These appear as granulomatous proliferative mass-like lesions or as ulcers draining serosanguineous or purulent fluid (**Figs. 1.8, 1.9**).[17, 18] These lesions are typically located on the nasal planum, face and nail beds, while cats may develop large dermal abscesses. Solitary bone infections causing lameness can occur in up to 30% of infected dogs. These typically involve the distal limbs.

Diagnosis

Blastomycosis is diagnosed based on a history of being in an endemic area, consistent clinical signs, and confirmation through cytologic (or histopathologic) exam or fungal detection.

Laboratory findings

In dogs, CBC and serum biochemistry abnormalities are largely non-specific and may reflect chronic inflammation. Urinalysis is typically unremarkable; however, organisms may be noted in the urine, particularly in intact dogs.

Diagnostic imaging

Lung lesions may be clinically silent, and thoracic radiographs are recommended for suspected blastomycosis, even in dogs lacking respiratory signs. Findings are variable, with diffuse miliary to nodular interstitial and bronchointerstitial patterns being most common (**Fig. 1.10**).[19] Less often, lung lobe consolidation or a solitary mass within the lung parenchyma is identified. Hilar lymphadenopathy may occasionally be evident.

Lesions of fungal osteomyelitis appear osteolytic with periosteal proliferation and soft tissue swelling. Bone lesions require cytology or biopsy to distinguish between fungal and neoplastic disease.

Cytology

Confirmation of blastomycosis is most reliably accomplished by cytologic or histologic sampling (**Fig. 1.11**). Cytologic evaluation of fine-needle aspirates (FNA) from enlarged lymph nodes can yield the diagnosis in 67–82% of cases. When skin lesions are present, cytologic evaluation of exudates or aspirates from lesions yields positive results in 85–94% of cases.[17]

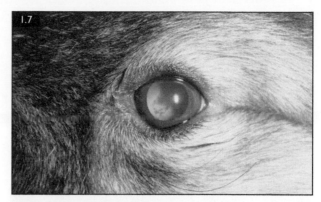

Fig. 1.7 Retinal granuloma in a dog with blastomycosis. (Courtesy of Dr Tony Carr)

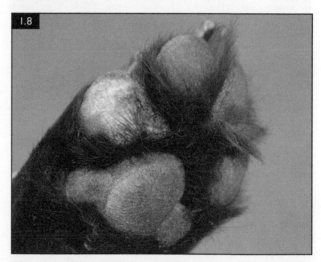

Fig. 1.8 Blastomycosis pododermatitis. (Courtesy of Dr Ryan Jennings)

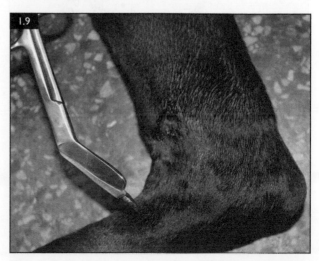

Fig. 1.9 Draining tract in a dog with blastomycosis.

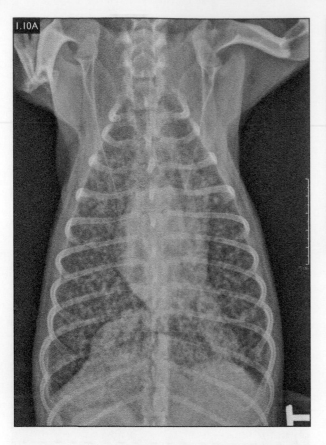

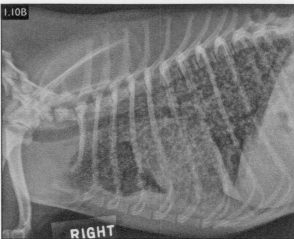

Fig. 1.10 Ventrodorsal (A) and lateral (B) thoracic radiographs of a dog with blastomycosis. (Courtesy of Stan Rubin)

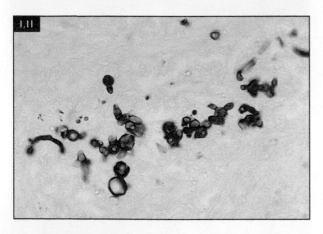

Fig. 1.11 Budding *Blastomyces dermatiditis* in the liver of a dog with blastomycosis (Gomori stain, 500× magnification). (Courtesy of National Center for Zoonotic, Vector-Borne, and Enteric Diseases (ZVED); Division of Foodborne, Bacterial and Mycotic Diseases (DFBMD), US Centers for Disease Control and Prevention)

Cytologic evaluation of samples obtained from the lung by transtracheal wash (TTW), bronchoalveolar lavage (BAL) and transthoracic lung aspiration (TLA) can be used in cases of pulmonary blastomycosis.[15, 20, 21]

Vitreal aspirates and subretinal aspirates have been recommended in cases that have only ocular involvement. However, these techniques may threaten vision in an eye that is not already blind and are not recommended as a first-line diagnostic test.[17]

Definitive diagnosis based on CSF analysis is rarely possible in dogs with blastomycosis involving the brain or spinal cord. *Blastomyces* organisms are almost never identified in CSF.

Histopathology may also be used but yeasts can be challenging to locate, and special stains are needed.

Immunoassays

Urine immunoassay is highly sensitive, detecting antigen in urine from 76–100% of dogs with systemic or pulmonary blastomycosis.[22] Cross-reactivity with other fungal agents (especially histoplasmosis) has been reported. Sensitivity and specificity for other samples, such as serum or BAL fluid, are low. Antigen testing is most useful in patients with isolated pulmonary infection, whereas patients with disseminated or extrapulmonary disease have lower diagnostic success.

Serologic testing may also be performed. Agar gel immunodiffusion (AGID) testing has a reported sensitivity of 40–90% and specificity of 90–100%.[10, 14, 21] The low sensitivity and high likelihood of negative results (false negatives) early in the course of infection[14, 21] limit the utility of this test in diagnosis. AGID is not useful for monitoring response to treatment or recurrence.[23]

Culture and PCR

Fungal culture is rarely performed because of the enhanced biosafety requirements. PCR testing is available, but sensitivity and specificity are not well defined, making the diagnostic utility unknown at this time.

Therapy

Drugs most often recommended for the treatment of dogs with blastomycosis are the azole antifungals and amphotericin B (AMB).[14, 24, 25] Itraconazole (ITZ; 5–10 mg/kg PO q24h or divided q12h) is considered the treatment of choice, because it is as effective as AMB, can be given orally and is associated with fewer adverse effects.[12, 24] ITZ does not cross the normal blood–brain, blood–prostate or blood–ocular barriers (whereas fluconazole and voriconazole do). However, infections at these sites often respond well to treatment with ITZ, perhaps because of increased penetration of the drug when inflammation is present.[24] Fluconazole (2.5–5.0 mg/kg PO or IV q12h) achieves high concentrations in the urine,

CSF and ocular fluids, and may have a role in the treatment of CNS, prostatic and urinary blastomycosis. Recent evaluation suggests no significant difference in treatment success for dogs treated with ITZ vs. fluconazole.[26] Therapy with ketoconazole alone is effective in less than 50% of cases, and is commonly associated with relapse and adverse effects.

AMB may be chosen as the preferred treatment for patients with severe disease, when oral therapy is not possible, for patients that are unable to tolerate therapy with azole antifungals, and for patients that have failed treatment with other drugs. The major adverse effect of AMB is cumulative nephrotoxicity, therefore renal function should be monitored before each dose.[23] A lipid complexed formulation is 8 to 10 times less nephrotoxic than AMB deoxycholate, allowing higher cumulative doses to be administered.[13, 23, 24]

Duration of therapy is dependent on resolution of clinical disease and radiographic signs, and potentially antigen testing. Three to six months of therapy are required and the duration may be longer in some cases.

Urine antigen testing may be useful for monitoring therapy and detecting clinical relapse. Dogs with higher initial antigen results have been reported to take longer to reach clinical remission. Urine antigen levels decrease significantly from baseline after 2–4 months of therapy and at the time of clinical remission. Testing will again become positive in 71% of patients that exhibit clinical relapse of disease.[27]

Prognosis/complications

An excellent prognosis is associated with appropriate therapy and when owners can commit to the time and cost of long-term treatment. Survival rates of 70–80% have been reported in response to treatment with ITZ, AMB or the two drugs in combination.[12, 14] It is important to communicate to owners that, even with appropriate duration of treatment, 20–25% of dogs will relapse after initial therapy. The likelihood of relapse is related to the severity of the initial lung disease, and it most often occurs within 6 months of cessation of therapy. Retreatment of a recurrence with an additional 60- to 90-day course of itraconazole has an 80% chance of a cure.

Most dogs with brain involvement will die. Dogs with severe diffuse pulmonary blastomycosis often deteriorate during the first 2–3 days of treatment, perhaps related to an inflammatory response directed against dying organisms in the lung.[12, 14] Fifty percent of these dogs will die within the first 7 days of therapy.

For ocular disease, rapid diagnosis and treatment are essential to preserve vision. Blind eyes that are severely affected with glaucoma or endophthalmitis are unlikely to become visual, and should probably be enucleated to prevent them from serving as a persistent focus of infection.[25]

BORDETELLA BRONCHISEPTICA
Michelle Evason

Definition
Bordetella bronchiseptica may cause rhinitis, tracheobronchitis and pneumonia in dogs and cats, as well as bronchitis in dogs. It is highly contagious, and infection is common in kittens with feline upper respiratory tract disease (FURTD) and puppies with canine infectious respiratory disease complex (CIRDC, "kennel cough").

Etiology and pathogenesis
Bordetella bronchiseptica is a motile, aerobic, gram-negative coccobacillus. Transmission is primarily via aerosol, direct contact with oral or nasal secretions, or through contact with contaminated fomites such as brushes, bedding, or food and water sources. The incubation period ranges from 2 to 10 days. Shedding from infected animals may occur for 1 month or more post-infection.

Incidence and risk factors
Reports of the incidence of disease and prevalence of *B. bronchiseptica* shedding are highly variable and depend on whether the animals were from high-density environments (e.g. shelters), their health status, geographic location (local and regional), and testing methods, such as the sampling site, sampling technique or test used for sampling (e.g. nasal

Prevention
Reducing exposure is difficult. Limiting exposure to rivers, lakes and excavated soil in endemic regions (where practical) may help to reduce risk. A modified live vaccine has been developed; however, it is not commercially available.

Public health and infection control
Blastomyces dermatitidis cannot be transmitted via aerosol means from animals to humans. Cutaneous inoculation via needle sticks and bites is possible.[7–9] Bandages should be changed frequently if used, as the mycelial phase of the organism can form in bandaged skin lesions, aerosolizing and theoretically infecting persons present during bandage changes.

vs. oropharyngeal vs. lower respiratory, PCR vs. culture).

Risk factors for disease in cats and dogs include younger age (<1 year) and living in a high-density group, e.g. kennel, at time of diagnosis or in recent history.[28–30] Infection in very young puppies (14 weeks or younger) has been associated with severe pneumonia.[28]

Common clinical signs
Examination findings are non-specific signs of respiratory disease (i.e. FURTD, CIRDC). Dogs with CIRDC may be presented with a honking cough (which can be severe), sneezing, stertor and serous to mucopurulent nasal discharge (**Fig. 1.12**). Owners may report vomiting; however, this is typically a productive cough. Cats with FURTD may have sneezing, stertor, and ocular and nasal discharge. Dogs and cats with bronchopneumonia may have a progressive cough, lethargy, respiratory distress or compromise, fever, anorexia and weight loss.[28, 29]

Diagnosis
Abnormalities with bordetellosis are non-specific, and frequently overlap with those of other pathogens. Similarly, testing methods may (or may not) assist with differentiating the presence of *B. bronchiseptica*

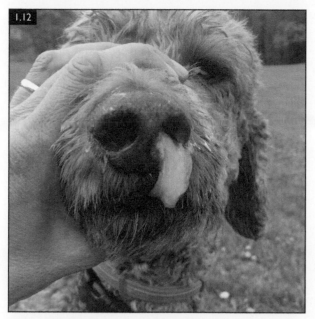

Fig. 1.12 Mucopurulent nasal discharge in a dog with *Bordetella bronchiseptica* infection. (Courtesy of Dr Kate Armstrong)

as part of the normal microbiota or as a cause of illness. Positive results may also occur with recent modified live vaccination.[31] Therefore, interpretation of test results and determining whether specific treatment is needed can be difficult. Specific pathogen testing is likely best reserved for outbreaks, high-risk populations (e.g. shelters), and severe or atypical presentations of disease.

Diagnostic imaging

Radiographs are typically normal with uncomplicated disease. Dogs or cats with pneumonia may have interstitial or alveolar changes. Lung lobe consolidation can occur.

Cytology

Cytologic exam of transtracheal wash (TTW), transtracheal lavage (TTL) or bronchoalveolar lavage (BAL) fluid may be normal or consistent with suppurative inflammation. Coccobacilli may be visible intra- or extracellularly.

Culture and susceptibility testing

Culture is not advised for routine acute FURTD or classic CIRDC because of the low diagnostic

value and low likelihood that antimicrobials will be required.[6]

Samples (swabs) are most practically obtained from the oropharyngeal cavity; however, nasal swabs, TTL, TTW and BAL samples can be successfully used for culture or PCR.[28] Lower airway samples (e.g. TTW, TTL and BAL) are ideal when possible, and if positive are considered more likely to be representative and aid diagnosis.[28] Interpretation of positive results from nasal or oropharyngeal samples (especially in high-density environments, e.g. shelters) is difficult because of the high prevalence.

PCR

PCR (DNA) testing of submitted swabs or lavage specimens is commonly used. Advantages include speed of detection and potential improved sensitivity over culture; however, sensitivity and specificity may vary with assay and lab. Intranasal or oral modified live vaccines may interfere with results[31] and false negatives may occur as with culture results.

Therapy

Most cases of FURTD- or CIRDC-related bordetellosis will be self-limiting and not require antimicrobials.[6] In patients with severe or prolonged disease, canine bronchitis, or bronchopneumonia where *B. bronchiseptica* infection is suspected, antimicrobial therapy (along with management of any concurrent disease) may be initiated before obtaining definitive test results. Typically, improvement is noted quickly (e.g. within 1 week) after antimicrobials and nursing care are initiated.[6]

Doxycycline is frequently recommended, in part owing to its efficacy against common co-infecting pathogens in CIRDC and FURTD.[6] In cats, doxycycline capsules and tablets should be coated for ease of swallowing, and followed by water or liquid, to help prevent esophageal strictures. Culture and susceptibility testing is advised for pneumonia cases, particularly those that appear refractory to therapy or progress rapidly.

Prognosis/complications

The prognosis with appropriate therapy is usually excellent. Most cases of CIRDC and FURTD resolve completely within 7–10 days.

Pneumonia cases usually require longer and more intensive therapy, which varies based on severity. In one study approximately 90% of dogs (puppies) survived.[28]

Prevention

Prevention centers on elimination of predisposing environmental conditions (e.g. overcrowding and stress) and underlying disease.

A variety of vaccines is available for dogs, including live mucosal (intranasal or oral) and inactivated parenteral. Greater efficacy of intranasal vs. oral vaccines, and superiority of both to parenteral vaccination, has been demonstrated.[32] Some vaccines are combined with other CIRDC pathogens (e.g. canine parainfluenza virus, adenovirus 2).

Mild-to-moderate respiratory signs may occur after vaccine administration. Importantly, vaccination may reduce disease severity, but it does not completely prevent infection or development of clinical signs.[33]

Infection control

The bacterium can survive in the environment for 10 days; however, most disinfectants will readily eliminate *B. bronchiseptica*.

Public health

Bordetella bronchiseptica infection has been described in immunocompromised humans who have contact with infected animals or modified live vaccines; however, human cases appear to be very rare.

CANINE ADENOVIRUS TYPE 2
J Scott Weese

Canine adenovirus type 2 (CAV-2) is one cause of canine infectious respiratory disease complex (CIRDC). As with other causes of respiratory disease, it is most common in dogs that have contact with many other dogs, such as those that frequent kennels, and can be found in a small percentage of clinically normal dogs.[34] It typically causes mild disease, characterized by cough and conjunctivitis. Severe disease is uncommon but can occur, as can secondary bacterial pneumonia. These presentations are most common in young puppies and when co-infection with other respiratory pathogens is present.

Diagnosis is most often performed via PCR testing of nasal or pharyngeal swabs. Treatment is supportive. Parenteral vaccination is common as this is a component of most core vaccines. Intranasal modified live vaccination is also available in a combination vaccine with *Bordetella bronchiseptica* and canine parainfluenza virus. Parenteral, but not intranasal, vaccination against CAV-2 provides cross-protection against hepatitis associated with canine adenovirus type 1. Intranasal vaccination can result in false-positive PCR results for up to 10 days after vaccination.[31]

CANINE INFECTIOUS RESPIRATORY DISEASE COMPLEX; KENNEL COUGH, INFECTIOUS TRACHEOBRONCHITIS
Michelle Evason

Definition

Canine infectious respiratory disease complex (CIRDC) is a common clinical syndrome, characterized by an acute onset of paroxysmal cough, sneezing, and ocular and nasal discharge. A variety of pathogens have been implicated, and co-infections (bacterial and viral) are common. Clinical signs are typically self-limiting in 7–10 days.

Pathogens

A variety of pathogens can be involved, either as sole agents or co-infections (**Fig. 1.13**). Specific information about individual pathogens can be found elsewhere in this chapter. Advances in technology are increasingly resulting in identification of novel viruses in dogs with respiratory tract disease; however, determination of whether these are pathogens

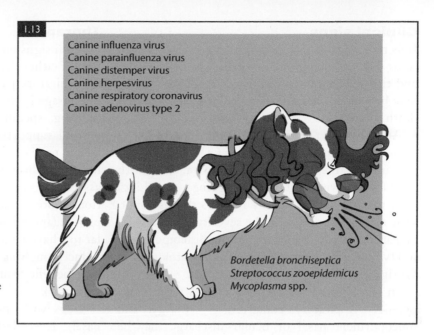

Canine influenza virus
Canine parainfluenza virus
Canine distemper virus
Canine herpesvirus
Canine respiratory coronavirus
Canine adenovirus type 2

Bordetella bronchiseptica
Streptococcus zooepidemicus
Mycoplasma spp.

Fig. 1.13 Leading causes of canine infectious respiratory disease complex (CIRDC).

or commensals is often difficult. These include canine pneumovirus, bocavirus, hepacivirus and canine reovirus.[35–37]

Etiology and pathogenesis

Clinically or subclinically infected dogs are the primary sources of infection. Risk of exposure and spread is increased with mingling of dogs, high-density housing or larger canine groups or events (e.g. shelter environment, dog park, veterinary clinic, breeding facility or kennel). Transmission is through aerosol, direct dog-to-dog contact or contaminated fomites (e.g. bedding, grooming equipment, human hands). Co-infection with multiple viruses or bacteria is common and may worsen disease severity.

Time to onset of clinical signs is typically 2–10 days after exposure. The respiratory tract (trachea, larynx, bronchi and sometimes nasal mucosa) is the primary site of infection. Gastrointestinal shedding of some pathogens (e.g. distemper virus, influenza virus) is possible. Shedding may begin before the onset of clinical signs. Infection with co-pathogens and immunosuppression affect shedding, incubation and severity of illness.

Geography

This syndrome is found worldwide. Prevalence and relative importance of different pathogens vary seasonally and geographically (globally, regionally and within cities in the same region).

Incidence and risk factors

CIRDC is common; however, the incidence is poorly defined. Infections may occur as sporadic disease, small clusters (e.g. a group of dogs associated with a kennel or dog park exposure), or large regional or national outbreaks.

Risk factors include a history of exposure to dog groups (e.g. shelter, pet store, dog show, dog park, puppy classes, canine athletic events, breeding, boarding or kennel facility). Increased duration and closeness of contact with other infected or shedding dogs increases risk of disease. Veterinary hospitals are a known source of infection.[35] All dogs are susceptible; however, puppies and immunocompromised dogs are at higher risk of complicated bacterial co-infection. Household pets with minimal contact with other dogs (or canine groups) are at lower risk.[38]

Clinical signs

Infection may be subclinical. The type and severity of signs will vary somewhat depending on co-infection and the dog's immune status. Although many dogs may become ill, few will have progressive signs and death is rare.

Acute harsh cough, classically described as "goose-honk", is the hallmark of CIRDC. Nasal or ocular discharges are frequently present, along with mild fever. Owners often note gagging (or retching) with mucoid froth and may refer to this as vomit. Other signs can vary with the severity of the disease or pathogen (e.g. dogs with canine distemper virus [CDV] infection may have ocular, dermatologic and GI signs).

In complicated or progressive cases fever, inappetence, respiratory compromise, lethargy, and mucopurulent nasal or ocular discharge may be present. Respiratory compromise (e.g. dyspnea) will occur with pneumonia.

Diagnosis

Diagnosis of CIRDC is syndromic and essentially involves identification of a likely infectious cause of respiratory tract disease. Diagnosis of specific etiologies can involve a range of tests (e.g. culture, PCR) but this is not usually indicated in sporadic cases because the results uncommonly impact treatment.[6] All pathogens involved in CIRDC are similar clinically, co-infections (viral, bacterial or both) are common and extensive diagnostics are of low yield. A further challenge for diagnosis is that some CIRDC pathogens may be present incidentally in dogs with respiratory disease of any etiology (e.g. colonization vs. infection).

Testing is indicated if there is evidence of pneumonia, when an outbreak is suspected or when clinical signs last longer than 7–10 days (or appear to be progressing). Testing may also be valuable in higher-risk environments such as shelters. During these times a combination of serology and PCR may aid diagnoses; however, both false negatives and false positives occur.

Radiographs are typically normal with uncomplicated CIRDC; however, dogs with pneumonia may have lobar consolidation and alveolar infiltrates.

Therapy

Clinical signs must be present prior to contemplation of either diagnostics or therapy, and running a "respiratory panel" in a clinically normal dog is discouraged. Given that CIRDC is typically self-limiting, specific therapy is not usually needed beyond supportive nursing care.[6] In cases where cough persists for longer than 10 days, remains harsh and hacking (vs. soft and productive) or is associated with complications (e.g. regurgitation, anorexia), a cough suppressant is advised for patient (and client) comfort. Switching from a collar to a harness or other restraint method may also reduce coughing. Dogs with herpesvirus keratitis may benefit from topical antivirals (idoxuride or cidofovir).

Dogs with mucopurulent discharge (ocular or nasal), fever, lethargy or anorexia warrant consideration of doxycycline antimicrobial therapy.[6] Persistent cough is not an indication for antimicrobials, but in dogs with progression to pneumonia antimicrobial therapy is indicated.[6]

Prognosis/complications

Most dogs have an excellent prognosis. Co-infections, immune suppression or diagnosis of CDV may complicate prognosis.

Prevention

Vaccination can be used to prevent (e.g. CDV) or reduce the likelihood and severity of disease (e.g. parainfluenza, adenovirus, H3N8 and H3N2 influenza virus, and *Bordetella*). However, vaccination does not prevent shedding of these pathogens (except CDV), and clinical signs may develop in vaccinated dogs. It is important to inform owners that vaccination is not completely protective, nor is there a vaccine for all CIRDC pathogens.

Reduction of overcrowding and subsequent stress, and awareness of immunosuppression, are required to decrease pathogen transmission. In suspected or confirmed outbreaks, early identification of ill dogs, proper infection control, quarantine, diagnosis of the cause and proper reporting are all needed to manage, ideally prevent and contain spread.

CANINE PARAINFLUENZA VIRUS
J Scott Weese

Definition
Canine parainfluenza virus (CPIV) is a highly transmissible RNA virus that is a common cause of canine infectious respiratory disease complex (CIRDC).

Etiology and pathogenesis
Dogs are exposed via respiratory mucous membranes, such as through inhalation of infectious aerosols, direct contact with infected dogs, or contact with contaminated fomites (e.g. bowls). After a 2- to 5-day incubation period, clinical signs develop. Viral shedding can start 24 hours before the onset of disease and tends to be of relatively short duration (4–6 days). Co-infection with other respiratory pathogens is common and can potentially exacerbate disease.[39]

Incidence and risk factors
CPIV is a commonly identified cause of CIRDC in some regions, being found in 6%–42% of cases.[38, 40–43] It can be identified in a smaller percentage of healthy dogs. Like other CIRDC pathogens, dogs exposed to group settings such as kennels and shelters are at higher risk.

Clinical signs
CPIV typically causes mild upper respiratory tract disease, characterized predominantly by coughing, which can be severe, often with nasal and/or ocular discharge. Fever, anorexia and lethargy may be present, but dogs are often bright, alert and coughing. When present, fever is usually mild. Secondary bacterial infection will usually result in more obvious systemic signs (e.g. greater elevation in temperature, lethargy, depression), as well as mucopurulent nasal and ocular discharges.

Diagnosis
PCR and serology are the two main tests. PCR has a quicker turnaround time and CPIV is a part of common PCR panels. Nasal or pharyngeal swabs may be tested. PCR is dependent on active CPIV shedding so diagnostic yield is highest in the first few days after the onset of disease. Later testing results in increasing risk of negative results.

Identification of a fourfold increase in serum antibody titer is also diagnostic. Because this requires paired testing of an acute sample and a convalescent sample collected 10–14 days later, it provides a retrospective diagnosis. It is most useful when a good PCR sample cannot be obtained or when testing is performed later in disease, when PCR results may be negative.

Therapy
There is no specific treatment for CPIV, but supportive care, particularly cough suppression, may be warranted. Uncommonly, secondary bacterial infections may develop and require antimicrobials.

Prognosis
Prognosis is excellent. Most dogs recover uneventfully within a few days.

Prevention
CPIV is included in common parenteral combination vaccines. However, parenteral vaccination confers limited protection and, although it is combined with core vaccine components (e.g. canine parvovirus), the CPIV component is considered a non-core vaccine.[44] Intranasal modified live vaccination is more effective.[45]

CANINE RESPIRATORY CORONAVIRUS
J Scott Weese

Canine respiratory coronavirus has been implicated as a cause of the canine infectious respiratory disease complex, but it is unclear whether it is an important primary cause of disease, relevant co-infection or harmless commensal. It has been reported in 7.7–9.4% of dogs with respiratory tract disease, but is rarely found in healthy dogs,[37, 41] supporting at least some role in disease. Seroprevalence rates can be high (40–50%),[37, 40] indicating that exposure is common. This virus appears to be highly contagious but tends to cause relatively mild and self-limiting disease.

Diagnosis is typically achieved via PCR testing of nasal or pharyngeal swabs. Serological testing can be performed; however, identification of a fourfold titer rise (in samples collected 2–4 weeks apart) is required to diagnose true clinical disease, given the relatively high prevalence of exposure (and seropositivity) in the dog population. Treatment is supportive. A vaccine is not currently available.

CHLAMYDIOSIS/*CHLAMYDIA* (FORMERLY *CHLAMYDOPHILA*) *FELIS*
Michelle Evason

Definition
Chlamydia felis infection is a common cause of conjunctivitis in cats, particularly those with feline upper respiratory tract disease (FURTD). Infection is typically associated with young age and high pet density environments (e.g. shelters, catteries, multi-cat households). Persistent infection can occur, and co-infection with other FURTD-causing pathogens is common.

Etiology and pathogenesis
Chlamydiae are obligate intracellular bacteria and cannot survive for more than a few days off their host. They are transmitted by direct contact with secretions (nasal, ocular), contact with shared fomites (e.g. grooming equipment, brushes, bedding) or possibly by aerosols. They persistently infect ocular and respiratory epithelial cells. Clinical signs develop within 2–5 days of infection, and infection may persist for months.[46, 47]

In cats, *C. felis* is a significant cause of conjunctivitis.[47–49] Co-infections with feline herpesvirus, calicivirus, *Bordetella* or *Mycoplasma* are common and may worsen disease severity and duration.[29, 47]

Geography
Worldwide; prevalence varies with location.

Incidence and risk factors
Highly variable shedding rates have been reported in cats. *Chlamydia felis* can be shed in the absence of identifiable disease, most often in shelter cats, where rates up to 59% have been reported.[47, 48] Shedding by healthy household cats is uncommon.[50] Risk factors for *C. felis* infection include younger age (1 year or less) and living in a high-density environment (e.g. multi-cat household, cattery, shelter).[46–49]

Common clinical signs
Clinical signs are non-specific and consistent with many other causes of FURTD. Cats with conjunctivitis may have serous to mucopurulent ocular discharge, chemosis (conjunctival edema) and blepharospasm (blinking due to pain or irritation) (**Fig. 1.14**). Signs of FURTD can include nasal discharge and sneezing. Most cats remain otherwise healthy, and systemic signs such as fever and cough are uncommon.

Diagnosis
Diagnostic results must be interpreted in light of the clinical signs because of the presence of *C. felis* in healthy cats. Signs of disease frequently overlap with those of other pathogens, and concurrent disease

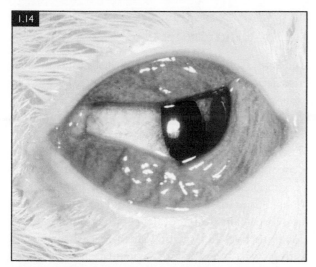

Fig. 1.14 Conjunctivitis associated with *Chlamydia felis* infection. (Courtesy of Dr Robert Sherding)

processes are common. PCR is most often used to confirm infection. However, *C. felis* is so common in some healthy populations that the diagnostic value of PCR in those groups (e.g. shelter animals) is limited. The appropriate sampling technique involves assertive conjunctival swabbing, in order to obtain sufficient numbers of bacteria.

Culture and serology

Culture is rarely performed outside of a research setting. Serology is not widely available, and acute and convalescent titers are needed.

PCR

PCR testing of conjunctival swabs or scrapings is most commonly used for confirmation of active infection. These tests offer a rapid turnaround; however, sensitivity and specificity may vary. Results must be interpreted in light of the clinical findings, because some cats may be non-clinical carriers, or have latent infection. If only one sample can be taken, the oropharynx is preferred; however, multiple samples will improve diagnosis.[51]

Therapy

Most cats with FURTD signs will have self-limiting disease. Supportive care includes hydration, meeting nutritional needs and nursing care.

Cats with chlamydial conjunctivitis are most often treated with doxycycline (5–10 mg/kg q12h for 3–4 weeks), which has been shown to clear infection after 42 days.[52] Amoxicillin–clavulanic acid (12.5–25 mg/kg PO q12h) or a fluoroquinolone is an option if doxycycline is contraindicated. Treatment duration is not well understood, and 7–10 to up to 42 days have been recommended for fluoroquinolones.[52, 53] A duration of 7–10 days is probably adequate in most cases. Concurrent topical therapy with tetracycline or chloramphenicol has also been used, but the additive efficacy is unknown.

Improvement is typically noted quickly (within 24–48 hours) after antimicrobials and nursing care are initiated. Catteries or multi-cat environments may require a longer duration of therapy, and treatment is advised for 2 weeks after resolution of clinical signs

Lack of response to therapy, or incomplete resolution, may be due to concurrent disease or persistent chlamydia infection and should prompt patient re-evaluation.

Prognosis/complications

Prognosis with appropriate therapy is typically rapid and excellent; however, some cats will have persistent infection.

Prevention

Prevention centers on elimination of predisposing environmental conditions (e.g. overcrowding, stress) and underlying disease. Good hygiene practices and disinfection will reduce infection rates.

A vaccine is available for cats. This is considered a non-core vaccine that may help reduce the severity of clinical signs in high-risk environments, together with appropriate environmental changes.[33] The vaccine is of limited use in household pets that do not have contact with high-risk populations.

CRENOSOMA VULPIS (FOX LUNGWORM)
Dennis Spann

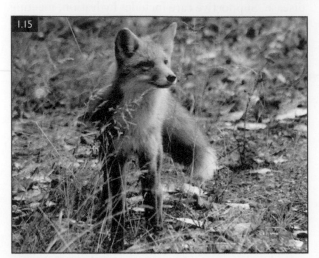

Fig. 1.15 Red foxes (*Vulpes vulpes*) are infected with *Crenosoma vulpis* at fairly high rates in some areas.

Definition
Fox lungworm infections occur in foxes, dogs and other carnivores that become infected by consuming snails and slugs containing the infective stage (L3) of *Crenosoma vulpis*. The adult parasites reside in the lungs and cause mild catarrhal inflammation and cough.

Etiology and pathogenesis
Crenosoma vulpis is the causative agent of fox lungworm. The red fox (*Vulpes vulpes*) is the definitive host (**Fig. 1.15**). Infected animals pass L1 larvae (**Fig. 1.16**) in feces. These larvae mature into L3 larvae in snails and slugs, and dogs become infected via ingestion of a slug or snail. After ingestion, the parasite is released into the intestines, penetrates the intestinal wall and migrates to the lungs via the liver and the vena cava. *Crenosoma* larvae penetrate the lungs and mature in the bronchi, bronchioles and trachea. Approximately 19–21 days after ingestion adult parasites pass infective L1 larvae. Adult parasites (**Fig. 1.17**) in the bronchi and bronchioles cause mild inflammation and coughing.

Geography
Crenosoma vulpis is endemic in many areas of Europe and North America, particularly the northeastern United States, Atlantic Canada, England, Ireland and central Europe. Dogs and other canids in close association with fox populations are at risk for infection with *C. vulpis*.

Incidence and risk factors
The prevalence of *Crenosoma* shedding and the incidence of disease are poorly defined and highly variable geographically. Rates can be high in some populations. For example, up to 23% of dogs were infected in a Baermann test prevalence study conducted on coughing dogs in Atlantic Canada.[54] Risk factors are eating snails and exposure to populations of foxes.

Clinical signs
Dogs infected with *C. vulpis* generally have minimal clinical signs but may have mild cough and retching. A chronic cough that is unresponsive to other therapies is a common clinical presentation.

Diagnosis
Eosinophilia, basophilia and monocytosis may be identified on a CBC.

Tracheal wash or bronchoalveolar lavage (BAL) will often identify eosinophilia, mixed neutrophilia and eosinophilic inflammation. L1 larvae are present in many cases. Baermann technique or zinc sulfate fecal float can be used to demonstrate L1 larvae in feces and may be the most sensitive technique.[55] Typically, three daily samples are tested.

The larvae have a conical head and pointed tail (**Fig. 1.16**). Adult *C. vulpis* females are 12–16 mm long; the males are 3.5–8 mm long. The anterior end of the body has cuticular folds that encircle the body, giving the worms their crenellated appearance (**Fig. 1.17**). The first-stage larvae shed in the feces are about 264–340 μm in length, with the oral ends bluntly conical and the tips of the tails tapering smoothly to the tip.

Thoracic radiography is usually normal, although a bronchiolar pattern may be present.

Therapy
A variety of treatments have been described (*Table 1.3*). Comparative efficacy is unclear. Prednisone (0.5–1 mg/kg) is sometimes used to reduce pneumonitis that may develop secondary to rapid parasite kill.

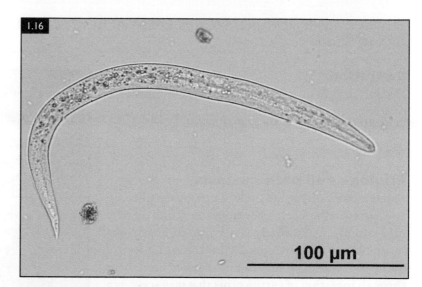

Fig. 1.16 L1 stage of *Crenosoma vulpis*. (Courtesy of Dr Gary Conboy)

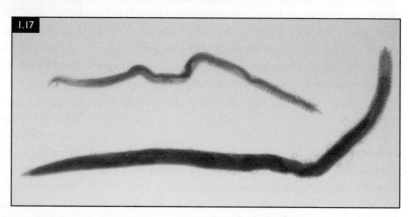

Fig. 1.17 Adult *Crenosoma vulpis*. (Courtesy of Dr Gary Conboy)

Table 1.3 **Treatment options for *Crenosoma vulpis***

DRUG	DOSE	DURATION
Ivermectin	0.2 mg/kg, once	Once
Fenbendazole	50 mg/kg PO	3–10 days
Moxidectin (2.5%) and imidicloprid (10%)		Once
Milbemycin oxime	0.5 mg/kg	Once
Praziquantel	50 mg/kg	Once daily for 7 days
Pyrantel	144 mg/kg	
Febantel	150 mg/kg	

Prognosis/complications

Prognosis is good even without treatment. Treatment is generally curative. Reinfection is possible.

Prevention

Mollusk control and routine monthly parasite control using milbemycin oxime or moxidectin may be used.

EUCOLEUS AEROPHILUS (*CAPILLARIA AEROPHILA*) (LUNGWORM)
Dennis Spann

Definition
Eucoleus aerophilus is a trichurid nematode parasite that lives in the tracheobronchial mucosa of dogs and cats. It causes local inflammation and chronic coughing.

Etiology and pathogenesis
Eucoleus has a direct life cycle. Eggs are coughed up and passed in the feces. They embryonate and become infective in approximately 40 days. *Eucoleus* eggs are resistant in many environments and remain infective for up to 1 year. The eggs can be ingested directly or through ingestion of earthworms that may serve as a paratenic transport hosts. Once ingested they hatch, and larvae migrate back to the lungs where, after a prepatent period of 20–35 days, adult worms begin shedding eggs. They are embedded in the mucosa of the trachea and large bronchioles. The presence of parasites causes an inflammatory reaction in the airways.

Geography
Worldwide distribution. Rates of infection vary but may be over 50% in foxes in some endemic areas.[56, 57]

Incidence and risk factors
The prevalence of infection in dogs and cats varies in studies and is generally low (e.g. <6%).[58] Higher rates may be found in some populations such as strays.[3]

Clinical signs
Subclinical infections are common. Clinical signs may be more severe with larger worm burdens and young age. Cough and increased bronchovesicular sounds are typically the earliest signs, or the only signs with mild disease. Increased respiratory rate may also be present. If the infection is very severe, the patient may have ill thrift and a thin body condition.[59] Rarely, bronchopneumonia or death may occur.

Diagnosis
Diagnosis is based on identification of 60- to 83-µm long by 25- to 40-µm wide, asymmetric, bipolar

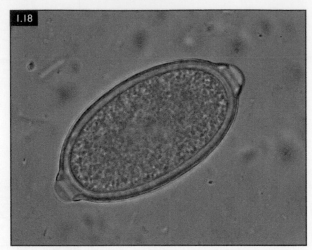

Fig. 1.18 *Eucoleus aerophilus* egg. Note the asymmetric bipolar operculated plugs. (Courtesy of Drs Donato Traversa and Angela Di Cesare)

plugged eggs in feces or tracheal mucus (**Fig. 1.18**). Similar appearing trichurid eggs may be present from *Eucoeus boehmi* infections or other trichurids passed in cat feces from prey species. Thoracic radiographs may identify increased airway markings and nodularity. Bronchoalveolar lavage can identify eosinophilic, neutrophilic or pleocellular inflammation.

PCR may be useful to assist with diagnosis when infections are light or when other trichurid eggs are present, complicating a definitive diagnosis.

Therapy
Fenbendazole (50 mg/kg PO q24h for 10–14 days) is most commonly used. Abamectin (0.3 mg/kg q24h for 1–2 doses) has been reported in a cat.[57] Eprinomectin has been used in cats to prevent egg shedding. Spot-on moxidectin/imidacloprid has also been effective in stopping egg shedding and in resolving clinical signs in cats.[4]

Prognosis/complications
The prognosis is good with therapy.

Prevention
Rapidly remove feces, and prevent coprophagy and geophagy.

FELINE CALICIVIRUS
Robert G Sherding

Definition

Feline calicivirus (FCV) is a highly contagious contributor to feline upper respiratory tract disease (FURTD) syndrome. Subclinical, latent or carrier states of infection are common, and affected cats usually have acute ocular and nasal disease, together with oral ulcers. History of high-density housing is frequent.

Etiology and pathogenesis

FCV is most commonly transmitted through direct cat-to-cat contact and fomites.[60] Virus is shed in oral, nasal and ocular secretions, and sometimes urine and feces. FCV remains infectious for up to 4 weeks in the environment and on fomites (e.g. cages, examination tables, food and water dishes, and human clothing). Uncommonly, aerosol transmission due to sneezing and coughing may occur.

FCV has an affinity for oropharyngeal and upper respiratory epithelium and pulmonary alveolar macrophages. Signs develop after an incubation period of 2–5 days.[61]

Geography

Worldwide, although the prevalence varies geographically.

Incidence and risk factors

FCV is very common and believed to account for up to 50% of feline upper respiratory tract infections.

The prevalence of subclinical carriers is 5–10% in the healthy pet cat population, 20% in show cats and 25–75% in cattery and shelter cats.[60, 61] The incidence of disease is poorly defined, but is highest in young kittens and unvaccinated cats.

Risk factors include history of stress, high-density group housing and close cat-to-cat contact in shelters, catteries and multi-cat households, especially where unvaccinated kittens are exposed to subclinical carrier adult cats.[62, 63] Recovered cats can remain subclinical carriers and shed infectious virus continuously for weeks, months or even years.

Clinical signs

Clinical signs vary with the virus strain and whether co-infection with another FURTD pathogen is present. However, FCV typically causes oral ulceration (tongue, palate, gingiva) (**Figs. 1.19, 1.20**), mild rhinitis (sneezing, nasal discharge) and conjunctivitis

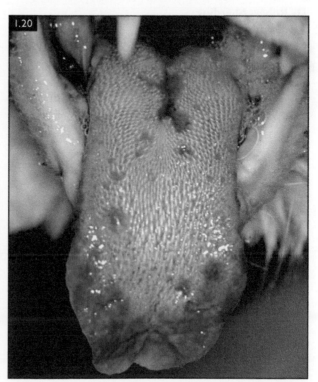

Fig. 1.20 Tongue ulcers caused by feline calicivirus. (Courtesy of Dr Robert Sherding)

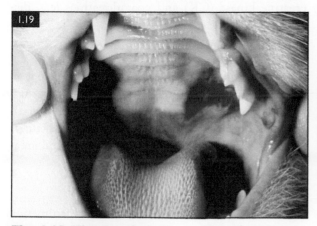

Fig. 1.19 Ulcers on the palate and lateral tongue margin caused by feline calicivirus. (Courtesy of Dr Robert Sherding)

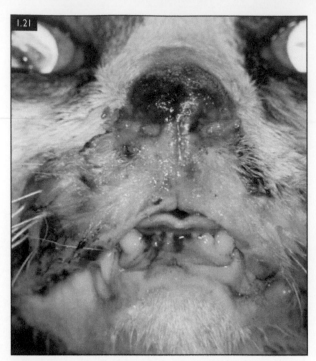

Fig. 1.21 Severe feline calicivirus infection in a cat, with ulcers on the nasal planum and lips, and profuse mucopurulent nasal discharge (rhinitis). (Courtesy of Dr Robert Sherding)

(ocular discharge), accompanied by an abrupt onset of inappetence, lethargy and fever. Illness is most severe in young kittens, and mild in previously vaccinated cats. In some cats, the tip of the nose (nasal planum) is ulcerated and crusted (**Fig. 1.21**). Clinical disease is usually self-limiting within 1–2 weeks. A subclinical or carrier state is common, and these cats often appear normal.

Viral pneumonia may occur in young kittens, which manifests as cough, labored breathing and secondary bacterial pneumonia. Transient synovitis, fever and joint pain (limping, reluctance to move), with or without concurrent respiratory signs, occur in some cats.

Highly virulent strains of FCV have emerged over the last decade in North America and Europe in sporadic outbreaks of severe virulent systemic disease with vasculitis, mostly in shelter cats.[64–67] Widespread vasculitis can cause epistaxis, GI bleeding, icterus, facial and limb edema, skin and footpad ulceration, abdominal pain, abdominal effusion and labored breathing (pulmonary edema,

pleural effusion). The mortality rate is up to 50%, and even healthy, well-vaccinated adult cats can succumb rapidly.

Persistent FCV infection is associated with chronic ulcerative–proliferative gingivostomatitis with signs of oral pain, dysphagia, halitosis, hypersalivation and bleeding.[68, 69]

Diagnosis

For individual infected cats, a presumptive diagnosis of "acute viral respiratory disease" or FURTD based on typical clinical signs and likelihood of exposure is usually adequate for patient management. Mucosal specimens evaluated by virus culture, PCR or direct immunofluorescence can establish a definitive diagnosis of FCV.[51] These tests are not routinely needed in most individual cases because infection is typically self-limiting in 2 weeks or less. However, confirmatory testing is useful for evaluating disease outbreaks in catteries and shelters, and for diagnosis in individual cats with severe or atypical clinical signs. Cats with severe or prolonged signs of FURTD should be tested for feline leukemia virus (FeLV) and feline immunodeficiency virus (FIV) as potential causes of immunosuppression.

Diagnostic testing

Hematology and urinalysis

Cats with the virulent systemic form of FCV can have anemia, neutrophilic leukocytosis, thrombocytopenia, hyperbilirubinema, hypoalbuminemia, increased serum liver enzymes, increased serum creatine kinase (CK) and coagulopathies (e.g. disseminated intravascular coagulation, DIC).[64, 67]

Radiology and imaging

Thoracic radiography is usually normal, except in severe cases with pneumonia. Uncomplicated viral pneumonia causes an unstructured bronchointerstitial infiltrate, whereas secondary bacterial pneumonia causes an alveolar infiltration pattern and areas of lung consolidation.

Cytology

Non-specific mucopurulent or mixed inflammation may be evident on samples from affected areas of the upper or lower respiratory tract. Identifiable viral inclusions are not observed in FCV infection. Oral lesions consistent with lymphoplasmacytic stomatitis should be confirmed by biopsy.

Virus culture

Virus isolation is considered the "gold standard" for confirming FCV, but is rarely performed.

PCR

PCR testing can be performed on oropharyngeal, nasal and conjunctival mucosal swabs or scrapings,[51] as well as airway lavage and lung specimens. PCR identification of FCV does not confirm causality of disease because non-clinical carriers can also be PCR positive. Therefore, results must be interpreted in conjunction with clinical signs and circumstances.

Direct immunofluorescence

FCV can sometimes be identified in swabs or scrapings of oropharyngeal, nasal or conjunctival mucosa submitted to a specialized lab. However, this is considered less reliable than virus isolation or PCR.

Treatment

In most cats, acute FURTD is self-limiting and the main treatment is supportive nursing and comfort care, such as gentle removal of ocular and nasal discharges.[60] Dehydration should be prevented to minimize drying and thickening of respiratory secretions, which can occlude airways.

Safe and effective antiviral drugs are not available for treating FCV. Antimicrobials may be considered in cats with mucopurulent ocular or nasal discharge, fever and lethargy, when secondary bacterial infection or co-infection is suspected. Typically doxycycline is chosen. Rarely, severe or complicated infections (mostly in young kittens) or prolonged anorexia may require additional care (e.g. parenteral fluid therapy, oxygen therapy, tube feeding or appetite stimulants). Life-threatening pneumonia or virulent systemic FCV may require intensive care at a facility with an isolation unit and oxygen support.

Treatment of FCV-associated chronic gingivostomatitis

This refractory condition can be treated by extraction of teeth near the lesions, followed by systemic antibiotics and chlorhexidine mouthwashes. Oromucosal administration of recombinant feline interferon-omega (0.1 MU q24h for 90 days) has also been shown to improve the condition.[69]

Prognosis/complications

With most FURTD cases, the prognosis is excellent and clinical signs resolve within 1–2 weeks. Recovered cats remain subclinical carriers and persistently shed virus for months to years. Bacterial pneumonia is a rare but serious complication in young kittens, and the prognosis is more guarded.

Outbreaks of virulent systemic FCV with vasculitis are rare, but in these cases the disease is much more severe and a mortality rate of up to 50% is expected, even in previously healthy, vaccinated adult cats.

Prevention

Vaccination against FCV is recommended as a "core vaccine" for all cats.[70] Vaccination is effective for preventing or minimizing clinical illness caused by FCV, but it does not completely prevent infection, eliminate the chronic carrier state or prevent virus shedding.[71] Modified live virus (MLV) injectable, inactivated (killed virus) injectable and MLV intranasal (IN) vaccines are available, and all are reasonably effective. IN vaccines induce faster and possibly better protection while avoiding adjuvant-related side effects, but mild sneezing and oculonasal discharge are common after IN vaccination.

FCV and other feline respiratory pathogens are highly contagious, so FCV infected cats should always be isolated from other cats to prevent the spread of infection. In addition, routine infection control measures combined with reducing stress and overcrowding help prevent the spread of respiratory disease in catteries and shelters.

FELINE HERPESVIRUS 1 (FELINE VIRAL RHINOTRACHEITIS)
Robert G Sherding

Definition
Feline herpesvirus 1 (FHV-1) is a common and highly contagious contributor to feline upper respiratory tract disease (FURTD), most commonly manifesting as acute rhinotracheitis and keratoconjunctivitis.

Etiology and pathogenesis
FHV-1 is an enveloped DNA virus that is endemic in the domestic cat population. It is most commonly transmitted through direct cat-to-cat contact and via fomites.[61] Virus is shed in oral, nasal and ocular secretions of acutely infected cats and those with recrudescence of latent infection. It remains infectious for up to 18 hours on fomites (e.g. cages, examination tables, food and water bowls, and human clothing). Less commonly, aerosol transmission occurs via sneezing and coughing.

FHV-1 has an affinity for conjunctival, corneal, nasal and laryngotracheal epithelium, where multifocal epithelial necrosis results in acute rhinitis, tracheitis, laryngitis and keratoconjunctivitis after an incubation period of 2–6 days. In some cats, FHV-1 also causes severe damage (necrosis and osteolysis) to the nasal turbinates. Rarely, FHV-1 has been associated with chronic ulcerative dermatitis and chronic corneal disease in cats.[72]

Nearly all cats that recover from FHV-1 infection become latent subclinical carriers for life. These latent carriers can shed FHV-1 intermittently, with or without episodic clinical signs, when reactivation is triggered by factors such as stress, parturition, lactation or glucocorticoid therapy.[73]

Geography
FHV-1 is prevalent in cats worldwide.

Incidence and risk factors
FHV-1 is common, and accounts for up to 40% of FURTD infections. The incidence of FHV-1 infection is highest in young kittens and unvaccinated cats. Risk factors include stress, high-density group housing and close cat-to-cat contact, as in shelters, catteries and multi-cat households, especially where unvaccinated kittens are exposed to subclinical carrier adult cats.[62, 63, 74] Shedding of FHV-1 is often triggered by parturition and lactation in latent carrier queens, which is an important source of infection in newborn kittens. The prevalence of subclinical carriers of FHV-1 in the healthy pet cat population ranges from 2% to 10%, but is up to 40% in shelter and cattery cats.[63, 74]

Clinical signs
FHV-1 typically causes acute FURTD with signs of inappetence, lethargy, fever, naso-ocular discharge (serous to mucopurulent), sneezing, stertor, coughing and hypersalivation (**Figs. 1.22, 1.23**). Corneal involvement causes keratitis and painful herpetic ulcers with lacrimation and blepharospasm (**Fig. 1.24**). Clinical disease is usually self-limiting within 1–2 weeks. Illness is most severe in young kittens and cats co-infected with other respiratory pathogens, and tends to be mild in previously vaccinated cats. Most recovered cats remain subclinical carriers for life, but usually appear healthy.

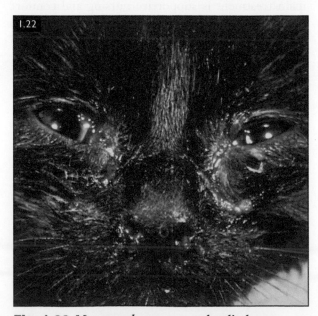

Fig. 1.22 Mucopurulent naso-ocular discharge and blepharospasm (squinting) in a kitten with acute rhinitis and conjunctivitis caused by feline herpesvirus-1. (Courtesy of Dr Robert Sherding)

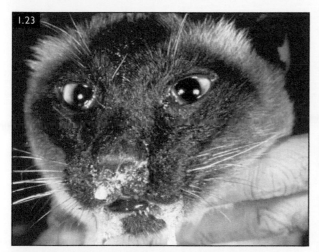

Fig. 1.23 Hypersalivation, nares obstructed with dried nasal discharge, and mucoid ocular discharge with prolapsed third eyelids in a cat infected with feline herpesvirus-1. (Courtesy of Dr Robert Sherding)

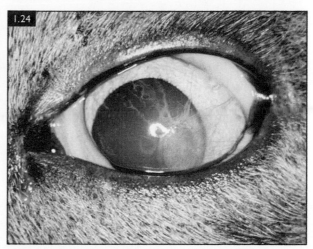

Fig. 1.24 A characteristic branching dendritic corneal ulcer stained with fluorescein on the left eye of a cat infected with feline herpesvirus-1. (Courtesy of Dr Robert Sherding)

Nasal turbinate damage can cause chronic obstructive rhinitis with fibrosis and stenosis of the nasal passages. Laryngitis can cause transient loss of voice or high-pitched vocal sounds (dysphonia). Secondary bacterial pneumonia causes tachypnea and dyspnea, especially in young kittens. Neonates may develop panophthalmitis (also called ophthalmia neonatorum), resulting in permanent blindness. Ulcerative skin lesions occasionally involve the facial area.

Diagnosis

For individual infected cats, a presumptive diagnosis of "acute infectious respiratory disease" or FURTD based on typical clinical signs and likelihood of exposure is usually adequate for patient management. Mucosal specimens evaluated by PCR, direct immunofluorescence or virus culture can establish a definitive diagnosis.[51, 75] These tests are not routinely needed in most individual cases because infection is typically self-limiting in 2 weeks or less. Confirmatory testing can be useful for evaluating disease outbreaks in catteries and shelters, and for diagnosis in individual cats with severe or atypical clinical signs.

Hematology and urinalysis

Routine tests are normal in most infected cats. Cats with secondary bacterial pneumonia may develop a neutrophilic leukocytosis. Cats with severe or prolonged signs of FURTD should be tested for feline leukemia virus (FeLV) and feline immunodeficiency virus (FIV) as potential causes of immunosuppression.

Radiology and imaging

Thoracic radiography is normal in most cats with FHV-1 infection, except in severe cases with pneumonia. Nasal CT and rhinoscopy are useful for evaluating cats with chronic nasal sequelae, such as frontal sinusitis, severe turbinate damage or nasopharyngeal stenosis, and to differentiate these from other causes of chronic nasal disease.

Cytology

Cytology from affected areas of the upper or lower respiratory tract shows non-specific mucopurulent or mixed inflammation. Intranuclear viral inclusions can occasionally be identified early in the disease in conjunctival scrapings or mucosal biopsies.

PCR

PCR testing can be performed on oropharyngeal, nasal, conjunctival and corneal swabs or scrapings, or airway lavage or lung specimens.[29, 51] PCR identification of FHV-1 does not confirm causality of disease because non-clinical carriers of FHV-1 infection can also be PCR positive. Results must be interpreted in conjunction with clinical signs and circumstances.

Direct immunofluorescence

FHV-1 can be identified in swabs or scrapings of nasal mucosa or conjunctiva submitted to a specialized lab, but this is less sensitive than PCR.

Viral culture

FHV-1 can be isolated in cell culture from swabs of the oropharynx, nasal cavity or conjunctiva submitted to a specialized lab, but this is less sensitive than PCR.

Serology

Measurement of FHV-1 serum antibodies is of limited use for diagnosis because most cats have antibody titers induced by prior vaccination or subclinical exposure.

Treatment

In most cats, acute FURTD is self-limiting and the main treatment is supportive nursing and comfort care, sometimes combined with antibiotics or antiviral therapy, depending on the severity.[73] FHV-1 disrupts the ocular tear film, so topical tear replacement eyedrops may be beneficial.[76] Dehydration should be prevented to minimize drying and thickening of respiratory secretions, which can occlude airways. Infectious respiratory disease should be treated on an outpatient basis whenever possible to prevent contamination of the veterinary facility and spread of infection to hospitalized cats. Rarely, severe or complicated infections (mostly in young kittens) or prolonged anorexia may require additional care (e.g. parenteral fluid therapy, oxygen therapy, tube feeding or appetite stimulants).

Antibiotics have no effect on FHV-1, and are not routinely needed in typical self-limiting viral respiratory infections, but antibiotics such as doxycycline may be considered in cats with mucopurulent naso-ocular discharge, fever and lethargy, if secondary bacterial infection or co-infection is suspected.

Oral L-lysine has been used to inhibit FHV-1 replication in herpes conjunctivitis and to reduce shedding of FHV-1. However, recent studies have concluded that lysine is not effective for prevention or treatment of FHV-1.[77–79]

Antiviral drugs are used when FHV-1 signs are severe, persistent or recurrent. Famciclovir (90 mg/kg PO q8–12h) is the most effective and well tolerated in kittens and adult cats for inhibiting FHV-1 replication, decreasing viral shedding, shortening recovery time, and treating both acute and chronic disease caused by FHV-1.[80] Other oral antiviral drugs used in human herpesvirus infection (e.g. acyclovir, valacyclovir) are less active against FHV-1 and are toxic for cats. Interferon has not been effective for treating FHV-1.

Topical ophthalmic antivirals are beneficial in cats with severe or refractory FHV-1 eye disease (e.g. keratitis, corneal ulcer, chronic keratopathies). These include cidofovir 0.5% (1 drop OU, q12h), idoxuridine 0.1% (1 drop OU, q4–6h) or vidarabine 3% (1 drop OU, q4–6h).[81] Eye irritation should be monitored as a potential side effect of ophthalmic antivirals. Topical corticosteroids should be avoided.

Prognosis/complications

The prognosis is usually excellent and clinical signs resolve within 1–2 weeks. Recovered cats remain latent subclinical carriers for life. Bacterial pneumonia is a rare but serious complication in young kittens, and the prognosis is more guarded. Uncommon chronic complications and sequelae of FHV-1 include chronic keratoconjunctivitis, chronic rhinosinusitis, nasal turbinate damage resulting in fibrosis and stenosis of nasal passages, and chronic ulcerative dermatitis.[61] Severe keratoconjunctivitis can result in adhesions of the conjunctiva to the cornea (symblepharon). In neonatal kittens, panophthalmitis (ophthalmia neonatorum) can cause irreversible blindness.

Prevention

Vaccination against FHV-1 is recommended as a "core vaccine" for all cats.[70] Vaccination is effective for preventing or minimizing clinical illness caused by FHV-1, but it does not completely prevent infection, eliminate the chronic carrier state or prevent virus shedding.

Modified live virus (MLV) injectable, inactivated (killed virus) injectable and MLV intranasal (IN) vaccines are available, and all are reasonably effective. IN vaccines induce faster and possibly better protection while avoiding adjuvant-related side effects, but mild sneezing and oculonasal discharge are common after IN vaccination. Commercial trivalent core vaccine products combine FHV-1 with feline calicivirus (FCV) and feline panleukopenia virus (FPV).

FHV-1 and other feline respiratory pathogens are highly contagious, so FHV-infected cats should always be isolated from other cats. In addition, routine infection control measures combined with reducing stress and overcrowding help prevent the spread of respiratory disease in catteries and shelters.

FELINE UPPER RESPIRATORY TRACT DISEASE
Michelle Evason and Robert G Sherding

Definition
Feline upper respiratory tract disease (FURTD) is a clinical syndrome. Affected cats usually have ocular and nasal discharge, sneezing and conjunctivitis. Clinical signs are typically self-limiting within 7–10 days.

Etiology and pathogenesis
A variety of pathogens may be involved, either individually or as co-infections. Most common are feline herpesvirus, feline calicivirus, *Bordetella bronchiseptica*, *Chlamydia felis*, *Streptococcus equi* subsp. *zooepidemicus* and *Mycoplasma* spp. (**Fig. 1.25**). Various other members of the commensal upper respiratory tract microbiota, such as *Staphylococcus* spp., *Streptococcus* spp., *Pasteurella multocida*, *Escherichia coli* and anaerobes,

can be detected in affected cats. However, their role in disease is often difficult to discern. Less commonly, organisms such as *Cryptococcus* spp., *Aspergillus* spp. or *Cuterebra* spp. are involved.

Infected cats are the primary sources of infection; this includes cats with subclinical, latent or carrier state infection. Therefore, any high-density housing or feline mingling increases risk of exposure and spread. Examples of these include shelters, veterinary clinics, breeding facilities or catteries, or feral or hoarding scenarios.

Transmission is through direct cat-to-cat contact, infectious aerosols or contaminated fomites, e.g. bedding, grooming equipment, human hands. Time from exposure to infection is typically days. The upper respiratory tract (nasal and oropharyngeal mucosa)

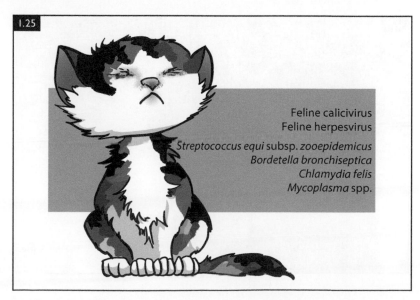

Feline calicivirus
Feline herpesvirus
Streptococcus equi subsp. *zooepidemicus*
Bordetella bronchiseptica
Chlamydia felis
Mycoplasma spp.

Fig. 1.25 Common causes of feline upper respiratory tract disease.

and ocular epithelium are the primary sites of infection. Shedding duration varies between pathogens and may occur before the onset of clinical signs. Organisms are shed in oral, nasal and ocular secretions.

Pathogens involved in FURTD may be present without clinical disease. This may be through colonization, carrier state or latency, e.g. herpesvirus reactivated by stress. As such, these pathogens may be incidental or a disease cause (or contributor) in upper respiratory disease of any etiology. A specific *single* pathogen is rarely identified as the causative agent of FURTD.[82]

Geography

Worldwide. Pathogens may vary geographically and seasonally.

Incidence and risk factors

FURTD is common; however, the incidence is poorly defined for most pathogens. Risk factors include history of exposure to feline groups (e.g. shelter cats). Increased duration and frequency of exposure increase risk of disease. Veterinary hospitals are a source of infection and transmission. Kittens and immunocompromised cats are at higher risk of severe bacterial co-infection and disease.

Clinical signs

The type and severity of clinical signs vary depending on the etiologic agent, co-infection and immune status. Most affected cats are bright and normally active with ocular and nasal discharge. Infection may be subclinical. Although many cats become ill, severe clinical disease or death is extremely rare. Onset may be acute or chronic (>10 days).

Conjunctivitis, sneezing, and bilateral or unilateral serous-to-mucopurulent ocular and nasal discharges are frequent (**Fig. 1.26**). Stertor, snorting and compromise of nasal airflow are common.[82–84] Epistaxis (intermittent or occasional) and vomiting may occur, along with mild fever, lethargy and inappetence. Keratitis, corneal ulceration, chorioretinitis or uveitis may be present depending on the causative pathogen (e.g. herpesvirus keratitis or *Chlamydia felis*-related conjunctivitis). Oral signs can range from mild to severe; these may include gingivostomatitis, hypersalivation and oral pain. Gagging may be seen with concurrent pharyngitis, and clients may report this as vomiting. A full oral exam performed under sedation is helpful, as lesions can be located at the base of the tongue where visualization is limited. Nasal, lingual and dermatologic lesions are most frequently associated with calicivirus and can be severe.

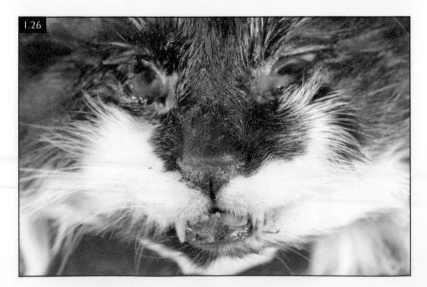

Fig. 1.26 Severe mucopurulent nasal and ocular discharge in a cat with feline upper respiratory tract disease. (Courtesy of Ryan Jennings)

In complicated or progressive FURTD, signs may include fever, anorexia, lethargy, and severe mucopurulent nasal or ocular discharge. Pneumonia may cause tachypnea and dyspnea with or without cough. Facial deformity is rare and suggestive of cryptococcosis.[82]

Diagnosis

Diagnosis is made through complete history and physical exam. Further diagnostics are based on whether disease is acute (<10 days) or chronic (>10 days). Type or location (i.e. unilateral or bilateral) of nasal discharge is unlikely to aid diagnosis.[82] Idiopathic feline rhinosinusitis ("feline snuffles") is a diagnosis of exclusion characterized histopathologically by lymphocytic–plasmacytic or mixed inflammation without identifiable cause.[84]

For acute (<10 days) disease, pursuit of diagnostics (e.g. nasal cytology, cultures, PCR panels) is not typically indicated, because the results uncommonly impact treatment. Testing is more important in outbreak situations (e.g. cattery, shelter or multi-cat household), or when disease occurs in a high risk (e.g. immune-compromised) cat.

Patient history should include information about vaccination status, exposure to other cats or dogs (*B. bronchiseptica*), indoor/outdoor status, potential intoxications (e.g. houseplants/irritants), and recent stress or changes in environment. Physical exam includes complete ocular, oral and otic exam, together with respiratory auscultation.

For chronic FURTD (particularly with prior therapy failure), testing is indicated. This should include assessment of feline leukemia virus (FeLV) and feline immunodeficiency virus (FIV) status, fungal disease and the multiple non-infectious causes of FURTD. Neoplasia may account for 25% of chronic nasal disease.[82] A thorough dental exam and probing for periodontal pockets is important for detection of oronasal communication.

Advanced imaging (MRI or CT) in combination with rhinoscopy, biopsy and histology may be needed for diagnosis of neoplasia, nasal foreign bodies, nasal stenosis, nasopharyngeal polyps, frontal sinusitis and mycotic rhinosinusitis. Additional diagnostics may include nasal lavage or brushing for cytology, culture and susceptibility testing and *Mycoplasma* spp. PCR or culture, along with fungal culture.

Culture and susceptibility testing, and cytology

Consultation may be helpful for decisions on obtaining nasal cultures, their interpretation and antimicrobial treatment. Differentiation of secondary bacterial infection from normal nasal microbiota is difficult. In acute FURTD nasal culture is not recommended owing to lack of diagnostic utility.[6] In chronic FURTD, culture of nasal flush, lavage or biopsy samples (or a combination of these) may be helpful for identification of *Mycoplasma* spp. and other bacterial pathogens.[84] However, the relevance of identification of *Mycoplasma* is questionable. Labs should be notified if *Mycoplasma* is suspected because of the specific culture needs.

Cytology of nasal samples (swab, lavage or brushing) may reveal a mixed inflammatory exudate.

Diagnostic imaging

Radiographs of the thoracic cavity are typically normal with uncomplicated disease. Cats with concurrent pneumonia may have lobar consolidation and alveolar infiltrates. Skull radiographs are non-diagnostic in most cases. Non-specific abnormalities can be found, such as increased nasal or sinus opacity, osteolytic or proliferative bony lesions, and evidence of underlying disease (e.g. tooth abscess, polyp or foreign body).

Diagnosis of chronic FURTD may be determined through a combination of advanced imaging (MRI, CT), rhinoscopy (visualizing the nasal passages) and procuring specimens for cytology, biopsy and culture. MRI or CT is typically abnormal, with evidence of nasal or sinus exudate. Any noted mass should be biopsied, particularly in older cats. Rhinoscopic collection of multiple samples and bilateral exam is advised because of the likelihood of diffuse disease. Findings on rhinoscopy may include discharge, mass, foreign body or a normal exam.[82] Histopathology may confirm a non-infectious diagnosis (e.g. neoplasia) or represent suppurative, lymphoplasmacytic or fibrotic inflammation, or a mixture. Detection of herpesvirus inclusions is rare.

Serology

Immunofluorescent assay (IFA), serum-neutralizing (SN) antibody and enzyme-linked immunosorbent assay (ELISA) antibody testing may confirm viral presence; however, this may (or may not) correlate with active clinical disease. Acute and convalescent titer testing are needed for determination of true clinical illness and may be most useful in an outbreak scenario. Latex agglutination tests for capsular antigen aid the presumptive diagnosis of cryptococcosis.

Virus detection

Virus isolation is most useful for investigating infectious disease outbreaks and to identify a new or emerging pathogen but is uncommonly performed. Specific sampling swabs and techniques may be needed, and diagnosis is improved with oropharyngeal swabs and sampling of multiple sites.

Nasal and pharyngeal swabs and conjunctival samples can be submitted for PCR or reverse transcriptase (RT)-PCR, alone or as part of panels. Viral PCR alone does not confirm causality of disease and must be interpreted with clinical signs and history.

Therapy

Acute FURTD is usually self-limiting within 10 days and specific therapy beyond nursing care is not needed for cats with normal appetite and attitude. In the absence of a specific cause noted on physical exam, the current recommendation is to monitor and observe without antimicrobial therapy.[6] Supportive nursing care provides both comfort and benefit to patients and owners.

Doxycycline should be considered in cats with mucopurulent discharge (ocular or nasal), fever or lethargy, or those who are not eating. Cats with herpesvirus keratitis may benefit from topical antivirals (idoxuridine or cidofovir), although efficacy data are limited. Oral famciclovir may improve clinical signs in cats with feline herpevirus infection.[80]

In chronic FURTD, therapy should be directed at the underlying cause (e.g. itraconazole for cryptococcosis or specific therapy for neoplasia, polyps or foreign bodies). If antimicrobials are needed, choice is ideally based on culture and susceptibility assessment. Optimal antimicrobial therapy duration in chronic FURTD is unknown. However, initial administration for 7 days while monitoring for clinical effect is the current recommendation. Cats with *Pseudomonas aeruginosa* identified on pure culture may require extensive nasal flushing to remove thickened secretions, and treatment with a combination of antimicrobials. Consultation is advised for antimicrobial selection based on nasal culture results because of difficulty in interpretation and therapy planning.

Prognosis/complications

Most cats with acute FURTD have an excellent prognosis and improvement should be noted within 10 days. In cats with chronic FURTD, prognosis is dependent on underlying disease. Prognosis is similarly difficult to estimate in cats diagnosed with chronic rhinosinusitis ("kitty snuffles"). For these cats, management of client expectations is required along with quality of life prioritization based on improvement (or stabilization) of clinical signs.

Prevention

Appropriate vaccination reduces disease severity for many viral pathogens involved in FURTD and can decrease shedding of herpesvirus. Feline calcivirus and herpesvirus are included among core vaccines; in higher-risk or multi-cat situations, a non-core vaccine such as *Chlamydia* sp. may be considered as part of a control program.[70] Importantly, vaccination does not prevent shedding of viral pathogens, eliminate the carrier or latent infection state, or completely protect against development of clinical signs. Similarly, while vaccination is beneficial in reduction of prevalence, there is not a vaccine for all pathogens.

Reduction of overcrowding, associated feline anxiety and immunosuppression are critical to decrease pathogen transmission and consequent infection. It is important to remember that all cats are a potential source of herpesvirus or calicivirus. Ideally cats are housed separately (with appropriate cage separation and lack of shared fomites) on entry to the veterinary hospital, unless they are from the same family/household. Effective quarantine, early identification of ill cats and diagnosis of the cause, together with proper infection control and reporting, are required to manage and ideally prevent (and contain) outbreaks.

FILARID LUNGWORMS: *FILAROIDES HIRTHI, OSLERUS (FILAROIDES) OSLERI*
Dennis Spann

Definition
Filarid lungworms, including *Oslerus osleri* and *Filaroides hirthi*, are parasites that infect the trachea, upper bronchi and lower respiratory tract of canids. *F. hirthi* infests the parenchyma of the lungs, causing secondary inflammation, airway inflammation and cough. *O. osleri* lives in nodules at the tracheal bifurcation and causes tracheal inflammation and coughing. These nodules can occasionally be mistaken for neoplastic masses radiographically.

Etiology and pathogenesis
Filaroides hirthi embeds deeply in the lung parenchyma. Eggs hatch in the airway and infective L1 larvae are transported up the trachea, swallowed and passed in vomitus or stool. These larvae are immediately infective, and dogs are infected when they eat the stool or vomitus. Young puppies are frequently infected when groomed by their mother. After ingestion, larvae migrate via the hepatic portal system to the lungs where they mature and cause clinical signs. The prepatent period is 32–35 days.

Oslerus osleri has a similar life cycle but lives in nodules in the trachea. The prepatent period is approximately 70 days.

Geography
Worldwide; however, higher infection rates are present in Israel and North Africa.

Incidence and risk factors
Both parasites are relatively uncommon. Younger dogs are more commonly affected.

Clinical signs
Filaroides hirthi and *O. osleri* infections are often subclinical. Clinically affected animals may have tachypnea, coughing, ill thrift and a coarse coat.[85, 86] Severely affected dogs can develop weight loss, ill thrift and exercise intolerance. Dogs that develop clinical disease related to *F. hirthi* typically have an underlying disease process or are immunosuppressed.

Diagnosis
Diagnosis is typically confirmed through a combination of suggestive clinical signs, fecal analyses, and/or airway evaluation and sampling (e.g. bronchoscopic identification of *O. oslerus* nodules, transtracheal wash samples) (**Figs. 1.27–1.30**).

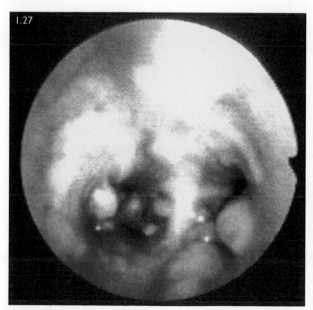

Fig. 1.27 Bronchoscopic view of nodules inhabited by filarid worms at the tracheal bifurcation. (Courtesy of Dr Sue Taylor)

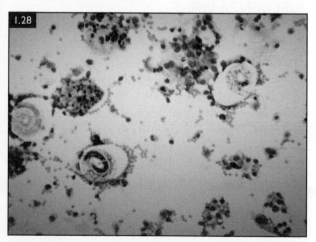

Fig. 1.28 Tracheal wash showing multiple coiled first stage larvae of *Oslerus osleri* organisms and mixed cellular inflammation. (Courtesy of Dr Sue Taylor)

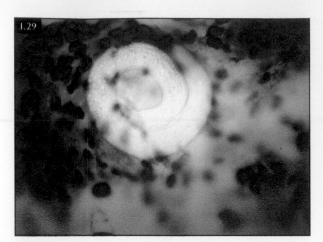

Fig. 1.29 Close-up image of L1 infective larvae of *O. osleri*. (Courtesy of Dr Sue Taylor)

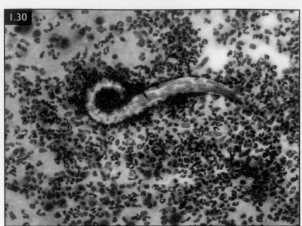

Fig. 1.30 *Filaroides hirthi* in an airway wash. (Courtesy of Dr Alicia Caro Vadillo)

Fecal analysis

Zinc sulfate flotation is more efficient than the Baermann technique for isolating infective larvae because the larvae have poor motility and are not readily detected by Baermann.[57] PCR has been developed but is not widely available.

Therapy

Fenbendazole (50 mg/kg PO q24h for 10–14 days) is commonly used. Ivermectin 0.2–0.4 mg/kg, single or repeated doses, is another option,[87] as is doramectin (0.4 mg/kg) injection.

Prognosis/complications

Prognosis is generally good. Immune-suppressed animals occasionally have severe infections resulting from autoinfection. Hypoadrenocorticism and distemper infection have been reported to be predisposing causes of hyperinfection.[88]

Prevention

Prevention of coprophagy is the main preventive measure.

INFLUENZA VIRUS
Michelle Evason and J Scott Weese

Definition

Influenza virus is an endemic pathogen in dogs in some regions, with occasional "spillover" of infection from humans or other animals to dogs and cats. Typically, dogs have non-specific signs of canine infectious respiratory disease complex (CIRDC) or pneumonia, which may (or may not) progress from mild to fatal disease. In cats, influenza is rare but most often characterized as mild feline upper respiratory tract disease (FURTD). Influenza viruses are high profile owing to concerns regarding zoonoses (human disease) and rapid spread across geographic areas (pandemics in humans or other animals).

The reservoirs of all variants of influenza A are wild birds, predominantly waterfowl. Some variants are able to infect other hosts, with marked differences in susceptibility of different species to infection and disease.

Dogs

Sporadic disease caused by H3N8 influenza of equine origin was noted periodically, with limited spread. However, adaptation of an equine H3N8 strain to dogs in Florida in the early 2000s resulted in the emergence of a true canine influenza virus (CIV).[89] Subsequently, avian-origin H3N2 CIV emerged in Asia and spread to North America.[90]

In addition to true CIV, sporadic direct human–dog infections with human influenza (e.g. H1N1) can occur.

Cats

There are no host-adapted (feline influenza virus) strains. However, cats are susceptible to many avian and human influenza viruses. Infections associated with a range of avian H3N2, H7N2 and H5N1, canine H3N2 and human H1N1 have been identified.[91–97] Most have been sporadic, but a large shelter outbreak with H7N2 has been documented.[91]

Etiology and pathogenesis

Influenza A may infect humans, birds and other animals, and reassortment of influenza viruses can result in the emergence of new types. Rapid changes (mutations or assortment) in both the hemagglutinin (H) and neuraminidase (N) glycoproteins of influenza A are referred to as "antigenic shifts". These rapid changes are responsible for past outbreaks and pandemic spread within the bird and human populations.

Transmission of influenza A is believed to occur through direct contact, inhalation or in some cases ingestion of infected birds. Viral shedding may occur through respiratory secretions (oral, ocular and nasal) and fecal routes. Shedding may occur before clinical signs. Incubation times are short (2–5 days) and this is when peak viral shedding is believed to occur. Antibody may be detected within 7 days. Viral shedding depends on strain, with H3N8 shed for a relatively limited period of time (<7 days), but H3N2 shedding is more prolonged (up to 3–4 weeks).[98] Shedding of non-host-adapted strains is likely short term. After exposure, the virus spreads to the lower respiratory tract and potentially the gastrointestinal tract.[99]

Geography

CIV is most widely documented in the USA and southeast Asia. Transmission of human variants could occur worldwide. The risk from avian influenza parallels its regional distribution, with the highest risk in southeast Asia.

Incidence and risk factors

The incidence of disease in dogs is ill defined and highly variable between and within regions. It seems to be an uncommon infection, with periodic small-to-large regional outbreaks. The prevalence of H3N8 has been reported from 0.5% to less than 5%, and up to 50% in dogs with CIRDC, although recent evidence would suggest that H3N8 CIV is now extremely rare. The prevalence differs based on housing environment (lower in pet dog vs. shelter environment) and geographic area. Variations are likely associated with outbreaks, and consequent increased awareness and testing. Reported risk factors for H3N8 CIV in the USA include group housing (shelter and kennel) and geographic area (Colorado, Florida, New York), dependent on year of illness.[100] There is increased risk of infection in dogs with close contact and stress (e.g. shelters, kennels, boarding or training facilities, veterinary hospitals and daycares).[36, 100] All ages and breeds of dogs may be affected; however, severe mortality due to pneumonia has been reported mainly in greyhounds.[89]

Limited prevalence data are available for cats, with most studies involving outbreaks. Infection is probably very uncommon.

Clinical signs

Clinical signs are indistinguishable from other causes of CIRDC and FURTD, as discussed in those sections. Cough, nasal and ocular discharge (conjunctivitis), fever and occasional vomiting predominate. Pneumonia can develop secondarily. Rarely, severe presentations such as hemorrhagic pneumonia can be encountered.

Physical examination

Exam findings can include a range of respiratory signs, and rarely systemic, neurologic and intestinal signs.

Diagnosis

Influenza is typically diagnosed via detection of virus shedding by PCR, along with suggestive clinical signs. Influenza is more likely to be present (and testing more valuable) when there are increased numbers of dogs or cats with respiratory disease in a specific geographic area, where multiple dogs or cats in a single household are ill, when affected animals have been imported from endemic regions (e.g. South Korea, China) or have been in contact with dogs from those regions, or when there has been contact with an animal with influenza.

Virus detection

Nasal or deep oropharyngeal swabs should be collected close to the onset of clinical signs (within 3–4 days). Conjunctival swabs may also be tested. PCR is widely available. Some assays are strain specific while others are broader, so it is important to ensure that the strain of concern is detected by the chosen test.

Although it is the "gold standard" for diagnosis, virus isolation is uncommonly performed diagnostically because of the time and expense. It is more commonly used for research or investigation of uncommon situations (e.g. outbreaks, atypical disease).

Serology

Demonstration of a fourfold or higher increase in antibody titer in paired samples (taken approximately 14 days apart) is diagnostic. Vaccination may interfere with test interpretation in dogs that have been vaccinated within the preceding few weeks. Serological testing is most useful when samples cannot be collected early in the disease and viral shedding may have already ceased.

Therapy

There is no specific treatment. Supportive care may be indicated, such as the use of cough suppressants. Antimicrobials may be indicated with more advanced disease, as is described under CIRDC. There is no evidence that antiviral medications are useful or needed.

Prognosis/complications

Prognosis is dependent on severity of presenting signs and capability of owners (e.g. supportive and isolation care needs and associated costs). Mild illness is common in many dogs and cats, and prognosis is excellent in these cases. Severely progressive respiratory, neurologic or systemic signs have a poor prognosis and death may result.

Prevention

Vaccines are available for both H3N8 and H3N2 CIV. They offer little to no cross-protection, and the vaccine strain must match the strain that is present in the area in order to be effective.

Currently available inactivated vaccines may reduce viral shedding and disease development.[32, 101, 102] Vaccines are non-core and should be considered for dogs at risk (e.g. before travel to endemic influenza areas or in group housing scenarios, such as boarding kennels).[70]

Public health and infection control

Current canine influenza viruses are not known to infect humans, but there is concern that they could recombine with another influenza virus and result in a strain that can affect people. Any novel influenza strain in an animal should be assumed to pose some risk to humans until proven otherwise. Cat-to-human transmission of influenza viruses can occur but is rare.[91, 103]

MYCOPLASMA SPP.
Michelle Evason

Definition

In dogs and cats, *Mycoplasma* spp. may cause infection of the mucous membranes of the respiratory, ocular, urinary or genital systems. *Mycoplasma* spp.-associated feline upper respiratory tract disease (FURTD) and canine infectious respiratory disease complex (CIRDC) are common in kittens and puppies in high-density environments (e.g. shelters). However, the relevance of *Mycoplasma* spp. in disease can be difficult to ascertain owing to its relatively high prevalence in healthy animals. *Mycoplasma* spp. are frequently present with other pathogens and may be opportunistic or incidental.

Etiology and pathogenesis

Mycoplasma spp. are cell wall-deficient bacteria that are dependent on their host for survival and energy. Transmission is through direct contact (e.g. cat to cat), or contact with shared fomites, such as brushes or bedding.

They may be opportunistic contributors (or compounders) of underlying infection or diseases. Lack of expected disease resolution and increased severity of clinical signs should raise the index of suspicion for concurrent *Mycoplasma* spp. infection. Relevance may vary among animal and *Mycoplasma* spp. In cats *M. felis* is considered a significant pathogen in conjunctivitis.[29, 30, 48, 50] *M. cynos* has been less convincingly associated with lower respiratory tract disease in dogs.[104, 105] Differentiating primary infection, co-infection and clinically irrelevant colonization is difficult.

Geography
Present worldwide.

Incidence and risk factors
Mycoplasma spp. can be found in a large percentage of healthy dogs and cats, as well as in those with disease. *M. cynos* may be more prevalent in dogs with respiratory disease and may increase the severity of clinical signs.[105] Risk factors for infection include younger age and high-density groups (e.g. kennels).[30, 48, 105, 106]

Risk factors for pneumonia and systemic disease include young age (<1 year), concurrent disease (other bacterium or virus), neoplasia or immunocompromise (e.g. ciliary dyskinesis or immune-compromising medications).[48, 104]

Clinical signs
Signs are consistent with CIRDC or FURTD.

Less commonly, urinary or reproductive disease can occur. Dogs with urinary or genital disease due to *Mycoplasma* spp. are frequently immunocompromised.[107] Clinical signs may be consistent with lower urinary tract infection or include systemic disease signs (e.g. fever, anorexia in severe prostatitis or epididymitis–orchitis).

Systemic infection may result in polyarthritis, with swollen painful joints and shifting limb lameness.

Infection of penetrating wounds (e.g. bites) may result in opportunistic abscesses, skin and soft tissue infection.

Diagnosis
Mycoplasma spp. infection can be challenging to diagnose conclusively and determine its relevance. Signs of disease are non-specific, and frequently overlap with those of other pathogens and concurrent disease processes. The high prevalence of some *Mycoplasma* spp. in healthy animals complicates test interpretation.

Diagnostic imaging
This is usually normal, except in pneumonia, where interstitial or alveolar lung patterns or lung lobe consolidation may be present.

Cytology
Cytologic examination of joint (synovial) fluid, CSF or bronchoalveolar lavage (BAL) fluid may be normal or consistent with suppurative inflammation. As with all suspected cases of polyarthritis, multiple joints should be tapped because not all may be affected. *Mycoplasma* spp. will not be visible on microscopic exam owing to their small size and lack of cell wall to take up stain.

Culture
Mycoplasma spp. can be challenging to grow, and require longer time frames and special culture and transport medium. False-negative results are common. Samples and swabs from clinically affected sites (respiratory tract, BAL, urine, synovial fluid) are optimal for interpretation. Susceptibility testing is rarely performed.

PCR
PCR testing is most commonly used. Advantages include speed of detection and improved sensitivity vs. culture; however, sensitivity and specificity may vary. Results must be interpreted in the light of clinical findings.

Therapy
Most cases of FURTD or CIRDC will be self-limiting, and do not require antimicrobials. In patients with severe disease where *Mycoplasma* spp. infection is suspected (and owing to the challenges of culture), antimicrobial therapy (along with management of any concurrent disease) may be initiated before obtaining definitive results. Typically, improvement is noted quickly (e.g. within 1 week) after antimicrobials and nursing care are initiated.[52]

Mycoplasmas are inherently resistant to many antimicrobials, including beta-lactams (e.g. amoxicillin), trimethoprim sulfonamides, rifampin and some macrolides. Doxycycline is frequently used. Pradofloxacin may also be used in cats with FURTD, but fluoroquinolones are typically reserved as second-line options. Treatment for a minimum of 7–10 days for FURTD in cats has been recommended.[53]

Prognosis/complications

Prognosis is usually excellent with appropriate therapy. Most cases are self-limiting in 7–10 days. Cases of pneumonia, or urogenital or systemic disease (polyarthritis) will require longer and more intensive therapy.

PARAGONIMUS KELLICOTTI (LUNG FLUKE)
Dennis Spann

Definition

Paragonimus kellicotti is a trematode that creates cystic lesions in the lung parenchyma and frequently causes an eosinophilic granulomatous pneumonia. Dogs, cats, muskrats, minks, raccoons, foxes and rarely humans can be infected.

Etiology and pathogenesis

Paragonimus kellicotti has an indirect lifecycle that involves two intermediate hosts, an aquatic snail (**Fig. 1.31**) and crayfish (**Fig. 1.32**). The flukes infect the definitive host after the host eats affected raw crayfish. Rats may serve as paratenic hosts, whose predation may also lead to infection. Metacercaria excyst in the host's small intestine. Flukes then penetrate the intestinal wall, traversing the peritoneal cavity for 1–14 days before penetrating the diaphragm and entering the lungs. Hermaphroditic adult flukes (**Fig. 1.33**) are usually found paired within cysts in the lungs. Cysts containing mating pairs open to bronchioles, so that eggs laid in the cyst pass out into the bronchiole. The eggs pass up the ciliated airways with mucus, are swallowed and pass out with the feces. The prepatent period is 3–36 days. Eggs mature for 2–3 weeks in a freshwater environment and then hatch into miracidia. A miracidium finds and penetrates a snail. First sporocysts, and then rediae, develop in the snail. Cercariae develop in the rediae, and when mature emerge from the snail. The cercariae then infect a crayfish or crab. Consumption of the tissue results in

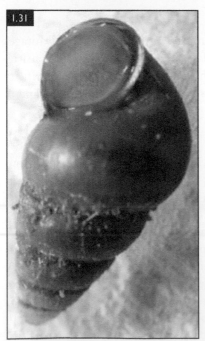

Fig. 1.31 *Pomatiopsis lapidaria* is the preferred first intermediate host for *Paragonimus kellicotti* throughout the Mississippi River drainage basin of the US midwest. (Courtesy of bioweb.uwlax.edu)

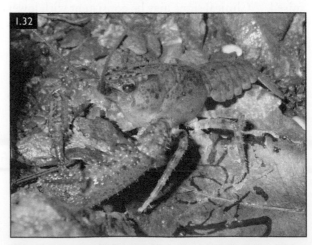

Fig. 1.32 Crayfish serve as an intermediate host for *Paragonimus kellicotti*.

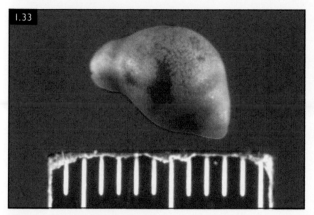

Fig. 1.33 *Paragonimus kellicotti* adult. (Courtesy of Dr Eleanor Hawkins)

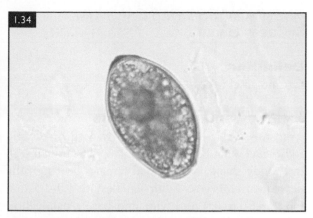

Fig. 1.34 *Paragonimus kellicotti* fluke egg. (Courtesy of Dr Eleanor Hawkins)

excystation of the metacercaria and repeat of the cycle. The fluke-containing cysts in the airways elicit an exuberant antiparasitic response, leading to cough, fever and eosinophilic granulomatous pneumonia.

Geography

Paragonimus spp. are prevalent worldwide where crayfish are found (e.g. southeastern and midwestern USA, particularly the Mississippi and Great Lakes drainage areas).

Incidence and risk factors

Incidence is variable and related to access to waterways and raw crustaceans. A high percentage of crayfish in the rivers of Missouri, Oklahoma and Ohio are infected.[108]

Clinical signs

Signs vary with the individual and the level of infection. Dogs may be clinically normal, or have fever, lethargy, and intermittent or persistent cough. With severe infections, ill thrift, hemoptysis and severe eosinophilic pneumonia occur. Ruptured cysts can occasionally lead to pneumothorax.

Diagnosis

Paragonimus kellicotti eggs (90 × 50 μm) can be recovered from feces by sugar flotation, sedimentation of feces or transtracheal wash, and identified by their size, seated operculum and a bump or flange on the end opposite the operculum (**Fig. 1.34**).

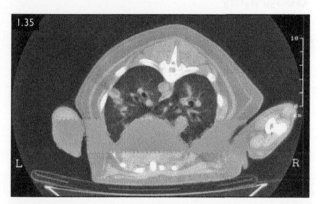

Fig. 1.35 CT scan of the lung of a dog infected with *Paragonimus kellicotti*. Multiple soft tissue density nodules are seen. (Courtesy of Dr Eleanor Hawkins)

Randomly located round nodules can be seen radiographically or on CT imaging. Bronchiectasis is occasionally seen (**Fig. 1.35**).

Therapy

Praziquantel (25 mg/kg PO q8h for 2–3 days) or fenbendazole (50 mg/kg PO q24h for 10–14 days) may be used.[109]

Prognosis/complications

Prognosis is generally good with diagnosis and treatment. Radiographic lesions can take weeks to months to resolve.[109, 110] Complications include rare reports of pneumothorax.

Prevention

Prevent access to raw crustaceans.

PNEUMONYSSOIDES CANINUM
M Casey Gaunt

Definition
Canine nasal mite.

Etiology and pathogenesis
Transmission is believed to be by both direct and indirect contact between dogs.[111, 112] The mite has an oval body shape, with gravid females bearing fully developed embryos. Adult females are 1.0–1.5 mm long and 0.6–0.9 mm wide and have a pale yellow color while alive.[113]

Geography
Worldwide distribution.

Incidence and risk factors
Dogs more than 3 years of age are more commonly infected than younger dogs and large breed dogs are infected more commonly than small breed dogs. No sex predilection has been identified. Dogs with endocrinopathies appear to be more likely to be infected with nasal mites.[114]

Clinical signs
Reverse sneezing is the most commonly reported sign, while rhinitis, sneezing, head shaking, epistaxis and impaired scenting ability have also been described.[115–117] Visualization of the mites on or around the nares may be possible. Serous nasal discharge may be present with severe disease; however, discharge from nasopharyngeal disease is usually swallowed.[118] Nasal mite infestation was identified as a risk factor for development of gastric dilation–volvulus in dogs in Norway.[119]

Diagnosis
Definitive diagnosis is made by visualizing the mites in or around the nares. This can be very difficult owing to the mite's location in the nasal sinuses and caudal nasal cavity. Rhinoscopy can be used to aid identification and may identify mites (**Fig. 1.36**) or follicular hyperplasia, which should raise suspicion.[118] Thorough nasal flushing may allow collection of mites in the fluid.[120]

A presumptive diagnosis can be made when appropriate clinical signs are identified, followed by response to treatment.[116, 118]

Therapy
Ivermectin was the first successful treatment reported.[121, 122] Given the potential complications associated with ivermectin treatment in some breeds, other macrocyclic lactones were investigated and found to be effective. Oral milbemycin (0.5–1 mg/kg PO every 7–10 days for 3 doses) and topical selamectin (6–24 mg/kg every 2 weeks for 3 doses) are also highly effective.[111, 116, 121]

Prognosis/complications
Excellent response to therapy has been reported with ivermectin, milbemycin and selamectin.[118] Temporary worsening after initial treatment has been encountered, potentially as a result of the inflammatory response to dying mites.[111] Treatment with a single anti-inflammatory dose of prednisolone (0.5 mg/kg PO) may be useful with the first treatment or if signs worsen after treatment is initiated.[118]

Prevention
It is logical to conclude that treatment with monthly anthelmintic therapy (milbemycin, ivermectin, selamectin) should prevent nasal mite infestation.

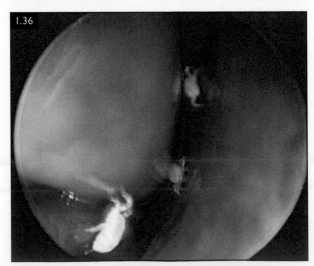

Fig. 1.36 *Pneumonyssoides caninum* **evident via rhinoscopy in a dog. (Courtesy of Dr Sue Taylor)**

PYOTHORAX
J Scott Weese

Definition
Pyothorax is an infection of the pleural cavity that results in accumulation of purulent pleural exudate.

Etiology and pathogenesis
There are many possible routes of entry for bacteria to gain access to the pleural space. Extension of pulmonary infection, foreign body migration or penetrating foreign body are most often implicated,[123, 124] but often an inciting cause is not identified.[125] Regardless of the origin, bacteria that gain access to the pleural cavity proliferate, initiating local and systemic inflammatory responses. A key part of this is the development of purulent effusion in the pleural space. A wide range of bacteria can be involved, predominantly oropharyngeal residents (*Table 1.4*).[126]

Risk factors
In both dogs and cats, pyothorax can occur as a sequel to upper respiratory infection and pneumonia. In cats, fighting is an important risk factor. Lifestyles and geography that predispose to exposure to potential foreign bodies such as grass awns also likely increase the risk (**Fig. 1.37**). Young animals are most often affected.[125]

Clinical signs
Clinical signs may be vague and non-specific, even with relatively advanced disease. Alterations in respiratory rate, effort and pattern are often present. Weight loss, lethargy, anorexia and cough may also be noted, particularly in more advanced cases. Fever may be present but is an inconsistent finding, particularly in cats. Signs relating to the underlying disease (e.g. pneumonia, trauma, wound) may be identified.

Lung and heart sounds may be muffled on auscultation. Pleural pain may also be noted when pressing on the chest during auscultation. Signs of systemic inflammation, including systemic inflammatory response syndrome or sepsis, may be present.

Diagnosis
Diagnostic imaging is critical. Radiographs (**Fig. 1.38**) and ultrasound can be used to identify pleural effusion. Radiographs or CT (**Fig. 1.39**) are important to help investigate the lung parenchyma, to assess severity of disease and help identify potential causes.

Pleural fluid aspiration is also critical to obtain fluid to confirm pyothorax and for culture. The fluid

Table 1.4 **Common pyothorax pathogens**	
CATS	**DOGS**
Actinomyces	Bacteroides
Bacteroides	Clostridium
Fusobacterium	Corynebacterium
Nocardia	Enterobacter
Pasteurella	Escherichia coli
Peptostreptococcus	Fusobacterium
Porphyromonas	Klebsiella
Prevotella	Pasteurella
Staphylococcus	Peptostreptococcus
Streptococcus	Prevotella
	Propionibacterium
	Staphylococcus
	Streptococcus

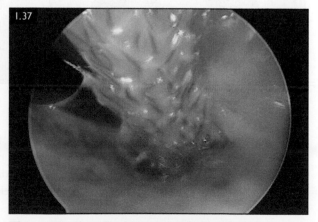

Fig. 1.37 Plant foreign material identified via thoracoscopy. (Courtesy of Dr Brigitte Brisson)

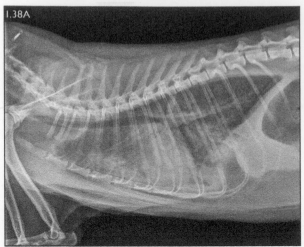

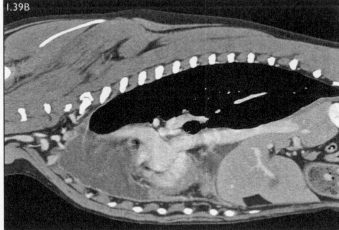

Fig. 1.38 Lateral (A) and ventrodorsal (B) thoracic radiographs of a cat with pyothorax secondary to a suspected cat-bite abscess. Note the pleural effusion and bronchointerstitial pattern. (Courtesy of Atlantic Veterinary College)

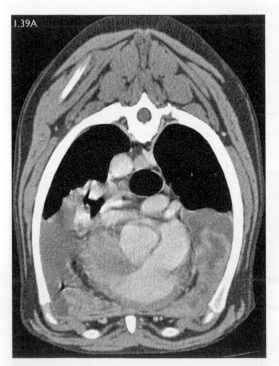

Fig. 1.39A, B Transverse and sagittal CT images of a dog with moderate bilateral pleural effusion, pleural thickening and thoracic lymphadenopathy due to pyothorax secondary to a stick foreign body.

is consistent with an exudate, with protein concentration greater than 30 mg/L and cell count greater than 5×10^9 cells/mL. Intracellular and extracellular bacteria are often identified, and white blood cells may have toxic changes. Cytology can also help identify potential involvement of pathogens such as *Actinomyces* (**Fig. 1.40**). Acid-fast stain should be considered to help detect acid-fast bacteria such as *Mycobacterium* and *Nocardia*. Aerobic and anaerobic culture should be performed.

Therapy

Treatment involves drainage, antimicrobials and supportive care. Drainage may be intermittent or continuous, with or without lavage, depending on the case and practical considerations (**Figs. 1.41, 1.42**).[126] Surgical intervention may be required in some cases, to facilitate drainage (particularly if an abscess is present), remove a foreign body or remove severely compromised lung tissue. The usefulness of intrapleural fibrinolytics is unclear.

Empirical antibiotic treatment should be broad spectrum, for example either ampicillin or clindamycin plus a fluoroquinolone, with de-escalation based on culture results.[126] Duration of antimicrobial treatment is not well understood, but 4–6 weeks is often used. Serial radiographs can be used to monitor lung pathology and pleural fluid production. Thoracic ultrasound is a convenient tool for monitoring fluid production and to evaluate the character

of fluid and debris in the pleural space. CT may be useful for identification of foreign bodies.

Prognosis

The prognosis is good if diagnosed and treated early in disease. Overall, survival rates of 60–80% are expected, with dogs at the higher end and cats at the lower end.[125, 127–129] More advanced disease, severe pulmonary involvement, pleural adhesions and an unidentified etiology can worsen the prognosis.

Prevention

Prevention of respiratory tract infections via vaccination, management, and keeping cats indoors to reduce fighting may reduce the risk of pyothorax.

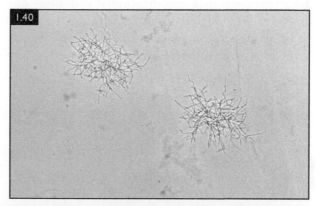

Fig. 1.40 Cytology showing the morphology of *Actinomyces* spp. (500× magnification). (Courtesy of Dr Lucille K Georg)

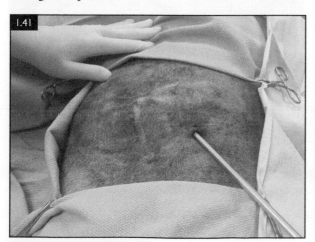

Fig. 1.41 Placement of a chest tube in a dog with pyothorax. (Courtesy of Dr Jim Dundas)

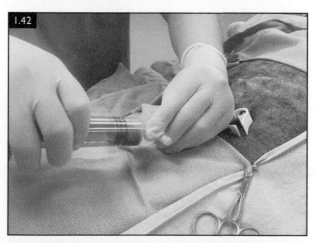

Fig. 1.42 Hemorrhagic, purulent exudate from the chest tube of a dog with pyothorax. (Courtesy of Dr Jim Dundas)

STREPTOCOCCUS ZOOEPIDEMICUS
J Scott Weese

Definition
Streptococcus equi subspecies *zooepidemicus* is a gram-positive bacterium that is an uncommon cause of potentially severe respiratory tract disease, otitis and meningitis in dogs and cats.

Etiology and pathogenesis
This bacterium is uncommonly found in healthy dogs and cats and it is unclear whether it is truly a canine and feline commensal. It is a common commensal in horses, but contact with horses is not required for it to be found in cats and dogs. Why this organism develops from a commensal to a pathogen in a specific animal is unclear but likely relates in part to concurrent diseases (e.g. viral upper respiratory tract infection) and factors that impact the immune system.

Incidence and risk factors
Streptococcus zooepidemicus can be found in the respiratory tract of a small percentage of healthy dogs (0–2%) and cats (0–1.5%).[40, 41, 43, 130] Disease is uncommon and occurs mainly in intensive housing such as shelters, kennels and hoarding situations. Outbreaks, some with high morbidity and mortality, can be encountered in those locations.[131, 132]

Clinical signs
Upper respiratory tract infections are characterized by purulent nasal discharge, coughing and sneezing, and can progress to rhinitis, sinusitis or pneumonia. These may be indistinguishable from those caused by other feline and canine upper respiratory tract pathogens.

Hemorrhagic pneumonia is more commonly reported in dogs[133, 134] and is often characterized by fulminant, rapidly fatal disease in shelters and kennels. Affected animals may be found dead in their cages with hemorrhagic nasal discharge.

In cats, progression beyond upper respiratory tract disease can include pneumonia and otitis.[132] There is increasing evidence of a role in otitis interna/media in cats (**Figs. 1.43, 1.44**), with the

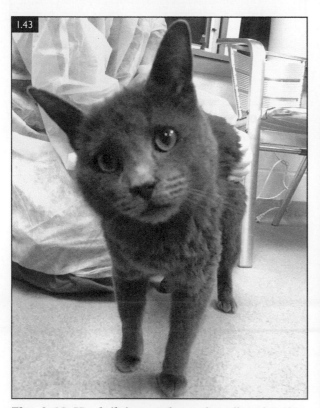

Fig. 1.43 Head tilt in a cat from a hoarding situation with otitis interna/media caused by *Streptococcus zooepidemicus*. (Courtesy of Dr Linda Jacobson)

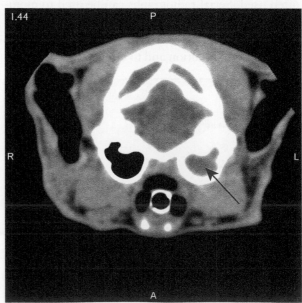

Fig. 1.44 CT image of a cat with left-sided otitis interna/media. Note the fluid-filled left bulla (arrow). (Courtesy of Dr Linda Jacobson)

potential for progression to meningoencephalitis.[135] Uncommon presentations in cats include myocarditis and endocarditis.[136]

Diagnosis

The bacterium can be readily detected by culture or PCR. Its relevance when identified from colonization sites (e.g. nose, mouth, pharynx, upper respiratory tract) can be hard to discern, particularly in populations where shedding is more common (e.g. shelters); however, positive cultures are strongly suggestive. Isolation of the bacterium from lower airways, the middle ear or otherwise sterile sites is diagnostic.

Therapy

Streptococci are almost always susceptible to penicillins (e.g. amoxicillin). Clavulanic acid is not required. Clindamycin and trimethoprim sulfonamide are other reasonable options. Doxycycline resistance is uncommon but has been identified.[131] Other components of treatment depend on the location and severity of disease.

Prognosis/complications

Prognosis is highly dependent on the type and location of infection. Acute hemorrhagic pneumonia carries a very guarded prognosis and affected animals may die rapidly. Chronic sequelae from rhinitis, sinusitis or chronic otitis externa can be difficult to manage.

Prevention

There is little information about prevention. Measures aimed at preventing and containing other upper respiratory tract pathogens likely apply equally to *S. zooepidemicus*. Although it can be found in healthy animals, isolation of clinically affected animals is reasonable because of the potential for high burdens of shedding.

Streptococcus zooepidemicus is a zoonotic bacterium, but the overall risk is quite low given the relatively large number of people who are routinely exposed to the bacterium (especially from horses) and the low incidence of disease. Transmission from a dog with upper respiratory tract infection to a handler has been reported.[137]

No clear preventive measures are available. Although restricting contact with horses and equine environments probably reduces the risk of exposure, most cases of *S. zooepidemicus* infection in dogs and cats do not have a history of horse contact.

REFERENCES

1   Pennisi, MG *et al.* (2015) Lungworm disease in cats: ABCD guidelines on prevention and management. *J Feline Med Surg* **17**:626–36.

2   Elsheikha, HM *et al.* (2016) Updates on feline aelurostrongylosis and research priorities for the next decade. *Parasit Vectors* **9**:389.

3   Knaus, M *et al.* (2011) Endoparasites of cats from the Tirana area and the first report on *Aelurostrongylus abstrusus* (Railliet, 1898) in Albania. *Wien Klin Wochenschr* **123**(Suppl 1): 31–5.

4   Traversa, D *et al.* (2009) Efficacy and safety of emodepside 2.1%/praziquantel 8.6% spot-on formulation in the treatment of feline aelurostrongylosis. *Parasitol Res* **105**(Suppl 1):S83–9.

5   Johnson, LR *et al.* (2013) Microbiologic and cytologic assessment of bronchoalveolar lavage fluid from dogs with lower respiratory tract infection: 105 cases (2001–2011). *J Vet Intern Med* **27**:259–67.

6   Lappin, MR *et al.* (2017) Antimicrobial use Guidelines for Treatment of Respiratory Tract Disease in Dogs and Cats: Antimicrobial Guidelines Working Group of the International Society for Companion Animal Infectious Diseases. *J Vet Intern Med* **31**:279–94.

7   Ramsey, DT (1994) Blastomycosis in a veterinarian. *J Am Vet Med Assoc* **205**:968.

8   Gnann, JW *et al.* (1983) Human blastomycosis after a dog bite. *Ann Intern Med* **98**:48–9.

9   Scott, MJ (1955) Cutaneous blastomycosis: report of case following dog bite. *Northwest Med* **54**:255–7.

10   Bromel, C *et al.* (2005) Epidemiology, diagnosis, and treatment of blastomycosis in dogs and cats. *Clin Tech Small Anim Pract* **20**:233–9.

11   Blondin, N *et al.* (2007) Blastomycosis in indoor cats: suburban Chicago, Illinois, USA. *Mycopathologia* **163**:59–66.

12   Legendre, AM *et al.* (1996) Treatment of blastomycosis with itraconazole in 112 dogs. *J Vet Intern Med* **10**:365–371.

13 Lloret, A *et al.* (2013) Rare systemic mycoses in cats: blastomycosis, histoplasmosis and coccidioidomycosis: ABCD guidelines on prevention and management. *J Feline Med Surg* **15**:624–7.

14 Kerl, ME (2003) Update on canine and feline fungal diseases. *Vet Clin North Am Small Anim Pract* **33**:721–47.

15 McMillan, CJ *et al.* (2008) Transtracheal aspiration in the diagnosis of pulmonary blastomycosis (17 cases: 2000–2005). *Can Vet J* **49**:53–5.

16 Saito, M *et al.* (2002) CT findings of intracranial blastomycosis in a dog. *Vet Radiol Ultrasound* **43**:16–21.

17 Garma-Avina, A (1995) Cytologic findings in 43 cases of blastomycosis diagnosed ante-mortem in naturally-infected dogs. *Mycopathologia* **131**:87–91.

18 Crews, LJ *et al.* (2008). Utility of diagnostic tests for and medical treatment of pulmonary blastomycosis in dogs: 125 cases (1989–2006). *J Am Vet Med Assoc* **232**:222–7.

19 Crews, LJ *et al.* (2008) Radiographic findings in dogs with pulmonary blastomycosis: 125 cases (1989–2006). *J Am Vet Med Assoc* **232**:215–21.

20 Wood, EF *et al.* (1998) Ultrasound-guided fine-needle aspiration of focal parenchymal lesions of the lung in dogs and cats. *J Vet Intern Med* **12**:338–42.

21 Hawkins, EC *et al.* (1990) Cytologic analysis of tracheal wash specimens and bronchoalveolar lavage fluid in the diagnosis of mycotic infections in dogs. *J Am Vet Med Assoc* **197**:79–83.

22 Frost, HM *et al.* (2015) *Blastomyces* antigen detection for diagnosis and management of blastomycosis. *J Clin Microbiol* **53**:3660–2.

23 Dial, SM (2007) Fungal diagnostics: current techniques and future trends. *Vet Clin North Am Small Anim Pract* **37**:373–92.

24 Grooters, AM *et al.* (2003) Update on antifungal therapy. *Vet Clin North Am Small Anim Pract* **33**:749–58.

25 Krohne, SG (2000) Canine systemic fungal infections. *Vet Clin North Am Small Anim Pract* **30**:1063–90.

26 Mazepa, AS *et al.* (2011) Retrospective comparison of the efficacy of fluconazole or itraconazole for the treatment of systemic blastomycosis in dogs. *J Vet Intern Med* **25**:440–5.

27 Foy, DS *et al.* (2014) Serum and urine *Blastomyces* antigen concentrations as markers of clinical remission in dogs treated for systemic blastomycosis. *J Vet Intern Med* **28**:305–10.

28 Radhakrishnan, A *et al.* (2007) Community-acquired infectious pneumonia in puppies: 65 cases (1993–2002). *J Am Vet Med Assoc* 230:1493–7.

29 Burns, RE *et al.* (2011) Histologic and molecular correlation in shelter cats with acute upper respiratory infection. *J Clin Microbiol* **49**:2454–60.

30 Litster, AL *et al.* (2012) Comparison of the efficacy of amoxicillin–clavulanic acid, cefovecin, and doxycycline in the treatment of upper respiratory tract disease in cats housed in an animal shelter. *J Am Vet Med Assoc* **241**:218–26.

31 Ruch-Gallie, R *et al.* (2016) Adenovirus 2, *Bordetella bronchiseptica*, and parainfluenza molecular diagnostic assay results in puppies after vaccination with modified live vaccines. *J Vet Intern Med* **30**:164–6.

32 Larson, LJ *et al.* (2011) Efficacy of the canine influenza virus H3N8 vaccine to decrease severity of clinical disease after co-challenge with canine influenza virus and *Streptococcus equi* subsp. *zooepidemicus*. *Clin Vaccine Immunol* **18**:559–64.

33 Anon (2016) WSAVA publishes updated guidance on vaccination of dogs and cats. *Vet Rec* **178**:56.

34 Lavan, R *et al.* (2015) Prevalence of canine infectious respiratory pathogens in asymptomatic dogs presented at US animal shelters. *J Small Anim Pract* **56**:572–6.

35 Weese, JS *et al.* (2013) Respiratory disease outbreak in a veterinary hospital associated with canine parainfluenza virus infection. *Can Vet J* **54**:79–82.

36 Priestnall, SL *et al.* (2014) New and emerging pathogens in canine infectious respiratory disease. *Vet Pathol* **51**:492–504.

37 Mitchell, JA *et al.* (2017) European surveillance of emerging pathogens associated with canine infectious respiratory disease. *Vet Microbiol* **212**:31–8.

38 Mochizuki, M *et al.* (2008) Etiologic study of upper respiratory infections of household dogs. *J Vet Med Sci* **70**:563–9.

39 Wagener, JS *et al.* (1984) Role of canine parainfluenza virus and *Bordetella bronchiseptica* in kennel cough. *Am J Vet Res* **45**:1862–6.

40 Sowman, HR *et al.* (2018) A survey of canine respiratory pathogens in New Zealand dogs. *N Z Vet J* **66**:236–42.

41 Joffe, DJ *et al.* (2016) Factors associated with development of canine infectious respiratory disease complex (CIRDC) in dogs in 5 Canadian small animal clinics. *Can Vet J* **57**:46–51.

42 Erles, K *et al.* (2005) Investigation into the causes of canine infectious respiratory disease: antibody responses to canine respiratory coronavirus and canine herpesvirus in two kennelled dog populations. *Arch Virol* **150**:1493–1504.

43 Decaro, N *et al.* (2016) Molecular surveillance of traditional and emerging pathogens associated with canine infectious respiratory disease. *Vet Microbiol* **192**:21–5.

44 Ford, RB *et al.* (2017) 2017 AAHA Canine Vaccination Guidelines. *J Am Anim Hosp Assoc* **53**:243–51.

45 Kontor, EJ *et al.* (1981) Canine infectious tracheobronchitis: effects of an intranasal live canine parainfluenza–*Bordetella bronchiseptica* vaccine on viral shedding and clinical tracheobronchitis (kennel cough). *Am J Vet Res* **42**:1694–8.

46 Greene, CE (2012) Chlamydial infections. In *Infectious Diseases of the Dog and Cat*, 4th ed. CE Greene, ed. Elsevier, St. Louis, MO, pp.270–6.

47 Sykes, J (2014) Chlamydial infections. In *Canine and Feline Infectious Diseases*, J Sykes, ed. Elsevier, St. Louis, MO, pp.326–33.

48 Hartmann, AD *et al.* (2010) Detection of bacterial and viral organisms from the conjunctiva of cats with conjunctivitis and upper respiratory tract disease. *J Feline Med Surg* **12**:775–82.

49 Veir, JK *et al.* (2008) Prevalence of selected infectious organisms and comparison of two anatomic sampling sites in shelter cats with upper respiratory tract disease. *J Feline Med Surg* **10**:551–7.

50 Low, HC *et al.* (2007) Prevalence of feline herpesvirus 1, *Chlamydophila felis*, and *Mycoplasma* spp DNA in conjunctival cells collected from cats with and without conjunctivitis. *Am J Vet Res* **68**:643–8.

51 Schulz, C *et al.* (2015) Sampling sites for detection of feline herpesvirus-1, feline calicivirus and *Chlamydia felis* in cats with feline upper respiratory tract disease. *J Feline Med Surg* **17**:1012–19.

52 Hartmann, AD *et al.* (2008) Efficacy of pradofloxacin in cats with feline upper respiratory tract disease due to *Chlamydophila felis* or *Mycoplasma* infections. *J Vet Intern Med* **22**:44–52.

53 Kompare, B *et al.* (2013) Randomized masked controlled clinical trial to compare 7-day and 14-day course length of doxycycline in the treatment of *Mycoplasma felis* infection in shelter cats. *Comp Immunol Microbiol Infect Dis* **36**:129–35.

54 Conboy, G (2004) Natural infections of *Crenosoma vulpis* and *Angiostrongylus vasorum* in dogs in Atlantic Canada and their treatment with milbemycin oxime. *Vet Rec* **155**:16–18.

55 Bihr, T *et al.* (1999) Lungworm (*Crenosoma vulpis*) infection in dogs on Prince Edward Island. *Can Vet J* **40**:555–9.

56 Nevarez, A *et al.* (2005) Distribution of *Crenosoma vulpis* and *Eucoleus aerophilus* in the lung of free-ranging red foxes (*Vulpes vulpes*). *J Vet Diagn Invest* **17**:486–9.

57 Traversa, D *et al.* (2010) Canine and feline cardiopulmonary parasitic nematodes in Europe: emerging and underestimated. *Parasit Vectors* **3**:62.

58 Traversa, D *et al.* (2009) Infection by *Eucoleus aerophilus* in dogs and cats: is another extra-intestinal parasitic nematode of pets emerging in Italy? *Res Vet Sci* **87**:270–2.

59 Burgess, H *et al.* (2008) *Eucoleus aerophilus* respiratory infection in a dog with Addison's disease. *Can Vet J* **49**:389–92.

60 Radford, AD *et al.* (2007) Feline calicivirus. *Vet Res* **38**:319–35.

61 Gaskell, RM *et al.* (2012) Feline respiratory diseases. In *Infectious Diseases of the Dog and Cat*, 4th ed. CE Greene, ed. Elsevier, St. Louis, MO, pp.151–62.

62 Binns, SH *et al.* (2000) A study of feline upper respiratory tract disease with reference to prevalence and risk factors for infection with feline calicivirus and feline herpesvirus. *J Feline Med Surg* **2**:123–33.

63 Helps, CR *et al.* (2005) Factors associated with upper respiratory tract disease caused by feline herpesvirus, feline calicivirus, *Chlamydophila felis* and *Bordetella bronchiseptica* in cats: experience from 218 European catteries. *Vet Rec* **156**:669–73.

64 Hurley, KE *et al.* (2004) An outbreak of virulent systemic feline calicivirus disease. *J Am Vet Med Assoc* **224**:241–9.

65 Pedersen, NC *et al.* (2000) An isolated epizootic of hemorrhagic-like fever in cats caused by a novel and highly virulent strain of feline calicivirus. *Vet Microbiol* **73**:281–300.

66 Pesavento, PA *et al.* (2004) Pathologic, immunohistochemical, and electron microscopic findings in naturally occurring virulent systemic feline calicivirus infection in cats. *Vet Pathol* **41**:257–63.

67 Reynolds, BS *et al.* (2009) A nosocomial outbreak of feline calicivirus associated virulent systemic disease in France. *J Feline Med Surg* **11**:633–44.

68 Dowers, KL *et al.* (2010) Association of *Bartonella* species, feline calicivirus, and feline herpesvirus 1 infection with gingivostomatitis in cats. *J Feline Med Surg* **12**:314–21.

69 Hennet, PR *et al.* (2011) Comparative efficacy of a recombinant feline interferon omega in refractory cases of calicivirus-positive cats with caudal stomatitis: a randomised, multi-centre, controlled, double-blind study in 39 cats. *J Feline Med Surg* **13**:577–87.

70 Day, MJ *et al.* (2016) WSAVA Guidelines for the vaccination of dogs and cats. **57**:E1–E45.

71 Pedersen, NC *et al.* (1995). Mechanisms for persistence of acute and chronic feline calicivirus infections in the face of vaccination. *Vet Microbiol* **47**:141–56.

72 Gould, D 2011. Feline herpesvirus-1: ocular manifestations, diagnosis and treatment options. *J Feline Med Surg* **13**:333–46.

73 Gaskell, R *et al.* (2007) Feline herpesvirus. *Vet Res* **38**:337–354.

74 Bannasch, MJ *et al.* (2005) Epidemiologic evaluation of multiple respiratory pathogens in cats in animal shelters. *J Feline Med Surg* **7**:109–19.

75 Burgesser, KM *et al.* (1999) Comparison of PCR, virus isolation, and indirect fluorescent antibody staining in the detection of naturally occurring feline herpesvirus infections. *J Vet Diagn Invest* **11**:122–6.

76 Lim, CC *et al.* (2009) Effects of feline herpesvirus type 1 on tear film break-up time, Schirmer tear test results, and conjunctival goblet cell density in experimentally infected cats. *Am J Vet Res* **70**:394–403.

77 Drazenovich, TL *et al.* (2009) Effects of dietary lysine supplementation on upper respiratory and ocular disease and detection of infectious organisms in cats within an animal shelter. *Am J Vet Res* **70**:1391–1400.

78 Bol, S *et al.* (2015) Lysine supplementation is not effective for the prevention or treatment of feline herpesvirus 1 infection in cats: a systematic review. *BMC Vet Res* **11**:284.

79 Rees, TM *et al.* (2008) Oral supplementation with L-lysine did not prevent upper respiratory infection in a shelter population of cats. *J Feline Med Surg* **10**:510–13.

80 Thomasy, SM *et al.* (2016) Oral administration of famciclovir for treatment of spontaneous ocular, respiratory, or dermatologic disease attributed to feline herpesvirus type 1: 59 cases (2006–2013). *J Am Vet Med Assoc* **249**:526–38.

81 Thomasy, SM *et al.* (2016) A review of antiviral drugs and other compounds with activity against feline herpesvirus type 1. *Vet Ophthalmol* **19**(Suppl 1):119–30.

82 Demko, JL *et al.* (2007) Chronic nasal discharge in cats: 75 cases (1993–2004). *J Am Vet Med Assoc* **230**:1032–37.

83 Scherk, M (2010) Snots and snuffles: rational approach to chronic feline upper respiratory syndromes. *J Feline Med Surg* **12**:548–57.

84 Johnson, LR *et al.* (2004) Correlation of rhinoscopic signs of inflammation with histologic findings in nasal biopsy specimens of cats with or without upper respiratory tract disease. *J Am Vet Med Assoc* **225**:395–400.

85 Yao, C *et al.* (2011) *Filaroides osleri (Oslerus osleri)*: two case reports and a review of canid infections in North America. *Vet Parasitol* **179**:123–9.

86 Conboy, G (2009) Helminth parasites of the canine and feline respiratory tract. *Vet Clin North Am Small Anim Pract* **39**:1109–26.

87 Outerbridge, CA *et al.* (1998) *Oslerus osleri* tracheobronchitis: treatment with ivermectin in 4 dogs. *Can Vet J* **39**:238–40.

88 Genta, RM *et al.* (1984) *Filaroides hirthi*: hyperinfective lungworm infection in immunosuppressed dogs. *Vet Pathol* **21**:349–54.

89 Crawford, PC *et al.* (2005) Transmission of equine influenza virus to dogs. *Science* **310**:482–5.

90 Voorhees, IEH *et al.* (2017) Spread of canine influenza A (H3N2) virus, United States. *Emerg Infect Dis* **23**:1950–7.

91 Lee, CT *et al.* (2017) Outbreak of influenza A (H7N2) among cats in an animal shelter with cat-to-human transmission – New York City, 2016. *Clin Infect Dis* **65**:1927–9.

92 Knight, CG *et al.* (2016) Pandemic H1N1 influenza virus infection in a Canadian cat. *Can Vet J* **57**:497–500.

93 Jeoung, H-Y *et al.* (2013) A novel canine influenza H3N2 virus isolated from cats in an animal shelter. *Vet Microbiol* **165**:281–6.

94 Kim, H *et al.* (2012) Inter- and intraspecies transmission of canine influenza virus (H3N2) in dogs, cats, and ferrets. *Influenza Other Respir Vir* **7**:265–70.

95 Pingret, JL *et al.* (2010) Epidemiological survey of H1N1 influenza virus in cats in France. *Vet Rec* **166**:307.

96 Sponseller, BA *et al.* (2010) Influenza A pandemic (H1N1) 2009 virus infection in domestic cats. *Emerg Infect Dis* **16**:534–7.

97 Marschall, J *et al.* (2008) Avian influenza A H5N1 infections in cats. *J Feline Med Surg* **10**:359–65.

98 Newbury, S *et al.* (2016) Prolonged intermittent virus shedding during an outbreak of canine influenza A H3N2 virus infection in dogs in three Chicago area shelters: 16 cases (March to May 2015). *J Am Vet Med Assoc* **248**:1022–6.

99 Klopfleisch, R *et al.* 2007. Distribution of lesions and antigen of highly pathogenic avian influenza virus A/Swan/Germany/R65/06 (H5N1) in domestic cats after presumptive infection by wild birds. *Vet Pathol* **44**:261–8.

100 Anderson, TC *et al.* (2013) Prevalence of and exposure factors for seropositivity to H3N8 canine influenza virus in dogs with influenza-like illness in the United States. *J Am Vet Med Assoc* **242**:209–16.

101 Rodriguez, L *et al.* (2017) A bivalent live-attenuated influenza vaccine for the control and prevention of H3N8 and H3N2 canine influenza viruses. *Vaccine* **35**:4374–81.

102 Rodriguez, L *et al.* (2017) A live-attenuated influenza vaccine for H3N2 canine influenza virus. *Virology* **504**:96–106.

103 Marinova-Petkova, A *et al.* (2017) Avian influenza A (H7N2) virus in humans exposed to sick cats, New York, USA, 2016. *Emerg Infect Dis* **23**:2046–9.

104 Chalker, VJ (2005) Canine mycoplasmas. *Res Vet Sci* **79**:1–8.

105 Chalker, VJ *et al.* (2004) Mycoplasmas associated with canine infectious respiratory disease. *Microbiology* **150**:3491–7.

106 Randolph, JF *et al.* (1993) Prevalence of mycoplasmal and ureaplasmal recovery from tracheobronchial lavages and prevalence of mycoplasmal recovery from pharyngeal swab specimens in dogs with or without pulmonary disease. *Am J Vet Res* **54**:387–91.

107 Ulgen, M *et al.* (2006) Urinary tract infections due to *Mycoplasma canis* in dogs. *J Vet Med A Physiol Pathol Clin Med* **53**:379–82.

108 Lane, MA *et al.* (2012) *Paragonimus kellicotti* flukes in Missouri, USA. *Emerg Infect Dis* **18**:1263–7.

109 Dubey, JP *et al.* (1979) Fenbendazole for treatment of *Paragonimus kellicotti* infection in dogs. *J Am Vet Med Assoc* **174**:835–7.

110 Peregrine, AS *et al.* (2014) Paragonimosis in a cat and the temporal progression of pulmonary radiographic lesions following treatment. *J Am Anim Hosp Assoc* **50**:356–60.

111 Gunnarsson, LK *et al.* (1999) Clinical efficacy of milbemycin oxime in the treatment of nasal mite infection in dogs. *J Am Anim Hosp Assoc* **35**:81–4.

112 Bredal, W (1996) Nesemidd hos hund. *Norsk Vet* **108**:11–17.

113 Chandler, WL *et al.* (1940) *Pneumonyssus caninum* n. sp., a mite from the frontal sinus of the dog. *J Parasitol* **26**:59–70.

114 Gunnarsson, LK *et al.* (2001) Prevalence of *Pneumonyssoides caninum* infection in dogs in Sweden. *J Am Anim Hosp Assoc* **37**:331–7.

115 Gunnarsson, L *et al.* (2000) Demonstration of circulating antibodies to *Pneumonyssoides caninum* in experimentally and naturally infected dogs. *Vet Parasitol* **94**:107–16.

116 Gunnarsson, L *et al.* (2004) Efficacy of selamectin in the treatment of nasal mite (*Pneumonyssoides caninum*) infection in dogs. *J Am Anim Hosp Assoc* **40**:400–4.

117 Marks, SL *et al.* (1994) *Pneumonyssoides caninum*: the canine nasal mite. *Comp Cont Educ Pract Vet* **16**:577–82.

118 Foster, SF *et al.* (2014) Nasopharyngeal disorders. In *Kirk's Current Veterinary Therapy XV*, JD Bonagura *et al.*, eds. Elsevier, St. Louis, MO.

119 Bredal, WP (1998) *Pneumonyssoides caninum* infection – a risk factor for gastric dilatation-volvulus in dogs. *Vet Res Commun* **22**:225–31.

120 Bredal, WP (1998) An epidemiological survey of therapy and diagnostic procedures used by Norwegian small animal practitioners in cases of nasal mite (*Pneumonyssoides caninum*) infection in dogs. *Vet Res Commun* **22**:389–99.

121 Bredal, W *et al.* (1998) Use of milbemycin oxime in the treatment of dogs with nasal mite (*Pneumonyssoides caninum*) infection. *J Small Anim Pract* **39**:126–30.

122 Brandt, RW (1988) *Pneumonyssus caninum* (nasal mite) in four golden retrievers. *Can Vet J* **29**:741.

123 Boyd, C *et al.* (2017) Survival of two dogs with pyothorax secondary to perforating oesophageal foreign body. *Aust Vet J* **95**:41–5.

124 Hicks, A *et al.* (2016) Epidemiological investigation of grass seed foreign body-related disease in dogs of the Riverina District of rural Australia. *Aust Vet J* **94**:67–75.

125 Stillion, JR *et al.* (2015) A clinical review of the pathophysiology, diagnosis, and treatment of pyothorax in dogs and cats. *J Vet Emerg Crit Care* **25**:113–29.

126 McFarland, LV *et al.* (1994) A randomized placebo-controlled trial of *Saccharomyces boulardii* in combination with standard antibiotics for *Clostridium difficile* disease. *JAMA* **271**:1913–18.

127 Boothe, HW *et al.* (2010) Evaluation of outcomes in dogs treated for pyothorax: 46 cases (1983–2001). *J Am Vet Med Assoc* **236**:657–63.

128 Rooney, MB *et al.* (2002) Medical and surgical treatment of pyothorax in dogs: 26 cases (1991–2001). *J Am Vet Med Assoc* **221**:86–92.

129 Waddell, LS *et al.* (2002) Risk factors, prognostic indicators, and outcome of pyothorax in cats: 80 cases (1986–1999). *J Am Vet Med Assoc* **221**:819–24.

130 Acke, E *et al.* (2015) Prevalence of *Streptococcus dysgalactiae* subsp. *equisimilis* and *S. equi* subsp. *zooepidemicus* in a sample of healthy dogs, cats and horses. *N Z Vet J* **63**:265–71.

131 Pesavento, PA *et al.* (2008) A clonal outbreak of acute fatal hemorrhagic pneumonia in intensively housed (shelter) dogs caused by *Streptococcus equi* subsp. *zooepidemicus*. *Vet Pathol* **45**:51–3.

132 Blum, S *et al.* (2010) Outbreak of *Streptococcus equi* subsp. *zooepidemicus* infections in cats. *Vet Microbiol* **144**:236–9.

133 Byun, JW *et al.* (2009) An outbreak of fatal hemorrhagic pneumonia caused by *Streptococcus equi* subsp. *zooepidemicus* in shelter dogs. *J Vet Sci* **10**:269–71.

134 FitzGerald, W *et al.* (2017) Acute fatal haemorrhagic pneumonia caused by *Streptococcus equi zooepidemicus* in greyhounds in Ireland with subsequent typing of the isolates. *Vet Rec* **181**:119.

135 Martin-Vaquero, P *et al.* (2011) Presumptive meningoencephalitis secondary to extension of otitis media/interna caused by *Streptococcus equi* subspecies *zooepidemicus* in a cat. *J Feline Med Surg* **13**:606–9.

136 Britton, AP *et al.* (2010) Rhinitis and meningitis in two shelter cats caused by *Streptococcus equi* subspecies *zooepidemicus*. *J Comp Pathol* **143**:70–4.

137 Abbott, Y *et al.* (2010) Zoonotic transmission of *Streptococcus equi* subsp. *zooepidemicus* from a dog to a handler. *J Med Microbiol* **59**:120–3.

CHAPTER 2

GASTROINTESTINAL DISEASES

BAYLISASCARIS PROCYONIS
J Scott Weese

Also known as the raccoon roundworm, *Baylisascaris procyonis* is highly prevalent in raccoons (definitive host) and uncommonly identified in fecal samples from dogs as an incidental finding on routine fecal flotation (**Fig. 2.1**). This can represent patent enteric infection or transient shedding of eggs that were ingested from the environment. PCR can be used to identify *B. procyonis* and differentiate it from *Toxocara canis*.

This roundworm likely causes little to no clinical disease in dogs, although encephalomyelitis from aberrant larval migration has been reported.[1] Diagnosis of neural migrans can be challenging and can be based on clinical signs, CSF eosinophilia, seropositivity and advanced imaging.

Shedding of this parasite by dogs raises human health concerns, as human disease is rare but potentially devastating. However, eggs are not immediately infective because 1–4 weeks in the environment are required for development of infective L2 larvae.

Routine dewormers that target *Toxocara canis* are effective against *B. procyonis*. Identification of

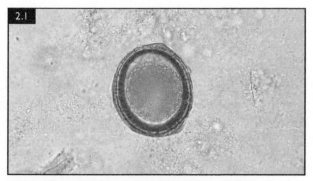

Fig. 2.1 *Baylisascaris procyonis* egg detected by zinc sulfate centrifugal flotation of feces from an infected dog. The normal definitive host is the raccoon; however, patent infections can also occur in dogs. Owing to similarities in appearance, these eggs are easily mistaken for those of *Toxocara canis*. They can be differentiated on the basis of a slightly smaller size (63–75 × 53–60 µm), and *B. procyonis* eggs lack the pronounced pitted, outer shell surface characteristic of *T. canis* eggs. (Courtesy of Gary Conboy)

B. procyonis should prompt discussion of ways to reduce exposure to raccoons and raccoon environments because of various infectious disease risks.

CAMPYLOBACTER
J Scott Weese

Definition
Campylobacter is a genus of microaerophilic bacteria, some species of which are important causes of enteric disease (diarrhea) in dogs and cats.

Etiology and pathogenesis
There are numerous *Campylobacter* species and only a subset are clear pathogens. *C. upsaliensis* is the main species found in healthy dogs and cats, and its role in disease is somewhat debatable. *C. jejuni* is less commonly identified but is more likely to be a cause of disease (and poses greater zoonotic risk). Various other species can be identified.

It is unclear whether disease develops from newly acquired *Campylobacter* or growth of *Campylobacter* already present in the gut. Regardless, the bacterium proliferates and produces a range of toxins that can result in intestinal mucosal damage, inflammation and secretion, with subsequent diarrhea.

Incidence and risk factors

Campylobacter shedding is common in some populations, particularly young dogs and cats. Animals in high-density environments, such as shelters, have shedding rates of 20% to over 90%.[2-4] In healthy adult household dogs and cats shedding is less common; however, rates of ~20% have been reported.[5-7] Risk is lower in dogs fed commercial dry diets.[8]

Disease is most commonly diagnosed in young animals.

Clinical signs

Diarrhea is the main sign. Blood or mucus may be present. Fever, vomiting, anorexia and lethargy are less common but can occur. Dehydration is more common in young or debilitated animals.

Diagnosis

Diagnosis can be a challenge because of the commonness of *Campylobacter* in some populations (e.g. young puppies and kittens, shelter animals) and differences in relevance of different species. Identification of *C. jejuni* or *C. coli* from a patient with diarrhea provides a presumptive diagnosis. Detection of *C. upsaliensis* is harder to interpret but could be relevant. Detection of other species is less convincing.

PCR

PCR is most commonly used, often as part of a testing panel. A limitation of some PCR assays is failure to speicate. This is because the relevance of *C. jejuni* or *C. coli* in an animal with diarrhea is likely greater than for other species.

Culture

Culture is the "gold standard" and has the advantage of providing isolates for speciation and antimicrobial susceptibility testing. It is less commonly used than PCR because of the slower turnaround time and variable ability of diagnostic laboratories to isolate and identify this fastidious bacterium accurately.

Fecal cytology

Cytology is not useful. Not all *Campylobacter* spp. are pathogenic, and some harmless bacteria have the same morphology as *Campylobacter* (**Fig. 2.2**).

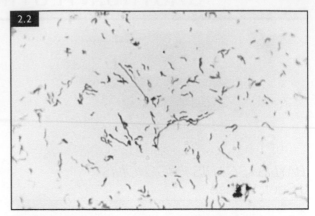

Fig. 2.2 Typical curved rod morphology of *Campylobacter* spp. (Courtesy of Robert Weaver)

Therapy

Supportive care may be required, depending on severity of disease. Antimicrobials are not always required as most cases are self-limiting. Antimicrobials are indicated in patients with chronic or severe disease. Macrolides (e.g. erythromycin) are the best first-line options, with other drugs typically reserved for refractory cases or where erythromycin resistance is present (*Table 2.1*). Duration of treatment is poorly understood but durations of 5–21 days have been used. Treatment aims to eliminate disease, not necessarily the bacterium, and shedding can persist post-treatment.

Prognosis/complications

The prognosis depends on the severity of disease and is usually excellent. Complications are rare. In humans, the autoimmune disorder Guillain–Barre syndrome has been associated with campylobacteriosis. It is unknown if this can develop in dogs and cats; however, an association between *Campylobacter* shedding and acute polyradiculoneuritis has been identified in dogs.[9]

Prevention

Prevention involves reducing fecal–oral exposure, particularly in high-group density environments such as kennels and shelters. Cleaning and disinfection, as well as appropriate fecal handling practices, may reduce the risk, but prevention of exposure is difficult.

Campylobacter is an important zoonotic pathogen and transmission to humans is most often associated with new puppies and kittens.[10-12] General hygiene practices are the key preventive measures.

Table 2.1 **Treatment options for campylobacteriosis**

DRUG	DOSE	COMMENTS
Erythromycin	10–15 mg/kg PO q8h	Typical first-line choice
Azithromycin	5–10 mg/kg PO q24h	Potential option in place of erythromycin but few reasons to use it ompirioally ovor orythromyoin
Tylosin	11 mg/kg PO q8h	Another potential macrolide option
Chloramphenicol	Cats: 10–15 mg/kg PO q12h Dogs: 25–50 mg/kg PO q8h	Human handling risks must be considered. Note the lower doses in cats
Enrofloxacin	Dogs: 10 mg/kg PO q24h	Effective but best reserved because of potential resistance emergence Avoid in cats and growing animals
Marbofloxacin	2.75–5.5 mg/kg PO q24h	Effective but best reserved because of potential resistance emergence
Pradofloxacin	Dogs*: 3–4.5 mg/kg PO q24h Cats: 7.5 mg/kg PO q24h	Avoid in growing animals
Orbifloxacin	2.5–7.5 mg/kg PO q24h	

* Only approved for dogs in some countries.

CANINE CIRCOVIRUS
J Scott Weese

Canine circovirus is a small, enveloped, single-stranded RNA virus that was initially suggested as being a cause of hemorrhagic diarrhea in dogs.[13] However, while an association of the presence of virus and diarrhea has been reported,[14] most studies have not supported a primary role in canine diarrhea.[15, 16] It may be relevant as a co-infection (especially with canine parvovirus) or it may simply be a commensal virus that can be found in healthy and diseased dogs alike.[15–17]

CANINE ENTERIC CORONAVIRUS
J Scott Weese

Canine enteric coronavirus (CECoV) has been implicated in sporadic enteric disease and outbreaks internationally. However, its role in disease is still difficult to discern. It has been found in 2–33% of healthy dogs,[18–22] particularly those in group housing, e.g. shelters, kennels.

Acute onset of diarrhea is the most commonly reported sign. Disease is self-limiting in most situations. However, fatalities have been reported when co-infections with canine parvovirus, canine distemper virus[23, 24] and pantropic canine coronavirus (strains closely related to CECoV) were present.[23, 25, 26]

Most often, CECoV is present incidentally (or as a complicating factor) in disease caused by other enteropathogens, as opposed to being a common primary pathogen.

PCR testing is available as part of some gastrointestinal panels. Caution should be used when interpreting results in dogs with sporadic, mild disease, because of the prevalence in healthy dogs.

Treatment is supportive. Since this virus usually causes mild-to-inapparent infection, vaccination is likely of limited use in most populations.

CLOSTRIDIUM DIFFICILE
J Scott Weese

Definition
Clostridium difficile is a gram-positive, spore-forming, anaerobic bacterium (**Fig. 2.3**) that is an important cause of enteric disease in various species. Its role in canine and feline disease remains unclear.

Etiology and pathogenesis
Clostridium difficile exerts its pathogenic effects primarily through the production of exotoxins. Toxins A and B are the main toxins, and some strains can also produce a binary toxin (CDT). The bacterium can be found in the intestinal tract of healthy individuals. Disease is most often associated with disruptions in the normal intestinal microbiota that allow *C. difficile* to proliferate and produce toxins. It is classically associated with antimicrobial treatment, but disease can occur in the absence of obvious risk factors.

Incidence and risk factors
A small percentage of healthy dogs and cats (usually <5%) shed *C. difficile* at any time.[27, 28] This can be higher in some populations, such as young animals or those receiving antimicrobial treatment. Contact with human hospitals and living with an immunocompromised person have been associated with increased risk of colonization. The role of *C. difficile* in disease is unclear in dogs and cats; however, an association between the presence of *C. difficile* toxins in feces and the presence of diarrhea has been reported.[29]

Clinical signs
C. difficile has been associated with various forms of gastrointestinal (GI) disease, including acute and chronic diarrhea. It is most commonly implicated in mild-to-moderate acute diarrhea. Vomiting, depression, lethargy, abdominal distension, bloating and other non-specific enteric signs may be present.

Diagnosis
Diagnosis is based on detection of the bacterium or its toxins in feces, along with consistent clinical signs.

Fecal enzyme-linked immunosorbent assay (ELISA)
Antigen ELISA targeting *C. difficile* "common antigen" is highly sensitive. The ELISA will also detect non-toxigenic strains, meaning that it will be positive in cases where the patient is simply colonized.

ELISAs targeting toxin A, toxin B or both toxins are also available. Positive results for toxins are more convincing as a cause of disease, because they indicate demonstrable levels of toxin in the gut. However, sensitivity is low,[30] so false-negative results can occur.

PCR
PCR targeting the toxin B gene is widely available and is a sensitive test. Specificity is a concern because of the baseline prevalence of *C. difficile* colonization in healthy dogs and cats. A positive PCR result in a patient with enteric disease is suggestive of *C. difficile* infection but is not definitive.

Culture
This bacterium can be challenging to isolate and culture is rarely available.

Fecal cytology
Cytology is not useful.

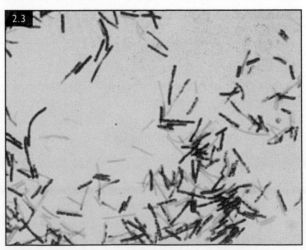

Fig. 2.3 Gram stain of *Clostridium difficile*.
Note the long, thin gram-positive (purple) rods (1,000× magnification).

Therapy

Supportive care is the mainstay of treatment. Disease is usually self-limiting, but metronidazole (10–15 mg/kg PO q12h for 5 days) is often used. Intravenous metronidazole (15 mg/kg IV q12h for 5 days) can be used if oral medications cannot be tolerated. In humans, vancomycin is most often recommended, but evidence indicating that this is effective or needed in dogs and cats is lacking.

Prognosis/complications

The prognosis depends on the severity of disease and is usually excellent.

Prevention

Exposure to *C. difficile* is likely common so preventive measures are aimed at limiting disruption of the gut microbiota. This may include prudent antimicrobial use, provision of a good diet, and limiting diet changes and other stressors.

CLOSTRIDIUM PERFRINGENS
J Scott Weese

Definition

Clostridium perfringens is a gram-positive, anaerobic, spore-forming bacterium (**Fig. 2.4**) that can cause enteric disease in a wide range of species. Less commonly, it can cause invasive infections, including severe disease such as clostridial myositis.

Etiology and pathogenesis

Clostridium perfringens exerts its pathogenic effects primarily through the production of exotoxins. The pathophysiology of disease is not well understood. However, it likely involves proliferation of *C. perfringens* and subsequent toxin production after an insult that perturbs the normal protective microbiota. Various toxins can be involved, and the role of different toxins is not well understood in dogs and cats (*Table 2.2*).

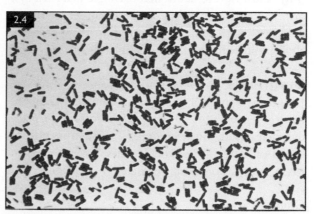

Fig. 2.4 Gram stain of *Clostridium perfringens* demonstrating the gram-positive, short rod nature of the bacterium (1,000× magnification). (Courtesy of Don Stalons)

Table 2.2 *Clostridium perfringens* toxin genes

TOXIN	COMMENT
Alpha	Found in all *C. perfringens* strains and likely plays little to no role in diarrhea in dogs and cats
Beta	Found in Type B and C isolates. Rarely found in dogs and cats and perhaps more likely associated with severe disease. Cause of serious disease in some other species
Epsilon	Found in Type B and D strains. Rare in dogs and cats. Role in disease unclear
Iota	Found in Type E strains. Rare in dogs and cats, and clinical relevance in those species is unclear
Enterotoxin (CPE)	Has been suggested as a cause of diarrhea in dogs and cats, but confirmation is lacking. ELISA to detect this toxin is available
NetF	More recently identified. May be associated with acute hemorrhagic diarrhea syndrome. Uncommon in healthy dogs and cats
Beta2 toxin	Relatively commonly found in isolates from dogs and cats. May play a role in diarrhea but can be found commonly in healthy animals

Incidence and risk factors

Clostridium perfringens is a normal gut commensal and can be found in a large percentage of healthy dogs (31–84%) and cats (20–50%[31]).[27, 32–35] Risk factors for disease are not well understood and likely involve various factors that can impact the gut microbiota (e.g. antimicrobials, diet change, stress).

There has been debate about a potential role in acute hemorrhagic diarrhea syndrome,[36] and recent evidence supports a role of NetF-producing strains.[37, 38]

Clinical signs

Diarrhea is the main clinical abnormality, with varying degrees of vomiting, anorexia and lethargy (**Fig. 2.5**). Severe acute hemorrhagic diarrhea syndrome is uncommon but can result in severe bloody diarrhea with rapid dehydration, hypotension, abdominal pain and signs of hypovolemic shock.

Diagnosis

Diagnosis can be a challenge because of the commensal nature of *C. perfringens*. Disease is probably overdiagnosed; however, presumptive diagnosis is based on detection of the organism, toxin genes or toxin, in addition to appropriate clinical signs.

Culture

Culture alone is of limited use because of the high prevalence in healthy animals. Testing isolates for certain toxin genes (e.g. *cpe*, *NetF*) can be more rewarding, but the diagnostic value is unclear.

Fecal enzyme-linked immunosorbent assay (ELISA)

ELISA has the advantage of detection of the toxins, not just the genetic potential to produce toxins; however, commercial assays are limited to an unvalidated test for one toxin (enterotoxin). Positive results are suggestive of disease but are not definitive.

PCR

PCR typically targets the alpha toxin gene, a gene that is found in all *C. perfringens*. Therefore, it is of limited use. Quantitative PCR for the alpha toxin gene is available and has been proposed as being diagnostic, but clear data are lacking. PCR can also be done for other genes, and positive results for genes more strongly associated with disease (e.g. *NetF*) can be useful.

Fecal cytology

Cytology is not useful.

Therapy

Disease can range from self-limiting to imminently life threatening, and supportive care can be critical. Metronidazole (10–15 mg/kg PO q12h for 5 days) is often used. Intravenous metronidazole (15 mg/kg IV q12h for 5 days) can be administered if oral medications cannot be tolerated. Other antimicrobials such as tylosin are likely effective.

Prognosis/complications

The prognosis depends mainly on the severity of disease and is usually excellent.

Prevention

Given that *C. perfringens* is a ubiquitous organism that is commonly found in healthy animals, prevention of disease mainly involves limiting (or avoiding) factors that can disrupt the protective microbiota (e.g. antibiotics and diet changes).

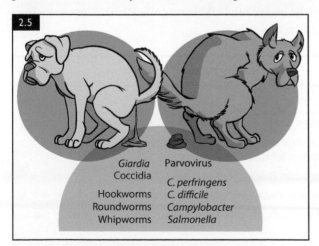

2.5

Giardia   Parvovirus
Coccidia
            C. perfringens
Hookworms   *C. difficile*
Roundworms *Campylobacter*
Whipworms   *Salmonella*

Fig. 2.5 Common parasitic, viral and coccidian causes of diarrhea in dogs.

CRYPTOSPORIDIUM
J Scott Weese

Definition
Cryptosporidium is a genus of coccidian (apicomplexan) parasites that can cause diarrhea in various species.

Etiology and pathogenesis
A wide range of *Cryptosporidium* spp. can be found. Most are fairly host adapted (i.e. *C. canis* is common in dogs, *C. felis* in cats), with limited crossover to other species. *C. parvum* can be found in dogs, cats, ruminants and humans, and probably represents the main clinical risk in dogs and cats, as well as the greatest zoonotic disease risk.

Infection is via the fecal–oral route. Unlike many parasites, the entire life cycle can be completed in the host and autoinfection within the gastrointestinal tract is an important part of the disease process. Diarrhea is thought to result from both hypersecretion and malabsorption.

Incidence and risk factors
Cryptosporidia can be found in a small percentage (<5%) of healthy dogs and cats, with higher rates in shelter animals.[18, 39–43] Studies have often failed to differentiate *Cryptosporidium* spp. and there are conflicting results regarding whether *C. parvum* or the more host-specific *C. canis* (dogs) and *C. felis* (cats) are most common. However, recent reports indicate that the host-specific species predominate in dogs and cats. Disease is most likely to occur in young, stressed or immunocompromised animals.

Clinical signs
Subclinical infections are common. When disease is present, it is usually small bowel diarrhea with few or no other clinical abnormalities. In compromised hosts, dehydration is of greater concern, but most affected dogs and cats have relatively minor disease with no serious systemic manifestations.

Diagnosis
The presence of *Cryptosporidium* spp. in healthy animals complicates diagnosis. Detection of the parasite in a diarrheic animal is suggestive at best.

In the absence of another identified cause, detection of *Cryptosporidium* spp., particularly high levels, is suggestive.

Various detection methods are available. Microscopy has limited sensitivity because of intermittent shedding and the difficulty that inexperienced personnel may have identifying *Cryptosporidium* spp. (**Figs. 2.6–2.8**). Use of concentration methods, such as zinc sulfate flotation and Sheather's sucrose

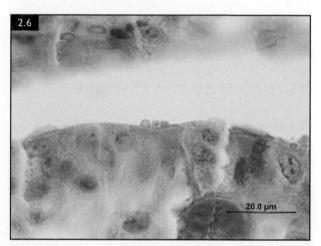

Fig. 2.6 Histologic section of intestine from a calf infected with *Cryptosporidium parvum* (stained with H&E). Although the oocysts appear on the surface, they are actually intracellular, residing within the plasma membrane of the intestinal cells. (Courtesy of Gary Conboy)

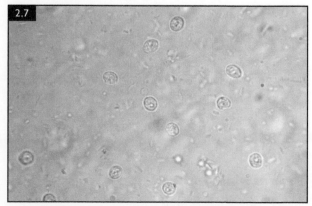

Fig. 2.7 Fecal microscopy demonstrating *Cryptosporidium* spp. (Courtesy of Peter Drotman)

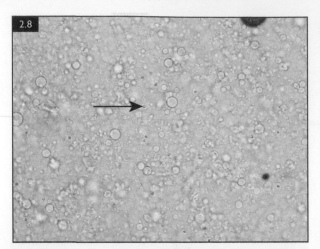

Fig. 2.8 *Cryptosporidium parvum* oocysts (arrow) detected on centrifugal fecal flotation. Note the small size (4–5 μm in diameter) and the slight pinkish hue in the oocyst cytoplasm. (Courtesy of Gary Conboy)

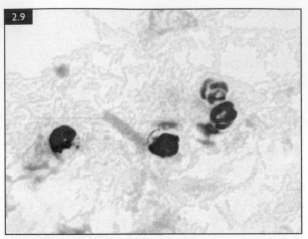

Fig. 2.9 *Cryptosporidium parvum* oocysts highlighted using modified acid-fast staining. (Courtesy of the Centers for Disease Control and Prevention)

flotation of saturated sodium chloride solution, can increase sensitivity. PCR testing is often available as part of PCR panels. The sensitivity of commercial assays is unclear, but PCR has the potential to be highly sensitive, if the DNA extraction methods are adequate for the relatively tough parasite. Fecal enzyme-linked immunosorbent assay (ELISA) can be used, with various sensitivity values, depending on the assay. Fluorescent antibody testing can be highly sensitive and specific but is less commonly available. Staining techniques can also be used to increase the sensitivity of microscopy but are not readily available (**Fig. 2.9**).

Therapy

Supportive care may be required, depending on severity of disease. Specific treatment is not usually needed nor is it very effective. Azithromycin, nitazoxanide, paromomycin and tylosin have been used in dogs and cats, but efficacy is limited or unclear (*Table 2.3*). Treatment is best reserved for severe cases or immunocompromised individuals, with limited expectation of efficacy.

Prognosis/complications

The prognosis is very good overall as this is usually a self-limiting disease in immunocompetent individuals.

Table 2.3 **Treatment options for *Cryptosporidium* spp.**

DRUG	SPECIES	DOSING
Azithromycin	Dogs	5–10 mg/kg PO q12h for 5–7 days
	Cats	7–15 mg/kg PO q24h for 5–21 days
Nitazoxanide	Dogs, cats	10–25 mg/kg PO q12–24h for up to 28 days
Paromomycin	Dogs, cats	150 mg/kg q24h for 5 days
Tylosin	Cats	10–15 mg/kg PO q8h for 14–21 days

Prevention

Prevention mainly involves reducing fecal–oral exposure. This can be a challenge because healthy animals can shed the parasite, and it is highly tolerant of environmental stressors and disinfectants. Cleaning of high-risk environments (e.g. shelters) and good general fecal handling will reduce the amount of exposure.

Cryptosporidium spp. are zoonotic but the role of dogs and cats in human disease is unclear. *C. parvum* presumably poses some risk, particularly in diarrheic animals. Evidence of zoonotic risk for *C. canis* and *C. felis* is limited, with greater concern about *C. canis*, but rare human infections with either species can occur.[44, 45]

CYSTOISOSPORA
J Scott Weese

Definition

Cystoisospora spp. are common coccidial pathogens in young dogs and cats. These obligate intracellular pathogens can be found in the intestinal tract, as both incidental findings and causes of disease.

Etiology and pathogenesis

Cystoisospora spp. are the most commonly found coccidians in dogs and cats. Not all species are pathogenic. *Cystoisospira* (formerly *Isospora*) *canis* and *C. ohioensis* are most commonly implicated in disease in dogs, whereas *C. felis* and *C. rivolta* are most common in cats.

Some coccidia, most notably *Eimeria*, may be found in the feces of dogs and cats that have ingested the feces or intestinal contents of prey. These are incidental findings.

Coccidia have a two-stage life cycle, with sexual and asexual cycles. Non-sporulated oocysts are produced in the intestinal tract of the definitive host and are excreted into the environment. To become infective, these oocysts must sporulate, which can occur over 9–12 hours under optimal temperature conditions (30–37°C).[46] The oocysts are environmentally tolerant and can persist in the environment. The next host is infected by ingestion of sporozoites from sporulated oocysts. Back in the intestinal tract, sporozoites excyst, and undergo sexual (gametes) or asexual (schizonts) stages (**Fig. 2.10**). Unsporulated oocysts are then produced and passed in feces, completing the life cycle. Infection of paratenic hosts such as rodents results in production of sporozoites or merozoites in extra-intestinal tissues. These are infective when ingested by the definitive host.

Canine and feline species are highly host specific and do not cross-infect. *Cystoisospora* shedding rates of 0.4–39% have been reported, with highest prevalence in shelters, pet stores and breeding kennels.[47–50]

Clinical signs

Subclinical infections are most common. Diarrhea, most often without blood or mucus, is the main clinical sign, unless complications such as dehydration and hypoglycemia have developed. Severe diarrhea is rare but can occur, particularly in very young or immunocompromised animals exposed to large coccidia burdens. Severe or persistent infections should prompt consideration of immunocompromise, concurrent disease or high burdens of exposure.

Diagnosis

Diagnosis is best achieved through detection of oocysts by centrifugal fecal flotation (**Fig. 2.11**). Shedding may be sporadic, so multiple tests may be required to rule out coccidiosis. However, with an experienced microscopist and an animal with active enteric disease, false-negative results are unlikely. The main coccidia can be differentiated on the basis of size, which is of most relevance for differentiating canine- or feline-specific coccidia from the transient passage of coccidia following ingestion of feces or prey.

Therapy

Infections are typically self-limiting and treatment is most often reserved for severe cases and compromised hosts. Supportive therapy is the mainstay of treatment because it is highly effective and anticoccidial therapies are of limited efficacy. Various drugs may be used against *Cystoisospora* spp., with varying degrees of success (*Table 2.4*) and licensed products vary by country. Ponazuril and sulfadimethoxine are likely the most commonly used drugs. Unfortunately, optimal duration of therapy has been

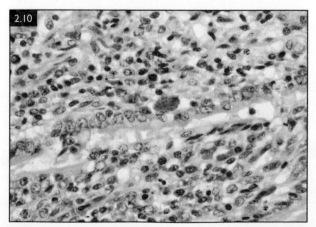

Fig. 2.10 *Cystoisospora* **schizont in the ileum of a dog.** (Courtesy of Ryan Jennings)

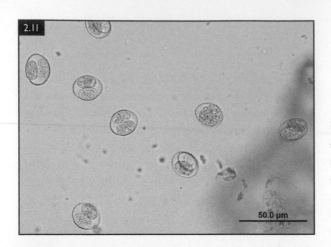

Fig. 2.11 *Cystoisospora* oocysts (17–51 × 15–39 μm depending on the species) detected by centrifugal sugar flotation of feces from a puppy. Freshly passed oocysts contain a single round sporoblast cell but relatively quickly undergo the first division and may be seen in the two-sporoblast-cell stage. (Courtesy of Gary Conboy)

Table 2.4 Treatment options for *Cystoisospora* spp.

DRUG	SPECIES	DOSING
Amprolium	Dogs	110–200 mg (total) PO q24h for 7–12 days
	Cats	60–100 mg/kg PO for 7 days
Emodepside + toltrazuril		≥0.45 mg/kg emodepside and 9 mg/kg toltrazuril PO single dose
Ponazuril	Dogs, cats	20 mg/kg PO q24h for 1–3 days
Sulfadimethoxine	Dog, cat	50–60 mg/kg PO q24h for 5–20 days
Toltrazuril	Dogs	10–30 mg/kg PO for 1–3 days
Trimethoprim sulfonamide	Dog, cat	30 mg/kg PO q12h for 6 days

poorly assessed. Environmental hygiene is important to reduce reinfection.

Prognosis/complications

Prognosis is excellent because coccidia rarely cause severe disease and infection is self-limiting. Control in dense housing situations may be more problematic.

Prevention

The main approach to prevention is use of good hygiene practices, especially in group situations where many young animals are present. Prompt and thorough cleaning of fecal contamination is most important. Coccidia are resistant to most disinfectants so physical removal is the key. *Cystoisospora* spp. are not a zoonotic disease concern.

ECHINOCOCCUS MULTILOCULARIS
J Scott Weese

Definition

Echinococcus multilocularis is a small tapeworm that causes sporadic canine disease in endemic areas and is of significant human health concern. Infections are rare in cats.

Etiology and pathogenesis

The life cycle involves canids as definitive hosts, and small mammals (mainly rodents) as intermediate hosts (**Fig. 2.12**). The main reservoirs are wild canids (foxes, coyotes) but patent intestinal infections in dogs can occur. Cats can also be infected but less commonly. Adult worms (**Fig. 2.13**) live within the gut of definitive hosts and eggs are passed in feces. Eggs are immediately infective and, when ingested by an intermediate host, larval stages migrate through tissue and result in the production of tumor-like lesions, particularly in the liver

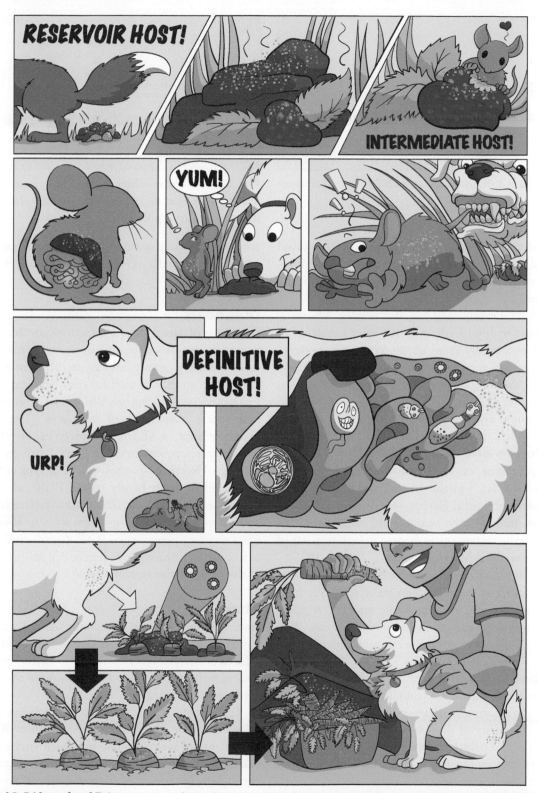

Fig. 2.12 Life cycle of *Echinococcus multilocularis* in a dog, showing reservoir, intermediate and definitive host stages with eggs passed in feces. Migration of larval stages may result in liver lesions of canine alveolar echinococcosis. This is a zoonosis.

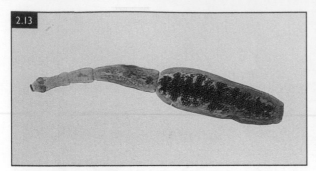

Fig. 2.13 Adult *Echinococcus multilocularis*. (Courtesy of Peter M Schantz)

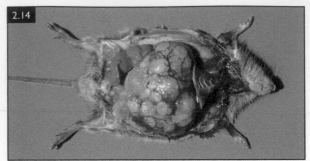

Fig. 2.14 Alveolar echinococcosis in a rat, an intermediate host for *Echinococcus multilocularis*. (Courtesy of Irving Kagan)

(alveolar echinococcosis [AE]) (**Fig. 2.14**). If a canid (or felid) ingests an infected intermediate host, gastrointestinal infection can develop, and the life cycle continues.

Dogs (and rarely cats) can also develop AE, similar to that in intermediate hosts, after ingestion of eggs or potentially from autoinfection when intestinal infection is present. Humans can be similarly affected, and AE is a serious zoonotic concern in some regions because it is often diagnosed late in disease and may be difficult to treat.

Incidence and risk factors

The prevalence of *E. multilocularis* in dogs (and humans) is related to the prevalence in wild canids. Some parts of central Europe (e.g. Switzerland) have had high rates of infection in wild canids, and this appears to be an emerging disease in various parts of Europe, Asia and North America.

Shedding of *E. multilocularis* eggs is uncommon in dogs in most areas but can be at relatively high prevalence (up to 20%)[51] in some endemic regions. Patent infections can occur in cats but are rare. The risk of AE in cats seems to be extremely low.

Clinical signs

Intestinal infections are subclinical. AE typically causes vague disease that mimics neoplasia. The type and severity of disease depend on the size and location of the parasitic mass, but abdominal distension is a common presenting complaint.[52] Most often liver lesions are present, so signs consistent with abdominal or thoracic masses and liver dysfunction are common. Lesions may be found incidentally at surgery or when diagnostic imaging is performed for other reasons.

Diagnosis

Diagnosis of patent enteric infections involves detection of *E. multilocularis* eggs in feces via fecal flotation or PCR. Eggs are not easy to differentiate from *Taenia* spp. so PCR is used for confirmation.

Diagnostic imaging usually identifies an abdominal mass, suggestive of neoplasia (**Fig. 2.15**). Differentiation of AE from neoplasia can involve surgical biopsies, percutaneous biopsies, cytology and/or serology. Definitive diagnosis of AE is typically made histologically from biopsy tissue. PCR can also be performed on tissues. Serological testing is available,[53] and seropositivity in a dog or cat with an abdominal mass is strongly supportive of AE. Cytological testing of fine-needle aspirates can also be diagnostic, as parts of the parasite may be identifiable.

Therapy

Enteric infections are effectively treated with praziquantel (5 mg/kg PO). Although single doses are effective,[54] repeated treatment is often given to patients with patent infections because of the significant zoonotic concerns.

Treatment of AE is difficult. Excision of the affected tissue is ideal, when possible. Medical treatment, either in conjunction with surgical debulking or as the sole approach, can be attempted through long-term or lifelong albendazole treatment (10 mg/kg PO q24h).

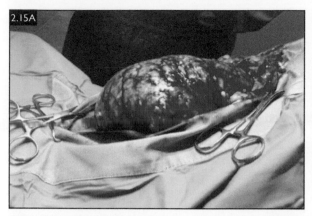
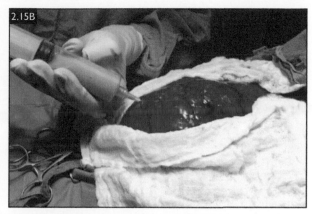

Fig. 2.15 Alveolar echinococcosis in a 4-year-old Boxer. The large (20 × 10 cm) mass (A) was in the cranial abdomen, attached to the liver and two smaller masses. Turbid, mildly hemorrhagic fluid (B) was aspirated from the mass. (Courtesy of Andrew Peregrine)

Prognosis/complications

The prognosis for enteric infections is excellent as they readily respond to treatment and do not cause clinical disease.

The prognosis for AE is poor, because complete excision of lesions is not usually possible, postoperative recurrence is common, and combinations of surgical and medical treatment rarely provide clinical cure. However, some dogs have survived for years with albendazole therapy.[52] Optimal approaches to management are unclear.[52]

Prevention

Praziquantel is an effective preventive. Monthly treatment should be considered in endemic areas, especially for dogs that may ingest small rodents. Methods to reduce exposure to wild canid feces and small rodents are warranted.

GIARDIOSIS
Margie Scherk

Definition

Infection by the protozoal parasite *Giardia duodenalis* can result in subclinical infection or diarrhea.

Species affected

Multiple mammalian and avian species including cats, dogs and humans.

Etiology and pathogenesis

Giardia duodenalis is a flagellate protozoal parasite. It has numerous genotypes or assemblages (*Table 2.5*). Some assemblages are zoonotic whereas others affect only non-human animals.

Giardia trophozoites colonize the small intestinal wall where they damage intestinal epithelial cells, resulting in inflammation and villus blunting. Both trophozoites and cysts are shed in the feces. Cysts can survive in the environment for several months and are immediately infective upon shedding. It takes only a few cysts transmitted via the fecal–oral route to cause infection. Transmission can be via direct contact with an infected host or indirectly through grooming feces-soiled fur or drinking contaminated water. The prepatent period is 3–10 days.

Incidence and risk factors

Giardia is commonly found in healthy dogs and cats. Meta-analysis of worldwide giardiasis found 15.2% prevalence in dogs and 12% prevalence in cats.[55] The high frequency of shedding by healthy animals complicates interpretation of results in diarrheic individuals. Puppies and kittens under 6 months of age are

Table 2.5 **Important *Giardia* assemblages and their common hosts**

ASSEMBLAGE	IMPORTANT HOSTS
A	Humans, dogs, cats, cattle, various wildlife
B	Humans, dogs, cattle, various wildlife
C	Dogs, cattle, pigs
D	Dogs, cattle
F	Cats

at greatest risk for clinical disease.[55] The population source plays a significant role in prevalence. In one study of dogs under 1 year of age, those from pet stores had the highest (100%) intestinal parasite burden, followed by those seen in veterinary clinics, and the lowest prevalence was found among dogs from an animal shelter.[39] Similarly, prevalence in cats from catteries but also from shelters/foster homes is higher than in other populations.[56, 57] Pet dogs and cats have the lowest prevalence.[55]

Clinical signs

Subclinical infection is most common. Acute or chronic small bowel diarrhea predominates, although large bowel diarrhea may also occur. In puppies and kittens, diarrhea occurs acutely and is characterized by soft, pale, foul-smelling stool that may contain fat or mucus. If infection is significantly diffuse, malabsorption with weight loss can occur.

Diagnosis

Testing should be reserved for diarrheic animals. Direct smear, saline wet mount and fecal flotation by centrifugation can be used to visualize *Giardia*. Fecal flotation by centrifugation is more sensitive than passive flotation: only 14.7% of *Giardia* cases were detected in dogs by the latter method.[58] Direct fecal smears, either by wet mount or by rectal cytology, may reveal cysts and motile piriform trophozoites. Different from *Tritrichomonas foetus*,

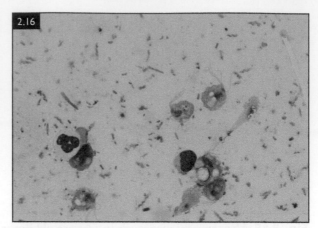

Fig. 2.16 Numerous *Tritrichomonas foetus* trophozoites showing undulating membrane and anterior flagellae with neutrophil and lymphocyte, spirochetes, chains of cocci and rods (Wright–Giemsa stain, 40× magnification). (Courtesy of Sally Lester)

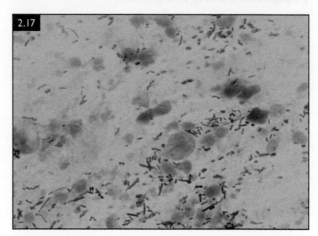

Fig. 2.17 *Giardia* trophozoite showing typical pear-shaped, dual nuclei in the broad anterior end. The multiple flagellae are not readily appreciated in this image. Spirochetes, rods, chains and single cocci are also present (Wright–Giemsa stain, 40x magnification). (Courtesy of Sally Lester)

these trophozoites move in a rolling, falling motion (*Table 2.6*, **Figs. 2.16, 2.17**). Because cysts and trophozoites are shed intermittently, multiple samples

Table 2.6 **Differentiation of *Giardia* spp. and *Tritrichomonas foetus***

TROPHOZOITE	*GIARDIA* SPP.	*TRITRICHOMONAS FOETUS*
Morphology	Concave ventral disc	Spindle-shaped, undulating membrane
Motility	Like a gently falling leaf	Jerky, forward movement

Table 2.7 **Treatment options for giardiasis**

DRUG	DOSE
Fenbendazole	50 mg/kg PO q24h × 3–5 days
Metronidazole	25 mg/kg PO q12h × 5–7 days
Ronidazole	Dogs: 30–50 mg/kg PO q12h × 7 days
	Cats: 20 mg/kg PO q12h or 30 mg/kg PO q24h × 14 days
Pyrantel, praziquantel, febantel	Dogs: label dose × 3 days
	Cats: 56 mg/kg (based on the febantel component) PO q24h × 5 days

may need to be assessed (three over 5–7 days) if using direct smear, saline wet mount or fecal floatation by centrifugation.

Several enzyme-linked immunosorbent assay (ELISA) tests are available including an in-clinic SNAP® test. This test is easier to use than direct fecal testing and is equally sensitive and specific to fecal flotation. Laboratory microplate assay is more sensitive and specific than the SNAP® test.[59] Fecal flotation combined with ELISA has a sensitivity of >97%.

Combination immunofluorescent assays (IFAs) are available at reference laboratories and have good sensitivity and specificity to detect both *Giardia* and *Cryptosporidium* spp. This test is superior to ELISA fecal antigen testing.

Polymerase chain reaction should be used only when genotyping is desired because PCR assays are less sensitive than other testing modalities.

Positive *Giardia* tests do not prove that the diarrhea is caused by the organism; nevertheless, treatment is warranted for these patients.

Therapy

Imidazoles are the cornerstone of treatment (*Table 2.7*). Fenbendazole or febantel is preferred, especially if there is evidence of concurrent nematode infection. Metronidazole is believed to be less effective, is more likely to result in adverse effects and is best avoided as initial therapy. Both metronidazole and fenbendazole may be used when the first agent is ineffective, or reinfection occurs. The goal of treatment is to stop diarrhea; elimination of infection or the carrier state is difficult. Healthy animals should not be treated.

Concurrent bathing (to remove cysts from the haircoat that might cause reinfection) and proper removal of feces may be indicated, particularly in apparently recurrent giardiasis. The role of fecal transplants and pro- or synbiotic therapy remains unclear.

Prognosis/complications

With treatment, most cases of giardiasis will resolve. Supportive care and additional attention to nutrition may be required for individuals while they recover from malabsorption. In cases in which diarrhea does not stop, concurrent disease or infection should be suspected. Infection with *Giardia* does not induce lasting immunity, and reinfection can occur.

Prevention

Prevention of infection requires good environmental hygiene, an uncontaminated water source (or boiling water), good nutrition and low-stress housing without crowding. Regular disposal of fecal matter is important to prevent fecal–oral transmission.

Public health and infection control

Zoonotic risk is very low in most regions. In developed regions, the types of *Giardia* sp. that are pathogenic for humans are unlikely to be acquired from dogs and cats. However, *Giardia* spp. should be considered potentially zoonotic in the absence of confirmation that an animal-species assemblage is involved.

GRANULOMATOUS COLITIS
Roger A Hostutler

Definition
Historically considered a condition solely of Boxers, granulomatous colitis has been reported in other breeds, e.g. French Bulldogs, Mastiffs and Mastiff derivatives. Large bowel diarrhea, usually with hematochezia, is the most common clinical sign.

Etiology and pathogenesis
Most recent evidence implicates a role for pathogenic bacteria, particularly *Escherichia coli*,[60] with development of an abundant immune response that results in granulomatous lesions.

Incidence and risk factors
Disease is most commonly reported in Boxer dogs younger than 4 years but has been seen in animals as young as 6 weeks of age, with no sex predilection. Given the breed specificity, granulomatous colitis is suspected to have a genetic basis related to increased susceptibility to *E. coli* invasion. No environmental or other risk factors have been identified.

Clinical signs
Clinical signs of large bowel diarrhea, including tenesmus, increased frequency and haematochezia, are most common. The hematochezia is thought to be more severe than with other forms of colitis. Dogs may exhibit signs attributable to small bowel disease (e.g. lethargy, weight loss).

Diagnosis
Clinicopathologic abnormalities may include anemia, either from blood loss or secondary to inflammatory disease. Hypoalbuminemia may be present either through shifts to acute phase protein production, loss of mucosal integrity, or as a component of blood loss.

Endoscopic biopsies of the colonic mucosa may provide histologic evidence of granulomatous colitis and should be obtained whenever possible. Endoscopic gross findings often include erythematous mucosa with erosions and/or a cobblestoned appearance (**Fig. 2.18**). Ulceration is sometimes observed. Histologically, the lesions are uniquely

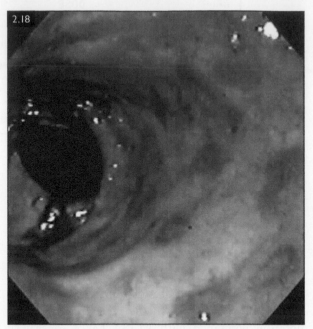
2.18

Fig. 2.18 Ulcerative lesions noted on lower gastrointestinal endoscopic evaluation of a Boxer with granulomatous colitis. (Courtesy of Roger Hostutler)

characterized by the depth of infiltration of periodic acid–Schiff (PAS)-positive macrophages into the lamina propria causing severe mucosal ulceration.[61] Definitive diagnosis is accomplished using FISH (fluorescent *in situ* hybridization). Culture and susceptibility testing are imperative in these animals.

Therapy
The cornerstone of therapy is reduction of invasive *E. coli* via antimicrobial treatment while allowing the mucosal ulceration to heal. Treatment with enrofloxacin (10 mg/kg PO q24h) alone has been associated with long-term remission; however, fluoroquinolone resistance is becoming a concern.[62] Evidence for efficacy of other fluoroquinolones such as marbofloxacin and pradofloxacin is lacking, but they may be selected based on clinician preference. Treatment for at least 6 weeks is recommended, although data regarding optimal durations are lacking.

If resistance to enrofloxacin is found, then alternative antibiotics known to have good macrophage penetration should be used based on susceptibility testing. Antibiotics with good macrophage penetration include chloramphenicol, florfenicol, trimethoprim sulfamethoxazole, tetracyclines and clarithromycin.[61]

Prognosis/complications

Prognosis is related to therapy response. If a good response to antibiotic treatment is seen then complete remission is possible. Ideally endoscopic biopsies should be obtained 10–14 days after completion of antibiotics to re-submit for histopathology, culture and susceptibility testing, and FISH analysis to confirm resolution of disease.

Prevention

Infection is thought to arise due to genetic susceptibility; prevention may become possible as the genetic basis is more fully understood.

HELICOBACTER SPP. (H. PYLORI AND NON-H. PYLORI HELICOBACTER SPP.)
Julie Armstrong

Definition

Helicobacter is a genus of fastidious spiral-shaped bacteria that contains *H. pylori*, as well as a variety of non-*Helicobacter pylori* helicobacter (NHPH). A clear causal link between *Helicobacter* infection and pathology (gastritis and follicular gland hyperplasia) and clinical signs in dogs and cats is lacking.[63–65] However, clinically dramatic responses to therapy have been noted. NHPH infection of dogs and cats is a consideration in patients with chronic vomiting and weight loss; however, most infected dogs and cats have no clinical signs.

Etiology and pathogenesis

Helicobacter spp. are gram-negative motile bacteria noted for their flagella and spiral shape. The larger of the species detected in dogs and cats are grouped into the category of gastric *Helicobacter*-like organisms (GHLOs) or more commonly NHPH species (**Fig. 2.19**).[64]

More than a dozen different NHPH species have been detected in the gastrointestinal tract (stomach and intestines) of dogs and cats, including *H. bizzozeronnii*, *H. salomonis*, *H. felis* and *candidatus*, and *H. heilmannii*. Of these *H. felis* and *H. heilmannii* have also been identified in cats. Healthy dogs and cats can have multiple species present within the stomach, unlike what is routinely noted in humans.

Pathologic changes noted in response to NHPH infection in dogs and cats include degeneration of gastric glands, with vacuolation and pyknosis and necrosis of parietal cells. This is noted more commonly in infected vs. uninfected dogs and cats.

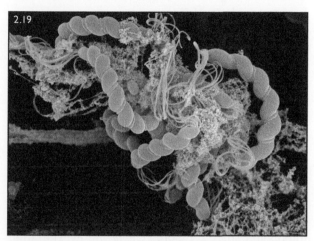

Fig. 2.19 Scanning electron micrograph image of *Helicobacter*-like organisms. (Courtesy of Michael Stoffel)

Mild-to-moderate monocytic gastric inflammation along with gastric lymphoid gland hyperplasia is also commonly noted. Gastric inflammation may be present in the absence of clinical signs.

The presence of NHPH in cats has been proposed as a plausible trigger in the development of feline lymphoma.[66] The presence of NHPH in the colon of dogs has been proposed as a connection with inflammatory bowel disease (IBD), but a causal association with diarrhea has not been established. The presence of organisms in the hepatobiliary system may also be noted, although the significance and relationship with hepatic pathology are uncertain.

Although *H. pylori* is an important human pathogen, causing gastritis, peptic ulceration and increased risk of gastric cancer, similar evidence of disease in dogs and cats is lacking.

Incidence and risk factors

Helicobacter spp. are abundant within healthy populations of dogs and cats. NHPH colonization is noted in up to 100% of healthy dogs and cats depending on the population, with highest rates in shelter and colony groups.[64] Close contact and greater fecal–oral exposure likely explain the high rates in shelters. There is some degree of geographic variation in the distribution of different NHPH species.[64, 65]

Clinical signs

In cats and dogs, *Helicobacter* spp. are most often an incidental finding unassociated with clinical signs. In some patients there may be chronic intermittent vomiting that may (or may not) occur together with weight loss, inappetence or diarrhea.

Diagnosis

Because *Helicobacter* spp. are extremely difficult to culture, diagnosis relies on either non-invasive or invasive testing such as histopathology, cytology and urease testing. Most often they are detected via histopathology performed on endoscopic or surgically obtained biopsies (**Fig. 2.20**) or cytology (brush/impression smear). Fluorescent *in situ* hybridization (FISH) utilizing biopsy samples allows direct visualization of the relationship between the bacteria and the mucosa as well as being more specific than silver stains.[63] However, a positive test result (with any modality) does not always equate with clinical disease.

Therapy

Specific antimicrobial therapy is not advised for dogs and cats, except in cases of biopsy-confirmed infection in clinically affected animals, with gastritis, that have undergone a thorough work-up to rule out concurrent disease. Effective therapy is generally ascertained by resolution of clinical signs. Ideally one would repeat testing to see whether the organisms have been eradicated, along with concomitant inflammation.

In general, triple drug therapy, consisting of two antibiotics along with an antacid, is advocated (*Table 2.8*).[63] It is believed that an extended course of

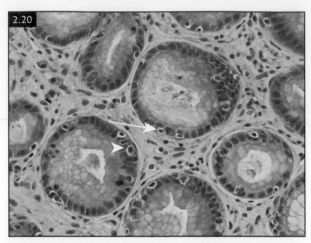

Fig. 2.20 *Helicobacter*. The arrowhead points to a globule leukocyte (lymphocyte), and several with orange granules are seen. The arrow indicates intraepithelial small lymphocytes. There are increased numbers of lymphocytes throughout the lamina propria. Spiral bacteria are seen within the lumen of a gastric gland (40× magnification, H&E stain; cross-section of glandular stomach [body of the stomach]). (Courtesy of Sally Lester)

Table 2.8 **Potential treatment protocols for *Helicobacter* spp.**
Metronidazole (11–15 mg/kg PO q12h) + amoxicillin (22 mg/kg PO q12h) + bismuth subsalicylate suspension (0.22 mL/kg q6–8h) for 21 days
Clarithromycin (7.5 mg/kg PO q12h) + amoxicillin (22 mg/kg PO q12h) + omeprazole/lansoprazole (1 mg/kg PO q24h for either drug) for 7–21days
Clarithromycin (7.5 mg/kg PO q12h) + amoxicillin (20 mg/kg PO q12h) + metronidazole (10 mg/kg PO q12h) for 21 days

therapy will improve the chance of eradicating the organism. Gastric ulceration is uncommon in dogs and cats, and the role of antacid therapy is debated. Famotidine was ineffective in one study,[67] but proton-pump inhibitors may have therapeutic effects. Although bismuth has been reportedly used in cats this must be considered with caution.

Prognosis/complications

Previous studies have demonstrated 80–90% clinical improvement with therapy (decreased frequency or resolved vomiting); however, recurrence of signs appears common. Complications such as gastric ulceration are unlikely.

NHPH infection commonly recurs,[68] making definitive treatment undefined. In human medicine the aim is for complete eradication of *H. pylori*, and antibiotic resistance has been noted. This has not been documented in veterinary medicine, apart from potential metronidazole resistance.[69]

Public health and infection control

Although dogs and cats are a risk factor associated with human colonization with NHPN, the overall zoonotic risk is low.

HETEROBILHARZIA AMERICANA (NORTH AMERICAN CANINE SCHISTOSOMIASIS)
Johanna Heseltine

Definition

Heterobilharzia americana is a trematode that infects the liver of dogs and deposits eggs in the intestinal wall and other organs, resulting in granulomatous inflammation and fibrosis. Acute or chronic large bowel diarrhea and protein-losing enteropathy are common presentations.

Etiology and pathogenesis

Raccoons and nutria are natural definitive hosts, but dogs can serve as a definitive host. Cercariae in freshwater penetrate the dog's skin during swimming or wading, then migrate through the lungs to the liver, where they mature into adults. Adults travel via the portal veins to the mesenteric veins, where they reproduce and lay eggs. These penetrate the mesenteric vein and intestinal mucosa to enter the intestinal lumen. Eggs (containing a miracidium) are shed into feces and, when exposed to freshwater, hatch a ciliated miracidium that swims to find the intermediate host, a lymnaeid snail (*Lymnaea cubensis* or *Pseudosuccinea* spp.). Sporocysts develop within the snail, within which cercariae form, and then emerge from the snail into water to find a canine host (**Fig. 2.21**).[70]

Patent infection occurs 68–121 days post-infection. In the dog, eggs deposited in the intestinal wall cause a granulomatous enterocolitis and fibrosis, whereas others disperse back to the liver or other organs, e.g. pancreas, lymph nodes, spleen, lung, kidney and rarely the brain. The severity of disease is dependent on the number of adult flukes, final location of the eggs, degree of inflammation and fibrosis, and severity of hypercalcemia.

Geography

H. americana is endemic to the Gulf coast and Atlantic region of the United States. It has been reported in Texas, Louisiana, Florida, North Carolina, South Carolina, Georgia, Oklahoma, Alabama, Virginia, Mississippi, Kansas and Indiana.

Incidence and risk factors

Young, large breed dogs housed indoors with occasional outdoor access have an increased incidence of the parasite. Multiple dogs in a household may exhibit clinical signs.[71, 72]

Clinical signs

Large bowel diarrhea is the most common clinical sign, often with weight loss and lethargy. Small intestinal diarrhea (often with melena) or a protein-losing enteropathy may occur. Vomiting, hyporexia and fever may present concurrently.

Polyuria/polydipsia may be present in infected dogs with hypercalcemia with (or without) acute kidney injury. Hepatic disease may be mild or severe. Some infected dogs are subclinically affected, and early signs may include cough or rash, but these signs are rarely noted.[70–72]

Diagnosis

Diagnosis may be based on fecal PCR testing, fecal saline sedimentation, or histopathology of affected tissues. Fecal PCR testing can detect $\geq$1–2 eggs/gram of feces. Eggs may be found on fecal saline sedimentation or a direct fecal smear (**Fig. 2.22**); however, routine fecal flotation is usually negative. It is recommended to test two to three fecal samples from different days, owing to the intermittent shedding of

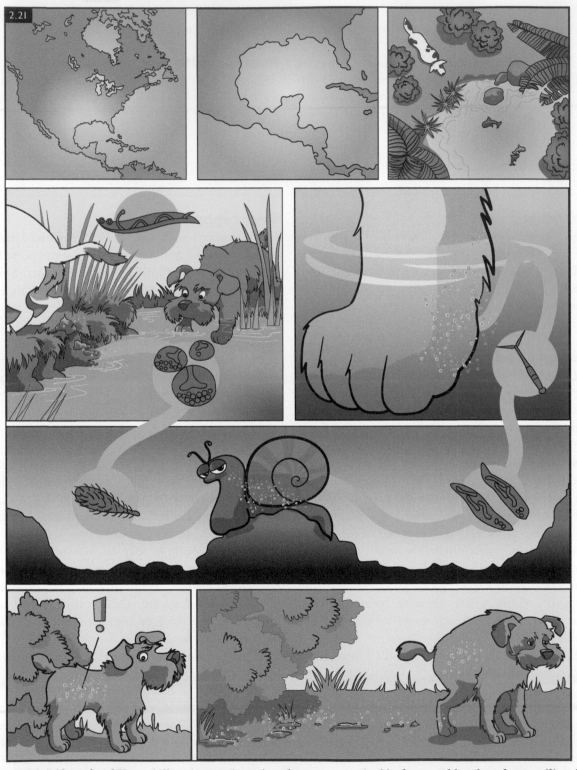

Fig. 2.21 Life cycle of *Heterobilharzia americana* in a dog: eggs are shed in feces and hatch to form a ciliated miracidium, which infects the intermediate host (snail). Sporocysts develop and cercariae emerge; these penetrate the skin of the definitive host (dog).

eggs. Granulomatous inflammation and eggs may be found on liver or intestinal biopsy.[72]

Laboratory abnormalities

Anemia or eosinophilia may be present.

Hypoalbuminemia and hyperglobulinemia are common. Liver enzymes may be elevated. Hypercalcemia is sometimes present, potentially due to overproduction of calcitriol by active macrophages in granulomatous inflammation, and may result in acute renal failure and azotemia.[70–72] Glomerulonephritis can also occur secondary to chronic antigenic stimulation from infection, resulting in proteinuria and possibly hypoalbuminemia.[72, 73]

Diagnostic imaging

Occasionally, abdominal radiographs show mineralization in the intestinal and/or gastric wall, splenomegaly or lack of serosal detail. Radiographs may be normal. Abdominal ultrasound may be normal or show thickening of the intestinal wall, sometimes with linear areas of mineralization in the submucosa or muscularis layers of the intestine (**Fig. 2.23**). The liver may appear coarse, heterogeneous, mottled, hyperechoic or hypoechoic. Splenomegaly, hyperechoic kidneys and abdominal lymphadenopathy may be found via ultrasound. At endoscopy, the intestinal mucosa may appear thickened and irregular (**Fig. 2.24**).[71, 74]

Histopathology, particularly of intestines or liver, may show granulomatous inflammation and fibrosis, sometimes containing eggs.[71] Less commonly, adult parasites may be found in tissue.[72] Dystrophic mineralization may occur in tissues.[75]

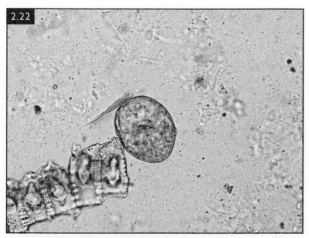

Fig. 2.22 *Heterobilharzia americana* egg (approximately 90 × 70 µm) containing a miracidium larva from a fecal saline sedimentation exam of a dog. (Courtesy of Jessica Rodriguez)

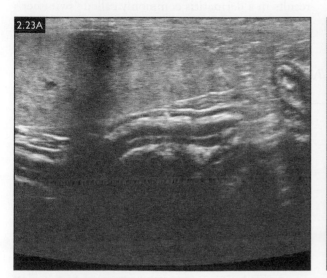 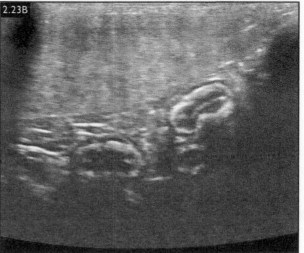

Fig. 2.23A, B Ultrasonographic images of the small intestine of a dog with *Heterobilharzia americana* infection, showing a hyperechoic submucosal layer with pinpoint hyperechogenicities due to eggs in the intestinal wall. (Courtesy of Jessica Rodriguez)

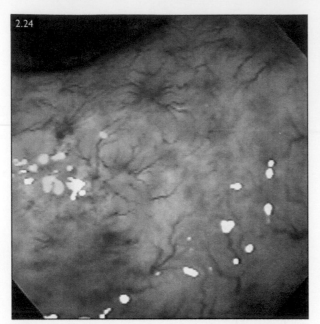

Fig. 2.24 Colonoscopy of a dog with *Heterobilharzia americana* showing severe changes with thickening of the colonic mucosa and increased vascularity. (Courtesy of Michael Willard)

Table 2.9 **Drugs for treating *Heterobilharzia americana* infection**	
DRUG	**DOSAGE**
Praziquantel	25 mg/kg PO q8h for 2–3 days
Fenbendazole	40 mg/kg PO q24h for 10 days

Therapy

Successful treatment has been reported with praziquantel, fenbendazole or a combination of both (*Table 2.9*).[71] Medical management of hypercalcemia is indicated, but calcium may not normalize until after the patient has been treated.[71] Acute kidney injury should be managed and monitored, if present.

Prognosis/complications

Treatment is not always successful. Prognosis is considered good for acute cases and guarded for chronic cases, and may depend on the severity of the granulomatous reaction and fibrosis. Evaluation of a fecal PCR or saline sedimentation is recommended 2 weeks post-treatment, but residual eggs may still be shed during this time, even if active infection is eliminated. In some dogs a second course of treatment is required to resolve clinical signs.[74]

Prevention

Freshwater sources should be avoided in endemic areas. Reinfection can occur. Testing of dogs that share the same environment may allow earlier therapy.[72, 74]

Public health and infection control

In humans, penetration of *H. americana* cercariae results in a dermatitis commonly called "swimmer's itch".

HOOKWORMS: *ANCYLOSTOMA* AND *UNCINARIA* SPP.
Michelle Evason

Definition

Ancylostoma (**Fig. 2.25**) and *Uncinaria* spp. (**Fig. 2.26**) are zoonotic nematodes that have a "hook-shaped" anterior end. Clinical signs in adult animals are usually mild. Large worm burdens in puppies or kittens may cause anemia, diarrhea or death in severe cases.

Etiology and pathogenesis

Dogs are infected by *A. caninum*, whereas *A. tubaeforme* infects cats. Both dogs and cats may be infected by *A. braziliense* and *U. stenocephala*.

Adult hookworms are found in the small intestine of their definitive hosts. Eggs are passed in feces. These become infective once they develop into third-stage larvae (after approximately 2–9 days). Dogs or cats are infected through direct ingestion of infected tissue (e.g. prey or environmental contamination), cutaneous larval penetration, ingestion of infected cockroaches or transmammary infection.

After infection, most larvae that reach the small intestine mature to adults (**Fig. 2.27**). Larvae that penetrate the skin pass through the blood to the

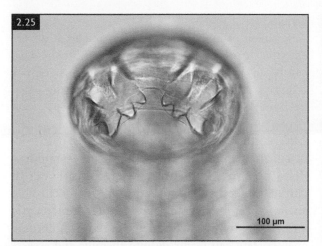

Fig. 2.25 Mouth of an adult female *Ancylostoma caninum* recovered from the small intestine of a dog. Note the prominent trifid teeth ("fangs") which the blood-feeding hookworms use to rip holes in the intestinal lining of the host so that they can feed at the bleeding wound site. (Courtesy of Gary Conboy)

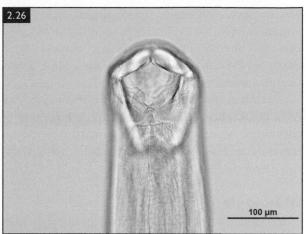

Fig. 2.26 Mouth of an adult female *Uncinaria stenocephala* recovered from the small intestine of a dog. The mouth opening is lined with a pair of cutting plates. Owing to its smaller size, *U. stenocephala* is less voracious a blood-feeder and therefore less pathogenic than *A. caninum*. (Courtesy of Gary Conboy)

Geography

Worldwide. Hookworms are more common in tropical and subtropical environments, particularly *A. braziliense*. *U. stenocephala* prefers cooler climates, such as the northern USA, Canada and Europe.

Incidence and risk factors

Prevalence varies with geography, lifestyle (prey consumption) and deworming history. In owned (well-cared-for) pets, prevalence ranges of 2.5–10% in dogs[76] and 0.5–7% in cats[76, 77] have been reported. Puppies that acquire infection while nursing contribute to ongoing rises in prevalence.

Infections are most common in young animals and those outdoors frequently, e.g. engaging in predator–prey behavior. High-density housing (shelters, breeding facilities) increases infection risk, particularly those with dirt flooring or environments that are not routinely cleaned.[76, 77]

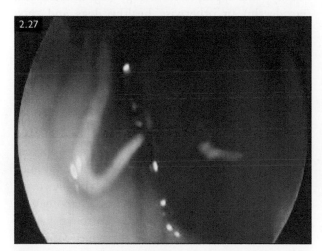

Fig. 2.27 Adult hookworm in the large intestine. (Courtesy of Johanna Heseltine)

lungs, where some larvae are coughed up and swallowed. Others can migrate to other body tissues and become dormant (arrested development). Once adult worms are removed (or killed) reactivation of larvae in the arrested development state occurs. Worms may live, attach and ingest blood from the small intestine for anywhere from 4 to 24 months. Eggs are typically shed within 2–3 weeks, but puppies infected while nursing may shed eggs 10–12 days after birth.

Clinical signs

Clinical disease is associated with worm burden and the voracity of hookworm blood-feeding. Healthy adult dogs and cats with few worms rarely develop clinical signs. Puppies and kittens infected with large burdens of *A. caninum* or *A. tubaeforme*, respectively, can be severely anemic, "poor doers", dehydrated and thin, and have dark tarry feces. Puppies infected through nursing may have severe clinical signs; death may result from the aggressive feeding habits of *A. caninum*.

Uncommonly, respiratory signs may develop, due to large numbers of hookworms migrating through the lungs, or severe anemia (hypoxia). Cutaneous larval migration can cause dermatitis, most commonly on the feet.

Diagnosis

Infection is diagnosed on the basis of history, clinical signs and fecal flotation. Fecal antigen tests (enzyme-linked immunosorbent assay, ELISA) may aid in diagnosis and can be used together with fecal flotation (**Fig. 2.28**).

Puppies that appear healthy, and then deteriorate rapidly in their second or third week of life, should raise the index of suspicion for infection. In these puppies, clinical signs can occur before egg release, thus identification and diagnosis cannot be made on fecal float, and empirical therapy is strongly urged.

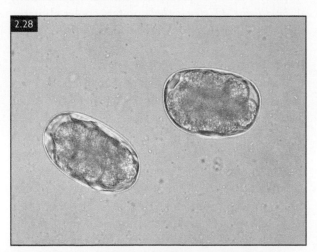

Fig. 2.28 *Uncinaria stenocephala* eggs detected on zinc sulfate centrifugal fecal flotation from an infected dog. The eggs are elliptical, 71–92 × 35–58 μm in size, with a clear, smooth shell wall, and contain a grape-like cluster of undifferentiated embryo cells (morula). Eggs of *Ancylostoma caninum* are identical in morphology but can be differentiated from those of *U. stenocephala* by their smaller size (52–79 × 28–58 μm). (Courtesy of Gary Conboy)

Cytology

Assessment of multiple fecal float samples at different times can aid diagnosis. In adult animals, eggs can be an "incidental" finding. Although therapy is required, continued search for an underlying diagnosis may be needed.

CBC, serum biochemistry

Anemia due to blood loss can occur in severe infections; this may be non-regenerative if early on. In chronic infections a normocytic, normochromic anemia progressing to hypochromic, microcytic anemia due to iron deficiency can result. A chronic anemia state can occur despite therapy, and assessment of iron levels is recommended. Eosinophilia may be present but is not sensitive or specific.

Therapy

Therapy is advised in all cases. Infection resolves rapidly with appropriate therapy (e.g. milbemycin, moxidectin) in otherwise healthy dogs and cats. However, third-stage larvae in arrested development will not be killed. Severely infected animals may require intensive hospitalization, IV fluid support, iron supplementation for anemia and potentially blood transfusion.

Nursing puppies are at risk of infection and should be dewormed. Deworming of the bitch does not remove hookworms in the arrested development state. Similarly, dormant larvae are reactivated once adult worms have been eradicated with deworming. Therefore, repeated rounds of therapy may be required. Therapy with fenbendazole from day 40 of gestation to day 14 of lactation will reduce activation of larvae.

Prognosis/complications

Prognosis is excellent with appropriate management. Severely infected animals may require more intensive therapy and can have chronic anemia. Severely affected puppies with acute *A. caninum* infection may die despite therapy.

Prevention

Regular testing of puppies, kittens, and adult dogs and cats for intestinal parasites is advised. Puppies and kittens should be checked more frequently in their first year of life. Routine deworming is effective in controlling infection. This is particularly important for hunting dogs, outdoor cats and breeding facilities, where infection (and reinfection) are likely, owing to lifestyle and transmammary transmission of *A. caninum* to pups. Puppies, kittens, and breeding bitches or queens should be treated when the young are 2, 4, 6 and 8 weeks of age, then moved

to a routine preventive program. Unfortunately, this deworming schedule is rarely utilized by breeders, or advised by veterinarians.

Environmental cleaning, prompt fecal removal and decontamination are integral parts of therapy and prevention of reinfection. Limiting predatory behavior (ingestion of infected tissue) and confining dogs to a fenced yard will help decrease risk of infection.

LIVER FLUKES: *PLATYNOSOMUM FASTOSUM, PLATYNOSOMUM CONCINNUM*
M Casey Gaunt

Definition
Platynosomum spp. are small trematodes (flukes) that may infect the gallbladder and biliary system (**Fig. 2.29**).[78] In cats, infection is typically subclinical, except in rare cases where vomiting, diarrhea and icterus may occur associated with heavy parasite burdens.

Etiology and pathogenesis
The life cycle is incompletely understood. Cats are definitive hosts. Intermediate hosts include land snails (e.g. *Subulina octona, Eulota similaris*), a variety of lizards (in Florida commonly *Anolis* sp.), the marine toad (*Bufo marinus*) and potentially cockroaches.[78, 79] Cats are infected through ingestion of cercariae present within lizards. After ingestion, the cercariae migrate to the gallbladder and bile ducts and develop into the adult stage (**Fig. 2.30**). Eggs are released into the bile and shed in cat feces at 8–12 weeks post-infection. These eggs are ingested by the first intermediate host (snail), which is then ingested by the second intermediate host (lizard, cockroach, isopod or toad), and finally transmitted to the cat through predator–prey behavior.[78]

Geography
This parasite is found widely in tropical and subtropical environments of North, Central and South America and the Caribbean, along with Asia (Russia, Thailand), Africa (Nigeria), Malaysia, Indonesia and Papua New Guinea.

Incidence and risk factors
The prevalence of *P. concinnum* infestation in cats in subtropical regions has varied between 15% and

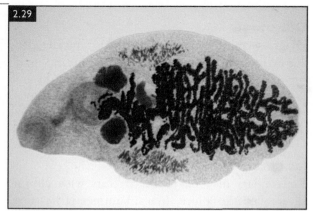

Fig. 2.29 Adult *Platynosomum fastosum* recovered from the gallbladder of a cat (Semichon's acetic-carmine stain). The fluke is 2.9–8.0 mm in length, dorsoventrally flattened with both an oral and a ventral sucker, with opposite testes anterior to the ovary and the loops of uterus filling most of the posterior portion of the body. (Courtesy of Gary Conboy)

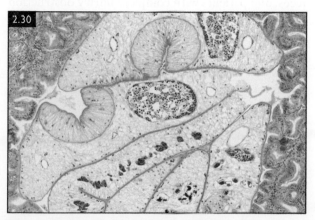

Fig. 2.30 Histological section of *Platynosomum fastosum* in a bile duct. (Courtesy of Ryan Jennings)

85%.[80] Accurate prevalence data are difficult to establish because infections are frequently subclinical and consequently undiagnosed.

Clinical signs

Infection is usually subclinical. Findings vary depending on trematode burden and the cat's immune response to the parasite. In severely affected patients, acute vomiting, lethargy and icterus may be present.[79] Cystic liver disease with progression to hepatic failure has been reported.[81] Cholangiocarcinomas have been associated with *P. fastosum* infestation.[82]

Diagnosis

Diagnosis may be challenging and is typically made through a combination of clinical signs and imaging in heavily infected cats. Confirmation is through fecal techniques or by locating flukes in the liver or biliary tract. Identification of *Platynosomum* spp. may occur incidentally in subclinically infested patients.[78]

Laboratory findings

Leukopenia may be noted. In cats with chronic severe hepatic failure, hypoalbuminemia has been reported.[81] Experimentally, heavily infected cats showed an eosinophilia that peaked at 4–5 months after infection, whereas AST (aspartate transaminase) and ALT (alanine aminotransferase) were transiently but substantially increased.[83]

Fecal examination

Diagnosis through fecal exam is difficult because the parasite has relatively low egg burdens per gram of feces, and patients with complete biliary obstruction may have no eggs found on fecal smear, sedimentation technique or zinc sulfate. High morphological variation between immature and mature eggs can complicate identification. The formalin–ether technique was reported as the most effective fecal diagnostic, identifying 100% of infected cats, whereas direct smear, zinc sulfate, sucrose and modified detergent flotation tests had 25–50% sensitivity.[84] Recently, the FLOTAC examination performed on fresh feces has shown promise, also identifying 100% of infected cats.[85] Serial testing may increase the likelihood of obtaining a positive sample and improve diagnostic sensitivity.

Cytology

Microscopic examination of bile may enable identification of fluke eggs.[79] Fine-needle aspiration of hepatic cysts has allowed diagnosis after recovery of live *P. fastosum* in the fluid.[81]

Diagnostic imaging

Ultrasound may reveal a tortuous, distended gallbladder and distended biliary ducts, suggesting a large number of parasites. This is considered a nonspecific finding that should lead to consideration of fecal exam to attempt confirmation of fluke diagnosis.

Therapy

Therapy is based on management of clinical signs and severity of hepatic disease (antiemetics, nutritional support, fluids), together with anti-parasitics. The most effective agent is praziquantel dosed at 20 mg/kg parenterally, once a day for 3–5 consecutive days. Treatment with praziquantel 5 mg/kg PO twice, given several weeks apart, reportedly resolved shedding of eggs in the feces in a mildly affected cat.[86] Concurrent treatment with prednisolone (1 mg/kg PO q24h) has been reported for management of concurrent hepatitis.[79] Surgery may be needed to relieve biliary obstruction.

Prognosis/complications

Most patients are subclinically infected; however, prognosis varies widely with clinical disease and should be considered guarded in severely affected cats. Death or euthanasia may occur following biliary obstruction,[79] whereas spontaneous recovery by 24 weeks was reported after experimental infection.[83]

Prevention

Routine prophylaxis with praziquantel would theoretically help to mitigate infection but prophylaxis is not routinely practiced in endemic regions.[78, 79] Limiting exposure to lizards may help reduce infestation if practical; however, indoor cats have reportedly been infected as well as outdoor cats.

PARASITIC GASTRITIS: *PHYSALOPTERA* SPP. AND *OLLULANUS TRICUSPIS*
Roger A Hostutler and Michelle Evason

Definition
The most common gastric parasites in cats and dogs are *Physaloptera* spp. and *Ollulanus tricuspis*. Infection usually manifests as chronic vomiting.

Species affected
Ollulanus tricuspis affects domestic and wild cats, and rarely dogs. *Physaloptera* spp. can infect domestic and wild dogs and cats.

Etiology and pathogenesis
Ollulanus tricuspis is a small nematode (0.7–1.0 mm) that infects the stomachs of cats. *O. tricuspis* is ovoviviparous, meaning the eggs hatch within the body and the young are born as L2 larvae. L2 larvae develop to maturity within the stomach and do not need a secondary host. This life cycle leads to ingestion of vomitus (where the parasite can live for up to 12 days) as the primary method of transmission, with a high rate of autoinfection.

Physaloptera spp. are larger helminths, with males measuring 2.5–3.0 cm and females from 3.0 to 6.0 cm in length (**Fig. 2.31**). Although wild carnivores

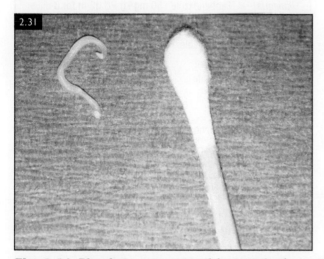

Fig. 2.31 *Physaloptera* sp. removed from a mixed-breed dog with a 2-3-month history of vomiting. This single worm was present within the pyloric antrum. Clinical signs resolved with removal and subsequent treatment with pyrantel pamoate. (Courtesy of Roger Hostutler)

such as the coyote are suspected to be the definitive hosts, the organism can infect the stomach and proximal duodenum of domesticated dogs and cats. Transmission begins when intermediate hosts such as beetles, crickets and cockroaches ingest eggs within the environment. The eggs hatch and develop into L3 larvae within the intermediate host. Ingestion of the intermediate host (or a paratenic host, e.g. a reptile, amphibian or mammal that has ingested an intermediate host) ultimately leads to further development into an adult and subsequent active infection. Clinical signs in dogs and cats are due to the attachment and blood-feeding on the gastric mucosa by the mature worms, causing inflamed lesions.

Geography
Ollulanus tricuspis occurs worldwide. *Physaloptera* spp. are most common in the midwestern United States.

Incidence and risk factors
Ollulanus tricuspis is much more common in catteries and in the stray cat population. Studies in central Europe have found an incidence of approximately 40% in the stray population and 6% in domesticated cats.

The incidence of *Physaloptera* spp. infection is unknown; however, it is comparatively infrequent.

Clinical signs
Ollulanus tricuspis most commonly causes chronic vomiting, with weight loss, decreased appetite and death in extreme circumstances.

Physaloptera spp. cause gastritis, with chronic vomiting being the most common clinical sign. Signs may be present with an extremely small worm burden. In severe cases, infection can lead to dehydration, malnutrition and subsequent weight loss.

Physical examination findings
For both *O. tricuspis* and *Physaloptera* spp., exam findings are not specific to primary infection but rather to chronic gastrointestinal disease, and include weight loss, generalized unthrifty condition, ptyalism and abdominal distension.

Diagnosis

Identification of adult *O. tricuspis* worms or larvae in vomitus or gastric contents, or via histologic identification is needed to obtain a definitive diagnosis. Fecal examination (Baermann testing) has a low sensitivity because the adults or larvae that pass into the intestines are mostly digested. Histologically, infection leads to mucosal ulceration with increased mucus production in the acute phase. However, in chronic cases mucosal hyperplasia with sclerosis can be identified.

Diagnosis of *Physaloptera* spp. can be difficult given that the eggs are often present in low numbers and generally do not float on routine fecal flotation or centrifugation. Larvated eggs may be found on direct fecal smear in higher numbers compared with flotation (**Fig. 2.32**). However, identification of the parasite via endoscopy or in vomitus is generally needed for a definitive diagnosis. Eosinophilia may be noted on CBC. Histologically, marked infections lead to gastric mucosal hyperplasia and edema that may exacerbate the clinical signs outlined above.

Therapy

See *Table 2.10*.

Prognosis/complications

Overall, the prognosis with *Ollulanus tricuspis* infection is good, given that natural eradication may be seen with a low burden of infection. In some cases, chronic vomiting may be persistent even after elimination of active infection. In the worst-case scenario, autoinfection can lead to an extreme worm burden and death.

Prognosis is typically favorable with *Physaloptera* infection, since the worm burden is often low, clinical signs are typically infrequent and response to therapy is excellent. However, with massive infection, dehydration, anorexia and malnourishment may develop and more intensive therapy is required.

Prevention

Ollulanus tricuspis

Given the method of transmission, isolation of individuals with the above clinical signs is highly recommended, especially in a cattery situation, while veterinary investigation is pursued. Once eradication

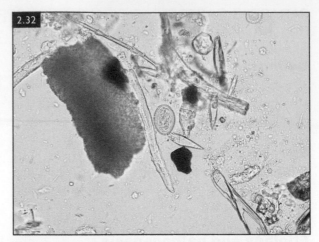

Fig. 2.32 *Physaloptera* sp. egg detected on sugar centrifugal fecal flotation examination from a skunk. The eggs are thick walled, 42–53 × 29–35 μm in size and contain a fully formed first-stage larva coiled inside. Fecal flotation has poor detection sensitivity; the detection method of choice would be fecal sedimentation. (Courtesy of Gary Conboy)

Table 2.10 **Treatment for *Ollulanus tricuspis* and *Physaloptera* spp.**

PARASITE	DRUG	DOSE
Ollulanus tricuspis	Fenbendazole	50 mg/kg PO q24h for 3 days
	Levamisole	5 mg/kg SC once
	Tetramisole	2.5% solution, 5 mg/kg once
Physaloptera spp.	Pyrantel pamoate	Dogs: 20 mg/kg PO q2 weeks for 3 months
		Cats: 5 mg/kg PO q2 weeks for 3 months
	Fenbendazole	50 mg/kg PO q24h for 3 days
	Endoscopic removal	

of clinical signs has been achieved, the disease should be self-limiting without long-term implications in the acute setting. Unfortunately, as stated above, the organism is often not identified on routine fecal examination and prophylactic deworming at routine intervals could be beneficial. Fenbendazole (50 mg/kg PO q24h for 3 days) and pyrantel (5–10 mg/kg PO once with a repeat dosage in 2–3 weeks) have both been advocated for this purpose.

Physaloptera spp.

Prevention of hunting paratenic hosts or ingestion of arthropod intermediate hosts is of utmost importance, as there are no approved pharmaceutical controls for *Physaloptera* spp. Prevention would additionally include strict sanitation and elimination of intermediate and paratenic hosts in kennel/cattery environments.

PARVOVIRUSES: CANINE PARVOVIRUS AND FELINE PANLEUKOPENIA VIRUS
Susan Kilborn

Definition

Canine parvovirus (CPV) and feline parvovirus (panleukopenia) virus (FPV) are related vaccine-preventable parvoviruses that can cause severe gastrointestinal and systemic disease.

Etiology and pathogenesis

Canine

CPV is a small, non-enveloped, single-stranded DNA virus. Parvoviral infection in dogs is a systemic disease that develops when variants of CPV-2 enter the body by oronasal transmission after exposure to virus in feces, vomit, or on environmental or animal surfaces. Viremia results in infection of rapidly dividing cells in the gastrointestinal (GI) tract (**Figs. 2.33, 2.34**), lymphoid tissue (**Fig. 2.35**) and bone marrow, which causes diarrhea, vomiting and leukopenia. Morbidity is high in unvaccinated dogs. The incubation period is 3–5 days. Virus is shed in feces 3 days after infection (several days before the onset of clinical signs), peaks on day 4–7 and declines by day 14.

Feline

FPV is a small, non-enveloped, single-stranded DNA virus that closely resembles mink enteritis virus and CPV-2. Panleukopenia in cats is a systemic disease that develops when FPV virus enters the body by fecal–oral transmission. Like CPV, the virus infects the bone marrow and gastrointestinal epithelial crypts (**Figs. 2.36, 2.37**). This results in diarrhea, vomiting, fever and mortality in untreated cats. The pathogenesis in cats older than 6 weeks is similar to that of CPV-2 in dogs. Infection *in utero*, and at up to 9 days of age, results in either fetal death or cerebellar hypoplasia.

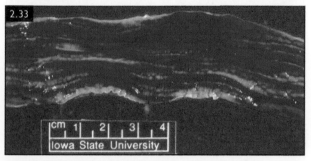

Fig. 2.33 Parvovirus enteritis, canine small intestine. (Courtesy of http://noahsarkive.cldavis.org–Texas A and M University–Read)

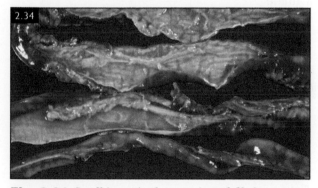

Fig. 2.34 Small intestinal necrosis and fibrin deposition in a puppy with severe canine parvovirus infection. (Courtesy of http://noahsarkive.cldavis.org–University of Alberta–Nation)

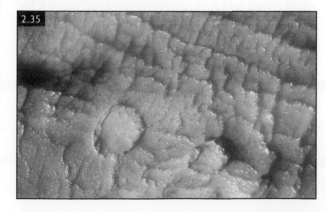

Fig. 2.35 Lymphoid depleted Peyer's patches in a dog with canine parvovirus infection. (Courtesy of http://noahsarkive.cldavis.org–The Ohio State University–Sagartz)

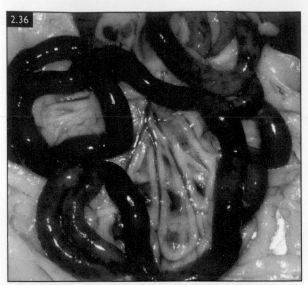

Fig. 2.36 Hemorrhagic small intestine in a cat with feline panleukopenia. (Courtesy of http://noahsarkive.cldavis.org–University of Georgia–Long)

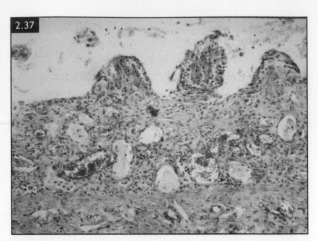

Fig. 2.37 Feline panleukopenia –histology of small intestine. (Courtesy of http://noahsarkive.cldavis.org–Mississippi State University–Ward)

Incidence and risk factors

Canine

There is a high incidence in unvaccinated dogs less than 6 months of age. Adults can be affected in outbreaks. Breeds at increased risk include Rottweilers, Doberman Pinschers, Labrador Retrievers, German Shepherd Dogs, Alaskan Sled dogs and Bull Terrier breeds. Concurrent parasitism or presence of pathogenic gastrointestinal bacteria (*Salmonella* spp., *Campylobacter* spp.) are additional risk factors in young dogs.

Feline

The incidence is unknown, but FPV is common in high-density, unvaccinated cat populations (e.g. shelters). Shedding of FPV is common in healthy shelter cats, and it is thought that shedding of CPV also occurs in healthy cats.

Clinical signs

Canine

Vomiting, nausea, hemorrhagic small bowel diarrhea, anorexia and lethargy are typical (**Fig. 2.38**). Dogs are depressed and weak, dehydrated, febrile, show abdominal pain on palpation, and may have hemorrhagic liquid feces on their perineum and on rectal exam. Some dogs may have pale mucous

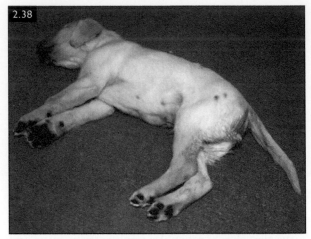

Fig. 2.38 Puppy with canine parvovirus infection. Note the abundant diarrhea staining around the perineum. (Courtesy of http://noahsarkive.cldavis.org–Michigan State University–Ramos-Vara)

membranes, hypothermia and signs of septic shock (from GI translocation of gram-negative bacteria) such as tachycardia, prolonged capillary refill time and poor pulse quality. Less common signs include neurologic signs such as seizures (due to hypoglycemia or disseminated intravascular coagulation [DIC] affecting the brain), and sudden death due to myocarditis in very young dogs (**Fig. 2.39**).

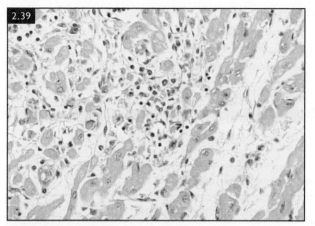

Fig. 2.39 Histology demonstrating myocarditis in a dog with canine parvovirus infection. (Courtesy of http://noahsarkive.cldavis.org–Oklahoma State University–Qualls)

Feline

Affected cats may have fever or hypothermia (if shock is present), dehydration, abdominal pain and coma, as well as petechial hemorrhages and other signs of DIC. Cats with cerebellar hypoplasia or other neurologic involvement show ataxia, hypermetria, intention tremors and retinal lesions.

Severe illness and mortality are highest between 3 and 5 months of age. Fetal or neonatal infection results in cerebellar ataxia or seizures.

Diagnosis

Diagnostic testing is summarized in *Table 2.11* for both species. Point-of-care, enzyme-linked immunosorbent assay (ELISA), fecal antigen detection is commonly used for testing in both species, but PCR testing is becoming more widely used.

Table 2.11 Diagnosis of canine parvovirus and feline panleukopenia virus

METHOD		DISEASE
Hematology	Canine	Lymphopenia, neutropenia, anemia (GI blood loss), thrombocytopenia (consumption due to DIC)
	Feline	As for canine
Biochemistry	Canine	Hypoalbuminemia, hypokalemia, hyponatremia, hypochloremia, hypomagnesemia, hypoglycemia
	Feline	As for canine. Azotemia may be present with severe dehydration
Acid–base	Canine	Metabolic acidosis (loss of bicarbonate) or metabolic alkalosis (severe vomiting)
	Feline	As for canine
Organism detection	Canine	**Fecal antigen (ELISA):** specificity very high; false positives can occur within 7–10 days of attenuated live vaccines. All three CPV-2 variants detected with ELISA testing
		PCR (feces, blood, tissue): very sensitive; interpret appropriately with other supportive evidence and recent MLV exposure. Real-time PCR can determine viral DNA load. May detect vaccine virus in feces for at least 2 weeks post-vaccination. Some assays discriminate between field and vaccine strains
	Feline	**Fecal antigen (ELISA):** ELISA-based fecal tests for CPV-2 variants will detect FPV. Same sensitivity issues (false negatives) as in the dog, due to transient shedding. Specificity high; false positives may occur (test dependent) within 2 weeks after MLV
		PCR (feces, blood, tissue): same issues as canine. Formalin-fixed tissue can be used for PCR
Pathology Gross	Canine	Thickening, distension and discoloration of the serosa and mucosa of the small intestine. Bloody, watery material within the GI tract
	Feline	Same as for canine. Pleural and peritoneal effusion may be present, small cerebellum in prenatal/neonatal kittens
Histopathology	Canine	Necrosis of the small intestinal crypt epithelium and depletion of all lymphoid tissue. Nuclear inclusions in crypt epithelium. Virus detected by *in situ* hybridization or quantitative PCR assays of tissues, including small intestinal mucosa
	Feline	Same as for canine. Cerebellum may show cell depletion

Abbreviations: DIC, disseminated intravascular coagulation; ELISA, enzyme-linked immunosorbent assay; GI, gastrointestinal; MLV, modified live vaccine; PCR, polymerase chain reaction

Serum antibody titers for both CPV-2 and FPV are not useful for diagnosis, owing to prior subclinical exposure or vaccination. Antibody measurement is useful to guide vaccination administration or to monitior protection in shelter environments.

Therapy

See *Table 2.12*.

Canine

Intravenous fluids, analgesia and antimicrobial therapy for secondary bacterial infections are the cornerstones of treatment. Antimicrobials should be considered for dogs with fever, hemorrhagic diarrhea, or signs of septic shock or systemic inflammatory response syndrome (SIRS) because of secondary bacteremia from translocation of gram-negative bacteria.

Table 2.12 **Treatment of canine parvovirus and feline panleukopenia virus infections**

THERAPY	SPECIES	DOSE	FREQUENCY/ROUTE	COMMENTS
Replacement crystalloid solution (LRS, PlasmaLyte, Normosol)	Canine	Deficit/6–24 h + maintenance (2–6 mL/kg/h) + fluid losses/hour	IV, SC fluids at 30 mL/kg q6h on outpatient basis	Potassium chloride (not >0.5 mEq/kg/h) Dextrose 2.5–5% (not SC) as required
	Feline	Same; maintenance at 2–3 mL/kg/h	IV	Same
Colloids	Canine	20 mL/kg (divide into 5 mL/kg boluses)	q24h, IV	If albumin <20 g/L
	Feline	10 mL/kg (divide into 2.5–3 mL/kg boluses)	q24h, IV	
Ampicillin	Canine	10–20 mg/kg	q8h, IV	Use with aminoglycoside
	Feline	15–20 mg/kg	q8h, IV	
Cefoxitin	Canine	15–30 mg/kg	q6–8h, IV	Can be used as a sole agent
	Feline	Same	Same	Same
Amikacin	Canine	20 mg/kg	q24h IV, SC	Rehydrate patient before aminoglycoside use. Fluoroquinolones off-label owing to cartilage damage in growing dogs
	Feline	10–15 mg/kg	q24h, IV	
Maropitant	Canine	1 mg/kg	q24h, SC × 5 days	Can use same dose IV over 2 min (dogs >4 months of age)
	Feline	1 mg/kg	q24h, SC or IV slowly × 5 days	Label dose >4 months of age
Ondansetron	Canine	0.1–0.2 mg/kg	q8–12h, IV	Use if maropitant is ineffective.
	Feline	0.1–0.22 mg/kg	q8–12h, IV	
Omeprazole or pantoprazole	Canine	1 mg/kg	q12h, IV or PO	To prevent reflux esophagitis
	Feline	0.5–1 mg/kg	q12h IV or PO	
Buprenorphine	Canine	0.02 mg/kg	q6–8h, IV	Butorphanol or hydromorphone is an alternative
	Feline	0.05–0.1 mg/kg	q8–12h, SC	Extra-label dosing: 0.03 mg/kg q6–8h IV or OTM
Feeding	Canine	RER (kcal) = 70 × (body weight in kg)$^{0.75}$; immediate feeding regardless of vomiting status	NE tube (liquid or blenderized diet) or oral feeding if eating	Increase kilocalorie delivery gradually over 2–3 days to avoid refeeding syndrome
	Feline	Same calculation. Benefits of early enteral nutrition are unproven	Same	

Abbreviations: LRS, lactated Ringer's solution; NE, nasoesophageal; OTM, oral transmucosal route; RER, resting energy requirement; SC, subcutaneous administration

Oral recuperation fluid administration may assist with more rapid return of appetite in some dogs.[87] Enteral nutrition started immediately (regardless of vomiting) results in weight gain and faster resolution of GI signs.[88]

Recombinant feline interferon-omega administered IV for three days is effective in reducing mortality in dogs with parvovirus.[89] The use of oseltamivir may reduce weight loss and leukopenia during illness, but no survival benefit has been proven.[90]

Outpatient treatment of dogs with once-daily subcutaneous fluids and antimicrobials may be reasonable when finances are limited, but some reduction in survival and more metabolic abnormalities result.[91]

Feline
See *Table 2.12*.

Prognosis/complications
Canine
Survival (in naturally occurring infections) when intravenous fluid, antimicrobial and antiemetic therapy was used is as high as 90%.[91] Mortality without therapy is as high. Complications and death typically occur due to SIRS, including hypothermia, bacterial endotoxemia and shock, hypoglycemia and edema due to GI protein loss.

Feline
Mortality rate in naturally occurring illness due to FPV (with supportive therapy provided) is approximately 50%.[92] Hypoalbuminemia and white blood cell count <1,000/μL are associated with increased risk of death.

Complications during acute illness are similar to those described in the dog. Cerebellar neurologic signs are a permanent complication of *in utero* or neonatal infection but are stable and may improve with time.

Prevention
Canine
Vaccination is highly effective. Vaccination with modified live (ML) CPV may result in fecal excretion of virus (in varying amounts) that causes PCR testing to be positive for up to 28 days after administration.[93] Point-of-care ELISA test kits to detect antibody have been validated in shelter and practice settings and may be useful to immediately guide vaccination decisions, but false-positive results from recent ML vaccination can also occur.

Feline
Vaccination is an important control tool. Vaccination of pregnant queens with ML vaccines should be avoided, except in high-risk shelter environments or outbreaks, because of the risk of cerebellar hypoplasia in the fetuses. Administration of a ML FPV vaccine results in protective immunity within 7 days of one dose that lasts for at least 3 years.[94]

SALMONELLA
J Scott Weese

Definition
Salmonella is a genus of gram-negative bacteria that can cause enteric and systemic disease in many species, including dogs and cats. They are important zoonotic pathogens.

Etiology and pathogenesis
There are many different serovars of *Salmonella enterica* subsp. *enterica*, and a wide range of these can affect dogs and cats. Infection is by the fecal–oral route. The infective dose is unknown and likely varies greatly by strain and based on the status of the gut microbiota. If *Salmonella* proliferates in the gut, it can attach to and invade enterocytes, and produce toxins. The combination of bacterial effects and the host immune response can cause epithelial cell injury, with subsequent fluid loss. Toxemia and bacterial translocation can develop depending on the degree of invasion and epithelial barrier damage. Effects are typically confined to the gastrointestinal (GI) tract; however, sepsis and infections of non-GI foci (e.g. bone, kidneys) can occur.

Risk factors
A small percentage of healthy dogs and cats carry *Salmonella* spp. at any time, typically <2% in animals

not fed raw meat.[5, 95, 96] In dogs and cats, raw meat diets and raw animal-based treats have been associated with increased risk of *Salmonella* shedding and have been implicated in sporadic cases of *Salmonella* sepsis.[97–100] Contaminated commercial dry diets have rarely been implicated in outbreaks. Outdoor cats are at increased risk from hunting infected birds, particularly songbirds. *Salmonella* spp. can be found in various foods and animals, so there is always some risk of exposure.

Clinical signs

Subclinical infections are most common. When disease is present, it can range from mild self-limiting diarrhea to severe GI disease and sepsis (**Fig. 2.40**). Gastrointestinal disease is impossible to distinguish from that due to other causes and results in diarrhea with varying degrees of lethargy, fever, anorexia, depression, vomiting and abdominal pain. Diarrhea may be bloody or include mucus.

Systemic complications from bacteremia and endotoxemia can result in more profound depression, hypotension, collapse, dehydration, tachycardia, tachypnea, and fever or hypothermia. Secondary organ dysfunction or disseminated intravascular coagulation (DIC) can develop. Disease can be rapidly progressive, with severe illness occurring shortly after (or even before) the onset of diarrhea.

Diagnosis

Culture and PCR are the two main methods. Culture has the advantage of yielding an isolate for susceptibility testing and typing but turnaround time is slower. PCR testing is often performed as part of PCR panels.

Therapy

Supportive care is the mainstay of treatment. Antibiotics are not indicated in most cases and are reserved for patients with evidence of sepsis or those

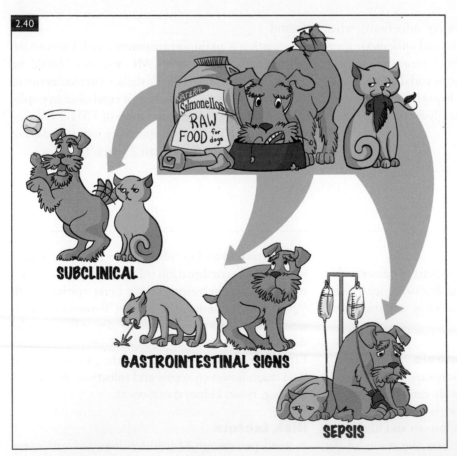

Fig. 2.40 Various routes of infection and clinical presentations of salmonellosis in dogs and cats.

at increased risk of serious consequences from bacterial translocation (e.g. neonates). Antibiotic therapy is not used to target enteric *Salmonella* spp., but rather to prevent or treat systemic manifestations from bacterial translocation. Restoration of the normal gut microbiota is probably a key factor for elimination of *Salmonella* spp. and unnecessary antibiotic use could theoretically prolong *Salmonella* shedding.

If antimicrobials are indicated, they are ideally chosen based on culture and susceptibility testing. Drugs that are typically effective against *Salmonella* spp. include second- and third-generation cephalosporins, fluoroquinolones and trimethoprim sulfonamides. Aminoglycosides are usually effective but must be used with caution in patients with dehydration or compromised renal function.

Prognosis/complications
The prognosis is very good unless serious systemic signs are present or rare secondary infections (e.g. osteomyelitis) develop.

Prevention
Avoiding high-risk foods (e.g. raw meat, raw animal-based treats), keeping pets away from livestock and preventing cats from hunting should reduce the risk.

TAPEWORMS: *TAENIA* SPP. AND *DIPYLIDIUM CANINUM*
Michelle Evason

Definition
Taenia spp. *and Dipylidium caninum* are cestode tapeworms found in dogs and cats. Clinical signs are typically non-existent to mild.

Species affected
Dogs, fox, coyotes, cats and humans are the definitive hosts. Intermediate hosts include cattle, pigs, rabbits, sheep, rodents and humans.

Etiology and pathogenesis
Taenia pisiformis (**Figs. 2.41, 2.42**), *T. multiceps*, *T. ovis*, *T. crassiceps* and *T. serialis* are found in dogs, whereas *T. taeniaeformis* is found in cats. *Dipylidium caninum* can infect both species.

Canids, cats and humans are the main definitive hosts for *Taenia* spp. Adult worms can be quite large and range to up to a meter in length, depending on the species. Eggs or proglottids (pregnant

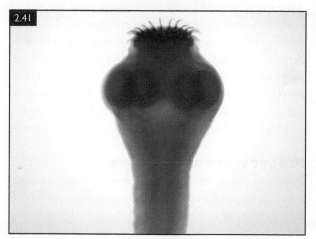

Fig. 2.41 Scolex of *Taenia pisiformis* recovered from the small intestine of a dog (Semichon's acetic–carmine stain). The scolex has four muscular suckers and an armed rostellum. (Courtesy of Gary Conboy)

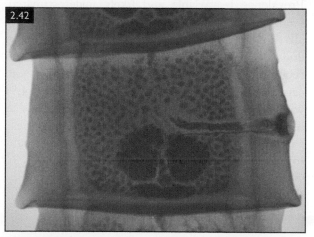

Fig. 2.42 Mature segment of *Taenia pisiformis* recovered from the small intestine of a dog (Semichon's acetic–carmine stain). Each segment contains both male and female reproductive organs. Note the single lateral genital pore. (Courtesy of Gary Conboy)

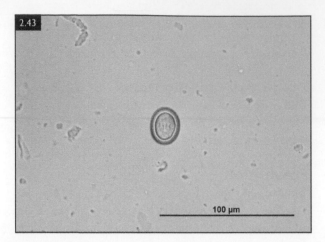

Fig. 2.43 *Taenia* sp. egg detected on centrifugal examination of feces from an infected dog. The brown, thick-walled eggs are 25–40 μm in diameter and contain a hexacanth embryo (i.e. there are six hooks). The eggs of *Taenia* spp. are identical in size and morphology to those of *Echinococcus* spp. (Courtesy of Gary Conboy)

worm segments) are passed in feces and are immediately infective. After ingestion by an intermediate host they hatch in the small intestine, and further development to second-stage larvae occurs. They can also migrate to other body areas (e.g. liver, muscle, brain or heart), and intermediate larval cyst-like structures may develop and cause disease, depending on size and location. Transmission is through direct ingestion of infected feces, tissue cysts found in prey, or through soil and environmental contamination.

Incidence and risk factors

Prevalence is variable and likely underestimated. Geography, lifestyle and deworming history are all thought to play a role. Ranges of 4–60% in dogs[101, 102] and 2–50% in cats[76, 102, 103] have been reported. Infections are most common in dogs and cats that show hunting (predator–prey) behavior,[102] young dogs and cats (<6 months),[77] or animals in high-density housing (shelters, breeding facilities), particularly those with dirt flooring or poor cleaning practice.

Clinical signs

Clinical disease is rare, and most dogs and cats have no clinical signs. Perianal irritation can cause "scooting" or anal itch, although this is more frequently due to anal gland impaction. Occasionally, eggs or proglottids can be found near the anus or attached to the fur.

Diagnosis

Infection is diagnosed based on fecal flotation or direct fecal exam for identification of eggs or proglottids. Pet owners frequently assist diagnosis because they are horrified at identifying motile worm segments.

Unfortunately, the sensitivity of fecal flotation is limited (**Fig. 2.43**). Assessment of multiple samples at different times can increase the sensitivity. Adhesive tape pressed to the perianal skin can reveal eggs or proglottid segments on direct exam.

Therapy

Therapy is advised in all cases, because of the risk of environmental contamination and spread. Infection resolves rapidly with appropriate therapy in otherwise healthy dogs and cats. Therapy should consist of treatment with anti-parasitic medications, such as praziquantel, epsiprantel or fenbendazole. Environmental decontamination should be performed concurrently.

Flea control is indicated when *D. caninum* is present.

Prognosis/complications

Prognosis is excellent with appropriate management. A concern in high-risk geographic areas is differentiation of *Echinococcus multilocularis* from *Taenia* spp., given the elevated animal and human health concerns with *E. multilocularis*. Unfortunately, these tapeworm eggs cannot be differentiated microscopically, and additional testing (e.g. PCR) is required for identification.

Prevention

Regular testing of puppies, kittens, adult dogs and cats for intestinal parasites is advised. Puppies and kittens should be checked more frequently in their first year of life. Intestinal tapeworm infections can be effectively eliminated; however, most products used for heartworm prevention or "routine" puppy and kitten deworming are not effective against tapeworms. Routine tapeworm treatment is particularly important for hunting dogs and outdoor cats, where infection (and reinfection) are likely due to lifestyle risks.

Prompt removal of feces to reduce egg and proglottid burden, limiting predatory behavior (ingestion of rodents, infected tissue cysts) and reduction of roaming will help decrease risk of infection. If *D. caninum* infection is diagnosed, flea control must be performed for all household pets.

Public health

Human *Taenia* and *Dipylidium* (**Fig. 2.44**) infections associated with dogs are rare. The ability to differentiate *Taenia* spp. from *Echinococcus* spp. is a much larger concern, because *Echinoccoccus* spp. pose a severe zoonotic risk.

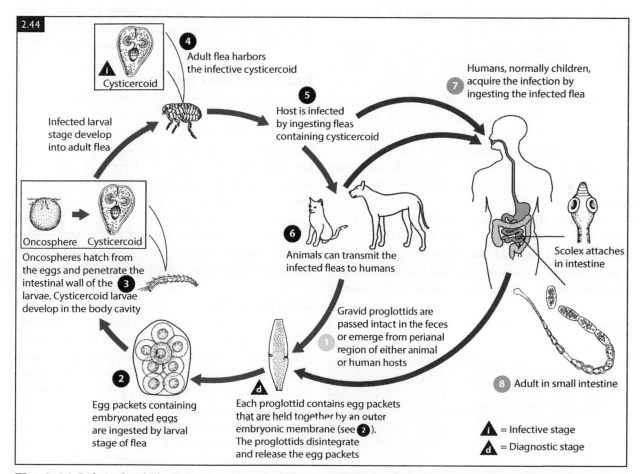

Fig. 2.44 Life cycle of *Dipylidium caninum*, including rare but potential transfer to humans. (Courtesy of the US Centers for Disease Control and Prevention)

TOXOCARA AND TOXASCARIS SPP. (ASCARIDS OR ROUNDWORMS)
Michelle Evason

Definition

Toxocara canis (dogs) and *T. cati* (cats) are the most common roundworms in dogs and cats. Infections in adult animals are usually subclinical. However, puppies or kittens with large worm burdens may fail to thrive and have a potbellied appearance.

Etiology and pathogenesis

Roundworms are large (>10–12 cm in dogs and 3–10 cm in cats) non-segmented nematodes (**Fig. 2.45**). *T. canis* is found in dogs, *T. cati (mystax)* and *T. malayiensis* are found in cats, and *Toxascaris leonina* can infect both species.

Adult roundworms live and reproduce in the small intestine of their definitive hosts. Eggs are excreted in feces and mature into third-stage larvae in the environment (soil). Two to four weeks are required for both *T. canis* and *T. cati* eggs to become infective, whereas *Toxascaris leonina* may be infective within a week. Dogs or cats are infected through direct ingestion of third-stage larvae from infected tissue found in prey or through consumption of eggs from their environment.

After ingestion of eggs by the definitive host, *T. canis* and *T. cati* pass through the small intestinal wall into the liver, and then to the lungs. Most larvae are coughed up, swallowed and mature into adult roundworms in the small intestine. Other larvae can migrate to body tissues and become dormant (arrested development). *Toxascaris leonina* does not leave the small intestine, and migration to other tissues does not occur.

Transplacental (*in utero*) infection with *T. canis* is an important route of infection, leading to disease in very young puppies. Transplacental infection is mainly due to reactivation of the larval arrested development stage in the bitch, which occurs during late pregnancy. Transmammary infection can occur in puppies and kittens. In cats, transmammary infection occurs only when a queen is infected late in pregnancy. In dogs, reinfection of the bitch can occur with ingestion of infected puppy feces.

Incidence and risk factors

Prevalence varies with age, geography, lifestyle (prey consumption, feral or shelter vs. owned pets) and deworming history. *In utero* or transmammary infections contribute to the high prevalence of shedding in young animals. Reported prevalence ranges in owned (well-cared for) pets are 2–13% in dogs[76, 101, 104] and up to 17% in cats.[101, 104]

Risk factors for infection include age (younger dogs and cats), outdoor lifestyle and predator–prey behavior (e.g. hunting dogs), along with high-density housing (shelters, breeding facilities).[76, 77, 104]

Clinical signs

Healthy adult dogs and cats are usually subclinically affected. Puppies (*T. canis*) or kittens (*T. cati*) can be "poor doers": unthrifty, failing to gain weight, with a poor haircoat and a potbellied appearance. Puppies with severe infection may vomit visible worms, initiating a prompt (horrified) owner reaction. Typically, kittens are older when infected and clinical disease is milder than in very young pups.

Coughing may be present with larval migration or pneumonia in heavy infections. Severe infection in few-day-old puppies can result in acute death.

Clinical disease with *Toxascaris leonina* appears rare and is typically found in conjunction with *T. canis* or *T. cati*.

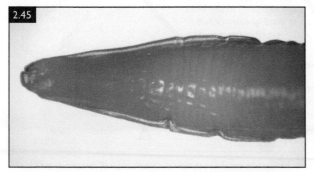

Fig. 2.45 Anterior end of an adult *Toxocara canis* recovered from the small intestine of a puppy. The lateral cervical alae give the head of the worm an "arrowhead" appearance. (Courtesy of Gary Conboy)

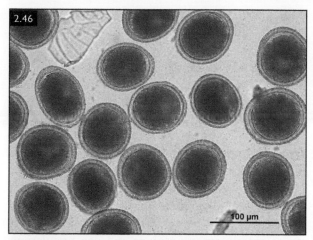

Fig. 2.46 *Toxocara canis* eggs detected by zinc sulfate centrifugal flotation of feces from an infected puppy. They are 85–90 × 75 μm in size with a thick pitted shell wall and contain a single, dark, round embryo cell. (Courtesy of Gary Conboy)

Diagnosis

Diagnosis is based on history (particularly lack of deworming), suggestive clinical signs and identification of eggs via fecal flotation with centrifugation, or adult worms in vomit (**Fig. 2.46**). Fecal antigen tests (enzyme-linked immunosorbent assay, ELISA) may aid diagnosis and can be used together with fecal float.

Fecal centrifugal flotation is recommended. Assessment of multiple samples at different times can aid diagnosis. In adult animals the presence of a few eggs is likely an "incidental" finding or weakly associated with an underlying disease process. Therefore, although therapy is required, continued search for an underlying diagnosis is needed.

Therapy

Therapy is advised in all cases. Every puppy or kitten should be considered infected and treated. Infection resolves rapidly with appropriate therapy in otherwise healthy dogs and cats. However, third-stage larvae in arrested development will not be killed and this can lead to recurrence of test positives and infection in heavily burdened dogs. Therapy in cats and dogs should consist of treatment with anti-parasitic medications, such as milbemycin oxime and moxidectin, fenbendazole, febantel or pyrantel pamoate. Most drugs used for monthly heartworm therapy are effective.

Prognosis/complications

Prognosis is usually excellent with appropriate management.

Prevention

Regular testing of puppies, kittens and adult animals for intestinal parasites is advised. Puppies and kittens should be checked more frequently in their first year of life.

Routine deworming is effective in controlling infection. Puppies and kittens should be treated at 2, 4, 6 and 8 weeks of age, then moved to a routine preventive program. Kittens do not need to be treated for ascarids until 6 weeks; however, owing to concern regarding hookworm infection, starting at 2 weeks is advised.

Deworming of the nursing bitch should occur at the same time as that of the puppies. However, deworming of the bitch does not remove worms in the arrested development state. Therapy with fenbendazole or ivermectin during pregnancy should be performed two to four times for bitches with prior litters with *T. canis* infection. Treatment of the bitch from day 40 of gestation to reduce activation of larvae should be performed.

Public health and infection control

Roundworms can cause visceral and ocular larval migrans in humans, which, although rare, can have severe consequences. Good fecal handling practices, covering children's sandboxes when not in use, wearing shoes and gloves while gardening, and hand washing after contact with outdoor environments will help reduce risk of infection.

TRICHURIS VULPIS (CANINE WHIPWORMS)
Michelle Evason

Definition
Trichuris vulpis is a whip-shaped nematode found in dogs. Clinical signs range from mild (subclinical) disease to severe diarrhea, with some cases "mimicking" Addison's disease.

Species affected
Dogs, wild dogs, foxes and coyotes can be affected, and rarely humans. Cats may be infected with *Trichuris* spp. in tropical areas; this is uncommon in North America.

Etiology and pathogenesis
Canids are the main definitive hosts. Eggs are passed in feces and are extremely resistant to drying and temperature extremes. Eggs are non-infective for 9–12 days in the environment; however, after this time, eggs ingested from the soil or feces hatch into larvae in the small intestine and penetrate the mucosa. Larvae move into the large intestine (cecum) and mature to adult worms (**Fig. 2.47**). Adult worms begin a proliferation of egg production between 74 and 90 days after infection.

Infection is spread by direct ingestion of feces, soil or environmental contamination. Clinical signs are due to the feeding habits and load of parasite burden in the cecum.

Incidence and risk factors
The prevalence is variable and likely impacted by geography, lifestyle and deworming history. Ranges of 1.2–10% are often reported in dogs presented to veterinary clinics,[76, 101] but the prevalence likely varies greatly among regions and dog populations (e.g. strays vs. household pets).

Infections are most common in young dogs (e.g. 6 months to 2 years),[76] or those in high-density housing (shelters, breeding facilities), particularly those with dirt flooring or poor cleaning practices.

Clinical signs
Many dogs are subclinically infected; however, some may have severe colitis with blood and mucus. Severe infections (particularly those in puppies) can result in weakness, weight loss, dehydration, anemia and bloody diarrhea.

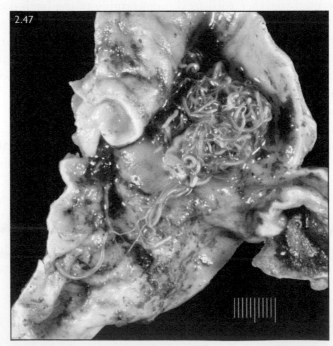

Fig. 2.47 Heavy *Trichuris* burden in the intestinal tract. (Courtesy of Ryan Jennings)

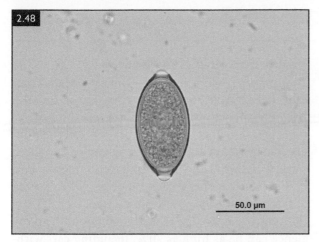

2.48

50.0 µm

Fig. 2.48 *Trichuris vulpis* egg detected on sugar centrifugal flotation examination of feces from a dog. The eggs are brown, bipolar plugged, 72–90 × 32–40 µm in size and contain undifferentiated embryo cells. The eggs tend to be symmetric about the plugs and there are lines visible in the shell wall at the insertion of the plugs, giving the appearance that the plugs are "threaded" into the wall. Detection sensitivity of *T. vulpis* eggs is greatly increased with the use of fecal flotation techniques that utilize centrifugation. (Courtesy of Gary Conboy)

Rarely, death due to blood loss, electrolyte imbalances (pseudohypoadrenocorticism) and dehydration can occur. Neurologic or cardiac signs due to electrolyte imbalances may occur.

Diagnosis

Infection is diagnosed based on history, clinical signs and centrifugal fecal flotation for identification of eggs (**Fig. 2.48**). Eggs must be differentiated from those of the lungworm *Eucoleus* spp. and urinary worm *Pearsonema* spp. Puppies may not shed eggs in feces until they are 3–6 months of age. Eggs may be shed intermittently, thus complicating diagnosis.

Fecal enzyme-linked immunosorbent assay (ELISA) detects antigen produced by mature and immature worms, which can be helpful to differentiate *T. vulpis* from other nematodes.[105]

CBC and serum biochemistry are typically normal; however, in severe cases anemia, hypoalbuminemia and hypoproteinemia due to blood loss can occur. Electrolyte imbalances can mimic Addison's disease with severe hyponatremia and hyperkalemia (e.g. Na^+/K^+ <27).

Endoscopy may reveal adult worms embedded in the colon. However, it is hoped that diagnosis (or trial therapy) would occur before selection of this diagnostic.

Therapy

Therapy is advised in all cases, owing to the risk of environmental contamination and spread. Typically, infection resolves quickly with appropriate therapy. Therapy should consist of treatment with anti-parasitic medications (praziquantel/pyrantel/febantel or fenbendazole) given once a month for a total of 3 months (three treatments). Follow-up fecal examination ensures successful eradication of infection.

Prognosis/complications

Prognosis is excellent with appropriate management. Clinical improvement is usually noted within a few days of therapy. Severely ill dogs may require intensive hospitalization and fluid therapy in addition to the above.

Treatment failures most commonly involve reinfection due to poor environmental cleaning and high pet densities, or inadequate treatment because of poor compliance or incorrect dosing.

Prevention

Regular testing of puppies and adult dogs for intestinal parasites (including *T. vulpis*) is advised. Puppies should be checked more frequently in their first year of life.

Anti-parasite programs should be individualized on the basis of risk (e.g. geography, travel) for all dogs. A variety of anthelmintic medications are effective for prevention of *T. vulpis* infection. These include milbemycin oxime (with or without praziquantel, spinosad and lufeneron), moxidectin and imidacloprid.

Environmental cleaning, prompt feces removal and decontamination are integral parts of therapy and prevention of reinfection. Eggs may persist in the environment for years.

TRITRICHOMONAS FOETUS COLITIS (TRICHOMONIASIS)
Margie Scherk

Definition

Tritrichomonas foetus (also known as *Tritrichomonas blagburni*) is a trichomonad protozoan that is an important cause of chronic large bowel diarrhea in cats (**Fig. 2.49**).

Etiology and pathogenesis

Transmission occurs via the fecal–oral route. Organisms survive for between 6 and 24 hours in feces at room temperature.[106] An Australian study has shown that slugs fed contaminated cat food shed viable *T. foetus*.[107]

Following ingestion, organisms proliferate in the ileum, cecum and colon as soon as 2–7 days post-inoculation in experimental studies[108] and cause lymphoplasmacytic and neutrophilic colitis. They are associated with the mucus on the epithelial surface and may also be found in colonic crypts.[109] Little is known about host immunity.

Co-infection with *Giardia* spp. is common.[57, 110] Other enteric pathogens may coexist with *T. foetus*, in particular *Cryptosporidium* spp. In naturally infected cats, co-infections do not appear to result in more severe disease.

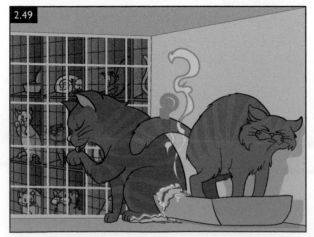

Fig. 2.49 Feline fecal–oral transmission of *Tritrichomonas foetus* in a group-housing setting.

Incidence and risk factors

Young cats living in high-density populations, especially purebred or show cats, are at greatest risk. Prevalence varies depending on the type of report (case report vs. clinic surveys) and the population included (all cats, diarrheic cats, shelter, cattery or show cats). Shedding rates of up to 39% in diarrheic cats have been reported. The method of testing can impact prevalence data.[111–113] When PCR testing is used to identify infection, the prevalence can be as high as 70%, including cats without clinical disease. Risk factors are presented in *Table 2.13*.[114, 115]

Clinical signs

Affected cats have good body condition and are active. Chronic or recurrent large bowel diarrhea that is malodorous is most common. Small amounts of soft-to-liquid stool are passed with increased frequency and straining, and may have increased mucus and hematochezia. Fecal incontinence and flatulence can occur. Subclinical infection occurs, and housemates of affected cats should be evaluated for shedding of trophozoites.

Although infection is typically self-limiting, the duration of disease can be lengthy. One study reported a median duration of 9 months (range 5–24 months) from the time of diagnosis,[116] with another reporting a median of 4.5 months (range 1 day to 7.9 years).[110] Up to 20% of cats may have systemic illness with anorexia, fever, vomiting and weight loss. These clinical signs may be a result of concurrent infection.[110]

Diagnosis

Direct microscopic evaluation, fecal culture, PCR and histopathology are methods available for diagnosing *T. foetus*. They are compared in *Table 2.14*.

Cytology

Samples must be no more than 2 hours old, preferably freshly collected in clinic because trichomonads do not survive refrigeration. With any technique, the preparation should be thin enough to read the

Table 2.13 Risk factors for *Tritrichomonas foetus* infection

PARAMETER	RISK FACTOR
Age	Under 12 months of age; older cats more likely to have subclinical infections
Breed	Purebred – including Siamese, Bengal, Norwegian Forest, Abyssinian
Housing density	Multi-cat environments, cat shows
History of diarrhea within previous 6 months	Self or other cats in household
Co-infection with other enteric pathogen	*Giardia* spp., *Cryptosporidium* spp.
Sex	No sex predisposition
Diet	Raw food in one study

Table 2.14 Comparison of tests available for *Tritrichomonas foetus*

TEST TYPE	SENSITIVITY	SPECIFICITY	COST	COMMENTS
Fecal flotation	0%	0%	$	No cyst stage
Direct fecal smear (wet mount/rectal cytology)	14.7%	Identify by shape and motility	$	Best if use fecal mucus False negatives common – multiple samples may be needed Difficult to differentiate from non-pathogenic *Pentatrichomonas hominis*
Fecal culture MDM/ InPouch TF	26.4%/58.8%	100%	$$	Up to 10 days
Histopathology	56%	High		Sensitivity increases with number of biopsies
PCR	90+%	High	$$$	Indicated when repeated direct exam and culture are negative

Abbreviations: MDM, modified Diamond's medium; InPouch TF Feline: BioMed Diagnostics, White City, Oregon

Table 2.15 Methods for diagnosis of *Tritrichomonas foetus*

Direct fecal smear	Place a rice grain/match head-sized amount of fresh, body temperature feces on a warm slide and mix with one drop of 0.9% saline
Rectal cytology	Gently insert a well-moistened, non-lubricated, cotton swab into the cat's colon. Rotate it quickly, withdraw it and roll it over multiple microscope slides
Colonic flush	Insert a red rubber catheter into the proximal colon, instill 10 mL of sterile saline and aspirate it. Place one drop on a microscope slide

text of a newspaper through it. After application of a coverslip, 40×, 100× and 400× magnification should be used to look for motile organisms (**Fig. 2.50**). Staining with a weak iodine solution facilitates morphological identification (*T. foetus, Pentatrichomonas hominis, Giardia* spp.) Methods to distinguish *T. foetus* from *Giardia* are shown in *Table 2.6*. Diagnostic and sample collection techniques are outlined in *Table 2.15*.

Culture

Fecal culture may be performed on samples that are freshly voided, digitally harvested, or collected by rectal swab or colon flush. The rice grain/match head-sized sample is placed in modified Diamond's medium (MDM) and submitted to the laboratory or placed in an InPouch TF Feline pouch (BioMed Diagnostics, White City, Oregon). The InPouch is incubated at room temperature in an upright

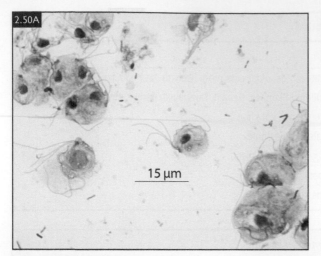

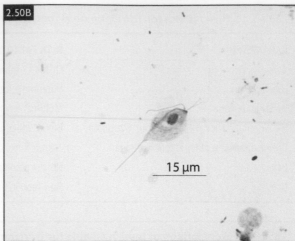

Fig. 2.50 *Tritrichomonas foetus.* (A) Note the undulating membrane and three anterior flagella (Wright–Giemsa stain). (B) While membrane is not as evident as in (A), the three anterior flagellae are noteworthy in this *T. foetus* trophozoite (Wright–Giemsa stain).

position in the dark (e.g. taped to the side of an unused drawer) and is examined microscopically for motile organisms every 48 hours for 10 days.

PCR

PCR is a potentially faster and more sensitive method. Samples must be fresh, free of litter, and ideally the cat should not have received antibiotics for 7 days. The sensitivity is twice as high as that of InPouch and turnaround time is faster than culture, but it is the most costly test.

Therapy

Although this is typically a self-limiting disease, ronidazole (30 mg/kg ideal weight PO q24h for 14 days) can speed response. It is not licensed for use in cats and must be compounded. Encapsulating the powder is preferable to other formulations as it is bitter. Relapses are possible at this dose and cats can continue to shed trophozoites even without diarrhea. Pregnant, nursing and very young kittens should not be given ronidazole.

Neither tinidazole nor metronidazole is effective in eliminating infection although they may provide transient benefit. Other antibiotics should not be used because they can affect the microbiota and may increase shedding of *T. foetus*.[117]

Prognosis/complications

Without treatment, the prognosis for resolution of diarrhea is good; however, relapses are common. Over half of the cats in remission are still PCR positive and may shed.[116] With ronidazole therapy, chance of clinical cure is very good.[117]

Prevention

The organisms do not form an environmentally stable cyst form and are killed by drying, refrigeration or temperatures >40°C (105 F). Following good hygiene and disinfection practices should prevent fecal–oral transmission. Although cats without diarrhea living in the same home as clinically affected cats may be shedding the organism, only cats that have been tested and shown to be positive should be treated.

REFERENCES

1   Thomas, JS (1988) Encephalomyelitis in a dog caused by *Baylisascaris* infection. *Vet Pathol* **25**:94–5.

2   Acke, E *et al.* (2006) Prevalence of thermophilic *Campylobacter* species in cats and dogs in two animal shelters in Ireland. *Vet Rec* **158**:51–4.

3   Sokolow, SH *et al.* (2005) Epidemiologic evaluation of diarrhea in dogs in an animal shelter. *Am J Vet Res* **66**:1018–24.

4 Leahy, AM *et al.* (2017) Faecal *Campylobacter* shedding among dogs in animal shelters across Texas. *Zoonoses Public Health* **64**:623–7.

5 Cave, NJ *et al.* (2002) Evaluation of a routine diagnostic fecal panel for dogs with diarrhea. *J Am Vet Med Assoc* **221**:52–9.

6 Baker, J *et al.* (1999) *Campylobacter* species in cats and dogs in South Australia. *Aust Vet J* **77**:662–6.

7 Leonard, EK *et al.* (2011) Factors related to *Campylobacter* spp. carriage in client-owned dogs visiting veterinary clinics in a region of Ontario, Canada. *Epidemiol Infect* **139**:1531–41.

8 Procter, TD *et al.* (2014) A cross-sectional study examining *Campylobacter* and other zoonotic enteric pathogens in dogs that frequent dog parks in three cities in South-Western Ontario and risk factors for shedding of *Campylobacter* spp. *Zoonoses Publ Health* **61**:208–18.

9 Martinez-Anton, L. *et al.* (2018) Investigation of the role of *Campylobacter* infection in suspected acute polyradiculoneuritis in dogs. *J Vet Intern Med* **32**:352–60.

10 Gillespie, IA *et al.* (2003) Point source outbreaks of *Campylobacter jejuni* infection – are they more common than we think and what might cause them? *Epidemiol Infect* **130**:367–75.

11 Tenkate, TD *et al.* (2001) Risk factors for *Campylobacter* infection in infants and young children: a matched case–control study. *Epidemiol Infect* **127**:399–404.

12 Oosterom, J *et al.* (1984) Epidemiological investigations on *Campylobacter jejuni* in households with a primary infection. *J Hygiene* **93**:325–32.

13 Decaro, N *et al.* (2014) Genomic characterization of a circovirus associated with fatal hemorrhagic enteritis in dog, Italy. *PLoS ONE* **9**:e105909.

14 Hsu, HS *et al.* (2016) High detection rate of dog circovirus in diarrheal dogs. *BMC Vet Res* **12**:116.

15 Anderson, A *et al.* (2017) Role of canine circovirus in dogs with acute haemorrhagic diarrhoea. *Vet Rec* **180**:542.

16 Dowgier, G *et al.* (2017) A molecular survey for selected viral enteropathogens revealed a limited role of Canine circovirus in the development of canine acute gastroenteritis. *Vet Microbiol* **204**:54–8.

17 Thaiwong, T. *et al.* (2016) Canine circovirus 1 (CaCV-1) and canine parvovirus 2 (CPV-2): recurrent dual infections in a Papillon breeding colony. *Vet Pathol* **53**:1204–9.

18 Tupler, T *et al.* (2012) Enteropathogens identified in dogs entering a Florida animal shelter with normal feces or diarrhea. *J Am Vet Med Assoc* **241**:338–43.

19 Stavisky, J *et al.* (2012) Cross sectional and longitudinal surveys of canine enteric coronavirus infection in kennelled dogs: a molecular marker for biosecurity. *Infect Genet Evol* **12**:1419–26.

20 Stavisky, J *et al.* (2010) Prevalence of canine enteric coronavirus in a cross-sectional survey of dogs presenting at veterinary practices. *Vet Microbiol* **140**:18–24.

21 Navarro, R *et al.* (2017) Molecular characterization of canine parvovirus and canine enteric coronavirus in diarrheic dogs on the island of St. Kitts: first report from the Caribbean region. *Virus Res* **240**:154–60.

22 Alves, C *et al.* (2018) Identification of enteric viruses circulating in a dog population with low vaccine coverage. *Braz J Microbiol* **49**:790–4.

23 Zicola, A *et al.* (2012) Fatal outbreaks in dogs associated with pantropic canine coronavirus in France and Belgium. *J Small Anim Pract* **53**:297–300.

24 Pratelli, A *et al.* (2001) Severe enteric disease in an animal shelter associated with dual infections by canine adenovirus type 1 and canine coronavirus. *J Vet Med B Infect Dis Vet Public Health* **48**:385–92.

25 Decaro, N *et al.* (2013) European surveillance for pantropic canine coronavirus. *J Clin Microbiol* **51**:83–8.

26 Pinto, LD *et al.* (2014) Characterization of pantropic canine coronavirus from Brazil. *Vet J* **202**:659–62.

27 Alvarez-Perez, S *et al.* (2017) Prevalence and characteristics of *Clostridium perfringens* and *Clostridium difficile* in dogs and cats attended in diverse veterinary clinics from the Madrid region. *Anaerobe* **48**:47–55.

28 Clooten, J *et al.* (2008) Prevalence and risk factors for *Clostridium difficile* colonization in dogs and cats hospitalized in an intensive care unit. *Vet Microbiol* **129**:209–14.

29 Weese, JS *et al.* (2001) The roles of *Clostridium difficile* and enterotoxigenic *Clostridium perfringens* in diarrhea in dogs. *J Vet Intern Med* **15**:374–8.

30 Chouicha, N *et al.* (2006) Evaluation of five enzyme immunoassays compared with the cytotoxicity assay for diagnosis of *Clostridium difficile*-associated diarrhea in dogs. *J Vet Diagn Invest* **18**:182–8.

31 Sabshin, SJ *et al.* (2012) Enteropathogens identified in cats entering a Florida animal shelter with normal feces or diarrhea. *J Am Vet Med Assoc* **241**:331–7.

32 Chon, JW *et al.* (2018) Prevalence, toxin gene profile, antibiotic resistance, and molecular characterization of *Clostridium perfringens* from diarrheic and non-diarrheic dogs in Korea. *J Vet Sci* **19**:368–74.

33 Silva, RO *et al.* (2013) Detection of toxins A/B and isolation of *Clostridium difficile* and *Clostridium perfringens* from dogs in Minas Gerais, Brazil. *Braz J Microbiol* **44**:133–7.

34 Goldstein, MR *et al.* (2012) Detection and characterization of *Clostridium perfringens* in the feces of healthy and diarrheic dogs. *Can J Vet Res* **76**:161–5.

35 Polak, KC *et al.* (2014) Infectious diseases in large-scale cat hoarding investigations. *Vet J* **201**:189–95.

36 Busch, K *et al.* (2015) *Clostridium perfringens* enterotoxin and *Clostridium difficile* toxin A/B do not play a role in acute haemorrhagic diarrhoea syndrome in dogs. *Vet Rec* **176**:253.

37 Leipig-Rudolph, M *et al.* (2018) Intestinal lesions in dogs with acute hemorrhagic diarrhea syndrome associated with netF-positive *Clostridium perfringens* type A. *J Vet Diagn Invest* **30**:495–503.

38 Mehdizadeh Gohari, I *et al.* (2015) A novel pore-forming toxin in type A *Clostridium perfringens* is associated with both fatal canine hemorrhagic gastroenteritis and fatal foal necrotizing enterocolitis. *PLoS ONE* **10**:e0122684.

39 Uehlinger, FD *et al.* (2013) Zoonotic potential of *Giardia duodenalis* and *Cryptosporidium* spp. and prevalence of intestinal parasites in young dogs from different populations on Prince Edward Island, Canada. *Vet Parasitol* **196**:509–14.

40 Gizzi, AB *et al.* (2014) Presence of infectious agents and co-infections in diarrheic dogs determined with a real-time polymerase chain reaction-based panel. *BMC Vet Res* **10**:23.

41 Osman, M *et al.* (2015) Prevalence and genetic diversity of the intestinal parasites *Blastocystis* sp. and *Cryptosporidium* spp. in household dogs in France and evaluation of zoonotic transmission risk. *Vet Parasitol* **214**:167–70.

42 de Lucio, A *et al.* (2017) No molecular epidemiological evidence supporting household transmission of zoonotic *Giardia duodenalis* and *Cryptosporidium* spp. from pet dogs and cats in the province of Alava, Northern Spain. *Acta Trop* **170**:48–56.

43. Scorza, AV *et al.* (2003) Polymerase chain reaction for the detection of *Cryptosporidium* spp. in cat feces. *J Parasitol* **89**:423–6.

44 Beser, J *et al.* (2015) Possible zoonotic transmission of *Cryptosporidium felis* in a household. *Infect Ecol Epidemiol* **5**:28463.

45 Gonzalez-Diaz, M *et al.* (2016) *Cryptosporidium canis* in two Mexican toddlers. *Pediatr Infect Dis J* **35**:1265–6.

46 Raza, A *et al.* (2018) Gastrointestinal parasites in shelter dogs: occurrence, pathology, treatment and risk to shelter workers. *Animals (Basel)* **8**:108.

47 Dupont, S *et al.* (2013) Enteropathogens in pups from pet shops and breeding facilities. *J Small Anim Pract* **54**:475–80.

48 Gaunt, MC *et al.* (2011) A survey of intestinal parasites in dogs from Saskatoon, Saskatchewan. *Can Vet J* **52**:497–500.

49 Grandi, G *et al.* (2017) Prevalence of helminth and coccidian parasites in Swedish outdoor cats and the first report of *Aelurostrongylus abstrusus* in Sweden: a coprological investigation. *Acta Vet Scand* **59**:19.

50 Hoopes, JH *et al.* (2013) A retrospective investigation of feline gastrointestinal parasites in western Canada. *Can Vet J* **54**:359–62.

51 Liu, CN *et al.* (2018) Estimating the prevalence of *Echinococcus* in domestic dogs is highly endemic for echinococcosis. *Infect Dis Poverty* **7**:77.

52 Corsini, M *et al.* (2015) Clinical presentation, diagnosis, therapy and outcome of alveolar echinococcosis in dogs. *Vet Rec* **177**:569.

53 Frey, CF *et al.* (2017) Dogs as victims of their own worms: serodiagnosis of canine alveolar echinococcosis. *Parasit Vectors* **10**:422.

54 Cvejic, D *et al.* (2016) Efficacy of a single dose of milbemycin oxime/praziquantel combination tablets, Milpro®, against adult *Echinococcus multilocularis* in dogs and both adult and immature *E. multilocularis* in young cats. *Parasitol Res* **115**:1195–1202.

55 Bouzid, M *et al.* (2015) The prevalence of *Giardia* infection in dogs and cats, a systematic review and meta-analysis of prevalence studies from stool samples. *Vet Parasitol* **207**:181–202.

56 Bissett, SA *et al.* (2008) Feline diarrhoea associated with *Tritrichomonas cf. foetus* and *Giardia* co-infection in an Australian cattery. *Aust Vet J* **86**:440–3.

57 Gookin, JL *et al.* (2004) Prevalence of and risk factors for feline *Tritrichomonas foetus* and *Giardia* infection. *J Clin Microbiol* **42**:2707–10.

58 Gates, MC *et al.* (2009) Comparison of passive fecal flotation run by veterinary students to zinc-sulfate centrifugation flotation run in a diagnostic parasitology laboratory. *J Parasitol* **95**:1213–14.

59 Barr, SC *et al.* (1992) Evaluation of two test procedures for diagnosis of giardiasis in dogs. *Am J Vet Res* **53**:2028–31.

60 Hostutler, RA *et al.* (2004) Antibiotic-responsive histiocytic ulcerative colitis in 9 dogs. *J Vet Intern Med* **18**:499–504.

61 Craven, M *et al.* (2011) Granulomatous colitis of boxer dogs. *Vet Clin North Am Small Anim Pract* **41**:433–45.

62 Craven, M *et al.* (2010) Antimicrobial resistance impacts clinical outcome of granulomatous colitis in boxer dogs. *J Vet Intern Med* **24**:819–24.

63 Jergens, AE *et al.* (2009) Fluorescence in situ hybridization confirms clearance of visible *Helicobacter* spp. associated with gastritis in dogs and cats. *J Vet Intern Med* **23**:16–23.

64 Amorim, I *et al.* (2015) Presence and significance of *Helicobacter* spp. in the gastric mucosa of Portuguese dogs. *Gut Pathog* **7**:12.

65 Simpson, K *et al.* 2000. The relationship of *Helicobacter* spp. infection to gastric disease in dogs and cats. *J Vet Intern Med* **14**:223–7.

66 Bridgeford, EC *et al.* (2008) Gastric *Helicobacter* species as a cause of feline gastric lymphoma: a viable hypothesis. *Vet Immunol Immunopathol* **123**:106–13.

67 Leib, MS *et al.* (2007) Triple antimicrobial therapy and acid suppression in dogs with chronic vomiting and gastric *Helicobacter* spp. *J Vet Intern Med* **21**:1185–92.

68 Anacleto, TP *et al.* (2011) Studies of distribution and recurrence of *Helicobacter* spp. gastric mucosa of dogs after triple therapy. *Acta Cir Bras* **26**:82–7.

69 Van den Bulck, K *et al.* (2005) In vitro antimicrobial susceptibility testing of *Helicobacter felis*, *H. bizzozeronii*, and *H. salomonis*. *Antimicrob Agents Chemother* **49**:2997–3000.

70 Johnson, EM (2010) Canine schistosomiasis in North America: an underdiagnosed disease with an expanding distribution. *Compend Contin Educ Vet* **32**:E1–4.

71 Fabrick, C *et al.* (2010) Clinical features and outcome of *Heterobilharzia americana* infection in dogs. *J Vet Intern Med* **24**:140–4.

72 Rodriguez, JY *et al.* (2014) Distribution and characterization of *Heterobilharzia americana* in dogs in Texas. *Vet Parasitol* **203**:35–42.

73 Ruth, J (2010) *Heterobilharzia americana* infection and glomerulonephritis in a dog. *J Am Anim Hosp Assoc* **46**:203–8.

74 Hanzlicek, AS *et al.* 2011. Canine schistosomiasis in Kansas: five cases (2000–2009). *J Am Anim Hosp Assoc* **47**:e95–102.

75 Corapi, WV *et al.* (2011) Multi-organ involvement of *Heterobilharzia americana* infection in a dog presented for systemic mineralization. *J Vet Diagn Invest* **23**:826–31.

76 Little, SE *et al.* (2009) Prevalence of intestinal parasites in pet dogs in the United States. *Vet Parasitol* **166**:144–52.

77 Gates, MC *et al.* (2009) Endoparasite prevalence and recurrence across different age groups of dogs and cats. *Vet Parasitol* **166**:153–8.

78 Basu, AK *et al.* (2014) A review of the cat liver fluke *Platynosomum fastosum* Kossack, 1910 (Trematoda: Dicrocoeliidae). *Vet Parasitol* **200**:1–7.

79 Haney, DR *et al.* (2006) Severe cholestatic liver disease secondary to liver fluke (*Platynosomum concinnum*) infection in three cats. *J Am Anim Hosp Assoc* **42**:234–7.

80 Rodriguez-Vivas, RI *et al.* (2004) Prevalence, abundance and risk factors of liver fluke (*Platynosomum concinnum*) infection in cats in Mexico. *Vet Rec* **154**:693–4.

81 Xavier, FG *et al.* (2007) Cystic liver disease related to high *Platynosomum fastosum* infection in a domestic cat. *J Feline Med Surg* **9**:51–5.

82 Andrade, RL *et al.* (2012) *Platynosomum fastosum*-induced cholangiocarcinomas in cats. *Vet Parasitol* **190**:277–80.

83 Taylor, D *et al.* (1977) Experimental infection of cats with the liver fluke *Platynosomum concinnum*. *Am J Vet Res* **38**:51–4.

84 Palumbo, NE *et al.* (1974) Cat liver fluke, *Platynosomum concinnum*, in Hawaii. *Am J Vet Res* **35**:1455.

85 Ramos, RA *et al.* (2016) New insights into diagnosis of *Platynosomum fastosum* (Trematoda: Dicrocoeliidae) in cats. *Parasitol Res* **115**:479–82.

86 Shell, L *et al.* (2015) Praziquantel treatment for *Platynosomum* species infection of a domestic cat on St Kitts, West Indies. *JFMS Open Rep* **1**:2055116915589834.

87 Tenne, R *et al.* (2016). Palatability and clinical effects of an oral recuperation fluid during the recovery of dogs with suspected parvoviral enteritis. *Top Companion Anim Med* **31**:68–72.

88 Mohr, AJ *et al.* (2003) Effect of early enteral nutrition on intestinal permeability, intestinal protein loss, and outcome in dogs with severe parvoviral enteritis. *J Vet Intern Med* **17**:791–8.

89 de Mari, K *et al.* (2003) Treatment of canine parvoviral enteritis with interferon-omega in a placebo-controlled field trial. *Vet Rec* **152**:105–8.

90 Savigny, MR *et al.* (2010) Use of oseltamivir in the treatment of canine parvoviral enteritis. *J Vet Emerg Crit Care* **20**:132–42.

91 Venn, EC *et al.* (2017) Evaluation of an outpatient protocol in the treatment of canine parvoviral enteritis. *J Vet Emerg Crit Care* **27**:52–65.

92 Kruse, BD *et al.* (2010). Prognostic factors in cats with feline panleukopenia. *J Vet Intern Med* **24**:1271–6.

93 Freisl, M *et al.* (2017) Faecal shedding of canine parvovirus after modified-live vaccination in healthy adult dogs. *Vet J* **219**:15–21.

94 Lappin, MR *et al.* (2009) Feline panleukopenia virus, feline herpesvirus-1, and feline calicivirus antibody responses in seronegative specific pathogen-free cats after a single administration of two different modified live FVRCP vaccines. *J Feline Med Surg* **11**:159–62.

95 Hackett, T *et al.* (2003) Prevalence of enteric pathogens in dogs of north-central Colorado. *J Am Anim Hosp Assoc* **39**:52–6.

96 Lefebvre, SL *et al.* (2006) Prevalence of zoonotic agents in dogs visiting hospitalized people in Ontario: implications for infection control. *J Hosp Infect* **62**:458–66.

97 Finley, R *et al.* (2007) The risk of salmonellae shedding by dogs fed *Salmonella*-contaminated commercial raw food diets. *Can Vet J* **48**:69–75.

98 Joffe, DJ *et al.* (2002). Preliminary assessment of the risk of *Salmonella* infection in dogs fed raw chicken diets. *Can Vet J* **43**:441–2.

99 Lefebvre, SL *et al.* (2008) Evaluation of the risks of shedding *Salmonellae* and other potential pathogens by therapy dogs fed raw diets in Ontario and Alberta. *Zoonoses Publ Health* **55**:470–80.

100 Stiver, SL *et al.* (2003) Septicemic salmonellosis in two cats fed a raw-meat diet. *J Am Anim Hosp Assoc* **39**:538–42.

101 Nolan, TJ *et al.* (1995) Time series analysis of the prevalence of endoparasitic infections in cats and dogs presented to a veterinary teaching hospital. *Vet Parasitol* **59**:87–96.

102 Conboy, G (2009) Cestodes of dogs and cats in North America. *Vet Clin North Am Small Anim Pract* **39**:1075–90, vi.

103 Little, S *et al.* (2015) High prevalence of covert infection with gastrointestinal helminths in cats. *J Am Anim Hosp Assoc* **51**:359–64.

104 Villeneuve, A *et al.* (2015) Parasite prevalence in fecal samples from shelter dogs and cats across the Canadian provinces. *Parasit Vectors* **8**:281.

105 Elsemore, DA *et al.* (2014) Enzyme-linked immunosorbent assay for coproantigen detection of *Trichuris vulpis* in dogs. *J Vet Diagn Invest* **26**:404–11.

106 Hale, S *et al.* (2009) Prolonged resilience of *Tritrichomonas foetus* in cat faeces at ambient temperature. *Vet Parasitol* **166**:60–5.

107 Van der Saag, M *et al.* (2011) Cat genotype *Tritrichomonas foetus* survives passage through the alimentary tract of two common slug species. *Vet Parasitol* **177**:262–6.

108 Gookin, JL *et al.* (2001) Experimental infection of cats with *Tritrichomonas foetus*. *Am J Vet Res* **62**:1690–7.

109 Yaeger, MJ *et al.* (2005) Histologic features associated with *Tritrichomonas foetus*-induced colitis in domestic cats. *Vet Pathol* **42**:797–804.

110 Xenoulis, PG *et al.* (2013) Intestinal *Tritrichomonas foetus* infection in cats: a retrospective study of 104 cases. *J Feline Med Surg* **15**:1098–1103.

111 Andersen, LA *et al.* (2018) Prevalence of enteropathogens in cats with and without diarrhea in four different management models for unowned cats in the southeast United States. *Vet J* **236**:49–55.

112 Arranz-Solís, D *et al.* (2016) *Tritrichomonas foetus* infection in cats with diarrhea from densely housed origins. *Vet Parasitol* **221**:118–22.

113 Paris, JK *et al.* (2014) Enteropathogen co-infection in UK cats with diarrhoea. *BMC Vet Res* **10**:13.

114 Yao, C *et al.* (2015) *Tritrichomonas foetus* infection, a cause of chronic diarrhea in the domestic cat. *Vet Res* **46**:35.

115 Hosein, A *et al.* (2013) Isolation of *Tritrichomonas foetus* from cats sampled at a cat clinic, cat shows and a humane society in southern Ontario. *J Feline Med Surg* **15**:706–11.

116 Foster, DM *et al.* (2004) Outcome of cats with diarrhea and *Tritrichomonas foetus* infection. *J Am Vet Med Assoc* **225**:888–92.

117 Gookin, JL *et al.* (2006) Efficacy of ronidazole for treatment of feline *Tritrichomonas foetus* infection. *J Vet Intern Med* **20**:536–43.

CHAPTER 3

NEUROLOGIC DISEASES

BACTERIAL MENINGITIS OR MENINGOENCEPHALITIS
Michelle Evason

Definition
Meningitis (or meningoencephalitis) can be due to myriad infectious (i.e. bacterial, fungal or viral) or non-infectious causes. Bacterial meningoencephalitis occurs after traumatic bacterial inoculation, extension of infection from the nasal cavity or ears, or via hematogenous dissemination. Clinical signs typically include fever, varying CNS signs and neck pain. Lack of therapy will lead to rapid decline and death.

Etiology and pathogenesis
Various species of bacteria may cause meningitis (inflammation of the pia and arachnoid) or meningoencephalitis (inflammation of the brain and spinal cord), including staphylococci, streptococci, *Pasteurella* spp., *Escherichia coli*, *Klebsiella*, *Nocardia* and *Actinomyces* spp. and, rarely, anaerobes.[1, 2] The bacteria spread to the meningeal space and cause inflammation of the meninges covering the brain and spinal cord. This can result in CNS (and/or CSF) invasion, vascular injury, thrombosis, edema and in some cases obstruction to CSF flow (hydrocephalus). Nerve root irritation may result in hyperesthesia, and further neurologic signs can develop with progressive disease (e.g. seizures).

Risk factors
Any age or breed of dog may be affected.[2] Risk factors include traumatic events and potentially immunocompromise (e.g. neonates).[1]

Clinical signs
Clinical signs are consistent with intracranial disease, and most commonly include a choppy gait, fever, stiffness, altered mentation, cranial nerve deficits, paresis, postural deficits, neck pain, ataxia, muscle spasms and reluctance to move.[2] Progressive neurologic decline, seizures and hyperesthesia can occur.[1, 2] Concurrent gastrointestinal and respiratory signs may be present.[2]

Diagnosis
Diagnosis is based on suggestive clinical signs and confirmatory CSF analysis. Typical CSF changes include increased protein, phagocytosed organisms and neutrophilic pleocytosis. Serum chemistry and CBC are frequently abnormal, with variable and non-specific changes.

Bacterial identification on CSF cytology, followed by culture and susceptibility testing, can confirm diagnosis and provide important information for therapy. Culture for aerobes and anaerobes should be performed; however, false negatives can occur due to low bacterial counts.[1, 2] The risk of brain herniation due to CSF sampling must be discussed with clients. Chronic infections may yield CSF samples containing monocytes, lymphocytes and eosinophils, in addition to neutrophils.

Meningeal lesions may be evident on CT or MRI.

Therapy
Therapy consists of supportive care, consideration of anti-inflammatory dose(s) of glucocorticoids and mannitol, and prompt antimicrobial therapy while CSF and culture results are pending. Although many antimicrobials may cross an inflamed blood–brain barrier, those that have better penetration, such as cefotaxime (20–50 mg/kg IV q6–8h) are advised. Fluoroquinolones may be useful.

Anticonvulsants, muscle relaxants and analgesia may be needed.

Prognosis/complications

The prognosis in dogs with acute presentation, minimal neurologic damage and early therapy is good. However, animals who present with severe neurologic complications have a more guarded prognosis. Long-term sequelae of neurologic disease can occur, such as head tilt, seizures and ataxia.

CANINE DISTEMPER VIRUS (DISTEMPER)
Michelle Evason and Susan Taylor

Definition

Canine distemper virus (CDV) is an important cause of respiratory, enteric and neurologic disease in puppies. It spreads rapidly through direct infected dog-to-dog contact. Clinical signs vary depending on virulence of the strain, dog age, immune status and presence of concurrent infections.

Species affected

Dogs and wild canids (e.g. coyote, fox, wolf) are the main hosts. Raccoons, pandas, ferrets, mink, skunks, otters, large wild cats, other carnivores and some non-human primates can be affected.[3] Domestic cats are clinically unaffected.[3]

Etiology and pathogenesis

CDV is an enveloped RNA morbillivirus of the family Paramyxoviridae. It is transmitted through contact with secretions from infected dogs (e.g. saliva, aerosols from cough, urine and feces) either through direct contact, or via objects/surfaces contaminated with these (e.g. water bowls or grooming tools). During the incubation period (3–6 days post-infection [PI]), direct viral destruction of lymphocytes results in lymphopenia and transient fever. Further spread to cells in the respiratory tract, gut, CNS, skin and urinary tract may occur (days 8–9 PI), depending on immune status and immune response. This viral dissemination is usually accompanied by a second stage of cell-associated viremia and fever. Viral shedding from either clinically or subclinically infected dogs may start as early as 5 days after infection and continue for months.[3, 4]

Depending on adequate antibody titers and cell-mediated immunity, one of three outcomes may occur: (1) infection may be eliminated, (2) classic acute distemper may occur, with subsequent death or recovery, or (3) there may be clinical resolution with viral persistence in the eye, lymphoid organs, footpads and CNS, creating the potential for late-onset sequelae, particularly ocular and neurologic disease.

Incidence and risk factors

CDV may be re-emerging, based on increases in reported cases. This may be due to decreased vaccination in some regions and establishment of CDV as endemic in wildlife (mainly raccoons).[3]

Young dogs (between 2 and 6 months) in kennels or other group settings have increased risk, and outbreaks may occur.[5, 6] Mature dogs and older puppies with incomplete vaccination protection may be more prone to developing disease when immunocompromised.[6] Disease is rare in properly vaccinated adult dogs.[7]

Clinical signs
Acute

Many dogs are subclinically affected or have transient signs such as fever, lethargy, decreased appetite and mild canine infectious respiratory disease complex (CIRDC). Occasionally CNS signs occur after subclinical infection (vs. 1–6 weeks after acute disease), resulting in pure neurologic distemper.[4]

Dogs with progressive acute CDV have fever, oculonasal discharge and persistent cough. Secondary bacterial infection often leads to bronchopneumonia and purulent nasal (**Figs. 3.1, 3.2**) and ocular discharge. Concurrent enteric signs include inappetence, occasional vomiting, diarrhea and dehydration. CDV immunosuppression invites development of opportunistic infections, and clinical signs vary, dependent on the pathogen.

Acute progressive neurologic signs occur 1–6 weeks after onset of systemic illness.[4] In some cases, respiratory and gastrointestinal (GI) signs will have completely resolved by the time neurologic

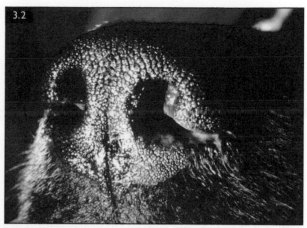

Fig. 3.2 Nasal erosion in a dog with distemper.

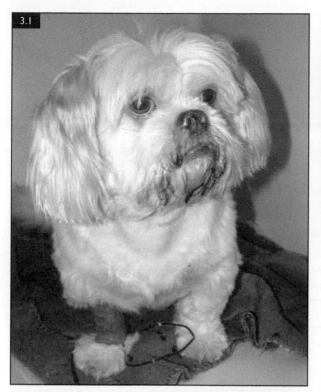

Fig. 3.1 Nasal discharge in a dog with distemper.

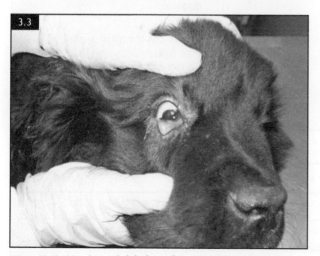

Fig. 3.3 Conjunctivitis in a dog with distemper.

disease develops. Neurologic signs may include seizures (especially in young dogs), abnormal mentation, apparent blindness, cerebellar and vestibular signs, paraparesis or tetraparesis, and myoclonus (involuntary rhythmic twitching of specific muscle groups). Focal "chewing gum" seizures localized to the head and jaws are common in puppies with

acute CDV. Neurologic signs rarely resolve and are typically progressive. Myoclonus may persist in dogs that seem to have otherwise recovered.

Depending on the stage of gestation when infected, unthrifty or weak pups, stillbirths and/ or abortion can occur. Transplacental infection occasionally leads to neurologic signs in the first 4–6 weeks of life.

Persistent CDV

Ocular signs may include conjunctivitis (**Fig. 3.3**) and subclinical anterior uveitis. Acute blindness due to optic neuritis, or transient or permanent keratoconjunctivitis sicca (KCS) can occur. Inactive "gold medallion" fundic lesions are considered characteristic of prior infection.[8]

Infection of the epithelium of the nose and footpads can lead to hyperkeratosis (**Fig. 3.4**). These changes are most evident in dogs that have developed neurologic signs, and can be an aid to diagnosis.[8]

Diagnosis

See *Tables 3.1, 3.2*. CDV infection is easily missed if the combination of respiratory, GI and CNS (particularly myoclonus) signs is lacking. Thorough vaccine and/or contact history, clinical signs, exclusion of differential diagnoses and awareness of concurrent disease is required for diagnosis. Diagnosis is made through a combination of tests and specimens from multiple different sampling sites in an individual dog.

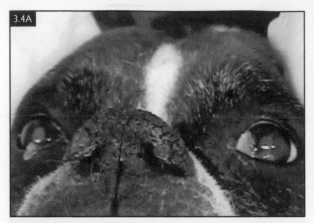
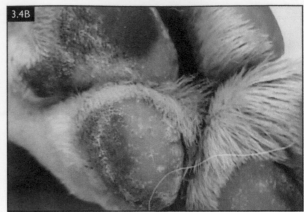

Fig. 3.4 Nasal (A) and footpad (B) hyperkeratosis in a dog with distemper.

Table 3.1 **Laboratory assays for diagnosis of canine distemper virus**

DIAGNOSTIC	SAMPLE	TARGET	OUTCOME/UTILITY
Immunofluorescent antibody (IFA)	Cytology smears (conjunctiva, tonsil, genital or respiratory epithelium) Whole cells (CSF, blood/buffy coat, urine sediment and bone marrow)	CDV antigen (Ag)	False negatives are common False positives can occur after vaccination
Immunohistochemistry (histopathology)	Frozen biopsy or necropsy samples (nasal mucosa, footpad and/or skin)	CDV Ag or CDV RNA	May be the most sensitive test for diagnosis
Reverse transcriptase (RT)-PCR	Urine, tonsils, conjunctival swabs, CSF and whole blood provide optimum samples	CDV RNA	Submission of multiple specimens from different body sites may improve diagnosis Both false negatives and positives can occur; considered more sensitive than IFA

Table 3.2 **Differential diagnoses for canine distemper virus infection**

RESPIRATORY SIGNS	ENTERIC SIGNS	NEUROLOGIC SIGNS
Canine influenza virus Canine parainfluenza virus Canine respiratory coronavirus *Bordetella bronchiseptica* *Streptococcus zooepidemicus* *Mycoplasma* spp. Canine adenovirus-2 Canine pneumovirus	Viral: canine parvovirus, coronavirus Bacterial GI disease (e.g. *Salmonella, Clostridium, Campylobacter*, etc.) Parasitic and/or protozoal disease (e.g. *Giardia, Cryptosporidium, Ancylostoma caninum, Toxacara canis, Toxascaris leonina*, etc.) Foreign body, dietary indiscretion and/or intussusception	Toxin: metaldehyde, strychnine, lead, ethylene glycol Metabolic: hypocalcemia, portosystemic shunt, hypoglycemia Non-infectious inflammatory: granulomatous meningoencephalitis, Pug encephalitis Infectious: rabies, toxoplasmosis, *Neospora, Cryptococcus*

Hematology and biochemistry

CBC and serum biochemistry may be normal or have non-specific changes that reflect inflammation, vomiting, diarrhea and dehydration. Intracytoplasmic distemper inclusions are uncommon, and their absence does not rule out disease.

Diagnostic imaging

An interstitial lung pattern may be seen in early infections. Dogs with secondary bacterial pneumonia may have an alveolar pattern (± consolidation). MRI can be normal or have changes suggesting inflammation and demyelination, which are non-specific for CDV.

CSF analyses

CSF can be normal, or consistent with subacute-to-chronic inflammation. The most common finding is a mild lymphocytic pleocytosis and increase in protein content. Intracytoplasmic inclusion bodies can sometimes be noted in CSF cells.

Serology

Diagnosis of acute CDV can be made through paired acute and convalescent titers. A fourfold rise in titer over a 2- to 4-week period in the absence of vaccination supports diagnosis. Increased anti-CDV antibody or positive reverse transcriptase (RT)-PCR in CSF is diagnostic. This may aid differentiation of vaccination from true CDV infection when compared with serum CDV antibody.[4]

In vaccinated dogs, higher CDV titers equate with reduced infection risk. Serum neutralizing (SN) titers of 1:16 to 1:20 correlate strongly with protection post-vaccination. Dogs that are unprotected or incompletely vaccinated have no CDV antibody titer (or very low titers) and are at high risk of infection. Vaccination is required for protection.

Therapy

Dogs with mild respiratory or GI signs, and no neurologic signs, typically recover with simple supportive care.

Increased severity of CDV-related illness requires more intensive nursing care (*Table 3.3*). Bronchopneumonia may result from secondary bacterial infection and antimicrobials are indicated, as for treatment of bacterial pneumonia.

Prognosis/complications

Prognosis is based on severity of presenting clinical signs and ability of owners to commit to extended care and cost. Some dogs with CDV infection have mild illness and recover without developing neurologic signs. Prognosis is excellent in these cases. Immunity (lifelong) occurs in most dogs after natural infection.

Approximately 30% of infected dogs develop neurologic signs acutely or as a sequela to CDV.[4] All owners need to be counseled from the outset about the risk of progressive irreversible neurologic signs developing weeks to months after apparent recovery.

Table 3.3 **Nursing care for canine distemper patients**
Clean, warm room that is free of drafts
Sedation or anxiolytics to reduce stress and fear may be considered
Nebulization and coupage for pneumonia as indicated
Intravenous fluid support to correct and prevent dehydration from systemic signs
Parenteral medications and antiemetics if vomiting and nausea are present
Nutritional support. This may need to be in the form of nasal or esophageal tubes to support requirements during recovery and also reduce risk of aspiration and resultant worsening of pneumonia. Force feeding is not advised owing to high risk of aspiration
Anticonvulsants to reduce seizures and risk of hyperthermia. Some dogs may benefit from a single anti-edema dose of dexamethasone. Suggested drugs to reduce seizures include benzodiazepines (diazepam or midazolam). Severely affected patients may require constant rate infusions of phenobarbital or propofol. Maintenance therapy with phenobarbital or potassium bromide may be required
Soft bedding, gentle cleaning and removal of ocular and nasal discharge, and ocular lubricant depending on patient need

When neurologic signs do occur, they rarely resolve and are often progressive. Poor quality of life often necessitates euthanasia. Dogs that develop mild myoclonus as their only neurologic sign can be maintained in the household as a functional pet.

Prevention

Distemper is a vaccine-preventable disease in dogs; however, vaccination protocols must be followed to establish full protective immunity. Distemper can develop in adult dogs that are inadequately vaccinated, exposed to high viral loads or immunocompromised. CDV titers may be helpful in scenarios where assessment of level of protection and possible risk of infection from CDV is needed (e.g. shelters).

CLOSTRIDIUM BOTULINUM/BOTULISM
Christine R Rutter

Definition

Botulism is a lower motor neuron (LMN) paralysis that occurs after exposure to neurotoxins produced by *Clostridium botulinum*.

Species affected

Botulism is uncommon in dogs and rare in cats.

Etiology and pathogenesis

C. botulinum is a gram-positive, anaerobic, spore-forming bacterium found ubiquitously in soil (**Fig. 3.5**). For growth, it prefers warm, low-acid, anaerobic environments with plentiful organic debris.

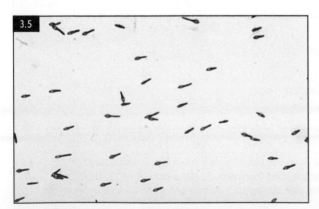

Fig. 3.5 Gram stain of *Clostridium botulinum*. Note the bulging spores.

Infection control

Dogs with suspected CDV infection must be isolated from others to eliminate risk of transmission. Given the long duration of viral shedding, isolation may be difficult in households. In veterinary clinics, affected dogs should be housed in isolation and handled using contact precautions. Effective isolation becomes even more difficult when intensive care (e.g. oxygen support) is required.

As an enveloped virus, CDV is easily inactivated by ultraviolet light, heat, drying and routine disinfection procedures. Cleaning of contaminated sites is important before disinfection, whenever possible. Below freezing the virus is stable for weeks to years.[8]

Spores are a dormant form resistant to environmental extremes.

Exposure to botulinum neurotoxin (BoNT) is most common after ingestion of preformed toxin in contaminated organic material (contaminated food, carrion or compost).[9, 10] The BoNT molecule does not cross the blood–brain barrier, limiting clinical signs to the peripheral nervous system.[11] The toxin rapidly and irreversibly binds presynaptic nerve terminals, preventing spontaneous and induced acetylcholine release at the neuromuscular junction, resulting in skeletal muscle and (to a lesser extent) autonomic paralysis.[12] Clinical signs develop from hours to 6 days after exposure.[9, 10] Development of clinical signs soon after exposure may be associated with more severe disease.

Geography

C. botulinum can be found worldwide in soil, and marine and freshwater sediments; however, the prevalence and distribution of different types vary among regions.

Incidence and risk factors

Cats are inherently more resistant to botulism than dogs, but the incidence in either species is low. Animals with exposure to carrion are most commonly affected.

Clinical signs

Affected dogs are typically alert, afebrile and in good body condition. Generalized LMN weakness and hyporeflexia, without hyperesthesia or abnormalities of the sensory or cognitive neurologic systems, can develop. Symmetric, ascending, hindlimb weakness that progresses to the forelimbs and cranial nerves but preserves the tail wag is common.

Cranial nerve deficits are expected and can include decreased palpebral reflex, decreased gag and weak jaw tone. Mydriasis, slow pupillary light response, pytalism, alterations in heart rate, megaesophagus, vocal changes, constipation, urinary atony or retention, keratoconjunctivitis sicca and respiratory distress may be present.[9, 10]

Canine patients are less likely to have hyperesthesia and more likely to have cranial nerve deficits (**Fig. 3.6**) and cholinergic signs than with other LMN disorders.[9, 13] Cats may be depressed, hypothermic, tachycardic and in respiratory distress. Symmetric, ascending, hindlimb weakness that progresses to the forelimbs is similar to that in dogs, but involvement of the cranial nerves has not been reported.[13]

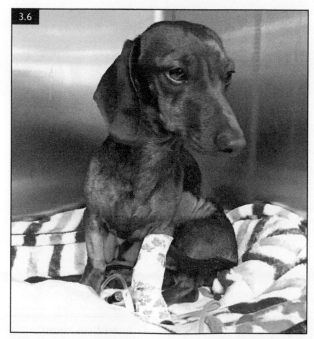

Fig. 3.6 Dog with botulism acquired from ingestion of a dead fish showing symmetric hindlimb weakness.

Diagnosis

Diagnosis is often based on a history of potential exposure and clinical presentation. The presence of typical clinical signs in multiple animals exposed to the same source or with exposure to the same carrion is highly suggestive of botulism. Complete blood count, blood chemistries, urinalysis, cerebrospinal fluid analysis and muscle biopsy are typically within normal limits.[9] Electromyography is consistent with LMN disease and conduction disturbance.[9]

Although difficult, identification of BoNT in serum, gastric contents, feces or food substrate is the gold standard for diagnosis. Samples should be collected early after patient exposure.[14] Culture or PCR can be used to identify the presence of the bacterium, but not BoNT itself, and the significance of culturing *C. botulinum* from gastric contents and feces is unknown, given the ubiquitous presence of the organism.[10] Measurement of BoNT antibody titer performed 3 weeks after exposure may help confirm a diagnosis in recovering animals.[9]

Therapy

Supportive care is the cornerstone of treatment (*Table 3.4*). Gastrointestinal decontamination may be helpful in acute exposure, though emesis increases the risk of aspiration. Cathartics containing magnesium could potentiate the effects of BoNT and should be avoided.[15] Unless otherwise indicated, antibiotic therapy is avoided to prevent further bacterial cell lysis (with corresponding BoNT release), and to preserve the intestinal microbiota to prevent *C. botulinum* overgrowth.[10] Aminoglycosides should be avoided, owing to their effects on neuromuscular transmission. Debridement and antibiotic therapy (e.g. penicillin, clindamycin) would be indicated for treatment of wound infection-associated botulism.[10] Recumbent patient care, nutritional management and urinary bladder management are fundamental. Severely affected patients may require nutritional support (e.g. feeding tube placement) or mechanical ventilation.

Antitoxin therapy is type specific and must be administered early in disease.[9] Most antitoxin products lack specific anti-BoNT/C antibodies. If available, an anti-BoNT/C product should be used in the absence of known involvement of another type of neurotoxin.

Table 3.4 **Treatment approach for botulism**
Nutritional support: nasal, esophageal or gastric tubes may be required to support energy requirements and avoid aspiration during the potentially prolonged recovery. Force feeding is contraindicated
Recumbent patient management including ample soft bedding, frequent repositioning and passive range of motion therapy
Elimination care: bladder expression, laxatives and enemas
Ocular lubricant and prevention of ocular trauma
Intravenous fluids to prevent dehydration
Respiratory monitoring for both hypoxia and hypoventilation

Prognosis/complications

Recovery occurs with formation of new neuromuscular junctions, which allows for complete resolution of clinical signs. The time to improvement in dogs ranges from 14 to 24 days,[9] starting with restoration of cranial nerve and forelimb function. Improvement has been noted in surviving cats 5–7 days post-ingestion.[13]

Severe cases can have weakness of the respiratory muscles, causing hypoventilation and hypercapnia. Megaesophagus puts affected patients at risk of aspiration and hypoxia. Mechanical ventilation carries a guarded prognosis but could be required due to hypoventilation, hypoxia or both.[16] Respiratory failure is the leading cause of natural death.[9]

Prevention

Botulinum toxin is destroyed by heating food to 80°C for 30 minutes or 100°C for 10 minutes. Proper handling of foodstuffs and preventing access to carrion is effective in preventing disease.

CLOSTRIDIUM TETANI/TETANUS
Michelle Evason and Christine R Rutter

Definition

Tetanus is a neurologic disease that develops when *Clostridium tetani* spores (**Fig. 3.7**) enter an open wound. The resultant bacterial growth and production of toxins can cause spastic paralysis and voluntary muscle rigidity. Tetanus can be localized to an affected limb or generalized.

Species affected

Dogs and cats can both be affected, although disease is rare in cats.

Etiology and pathogenesis

C. tetani is a gram-positive, anaerobic, spore-forming bacterium that is widely distributed as spores in the environment. Clostridial spores are highly resistant in the environment and can persist for years.

Spores enter the body via a wound and grow in the anaerobic conditions provided by necrotic tissue. Clinical signs develop a few days to a few weeks after

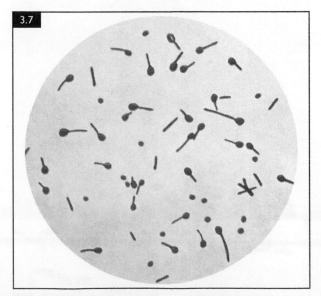

Fig. 3.7 Photomicrograph of *Clostridium tetani* spores stained with methylene blue. (Courtesy of US Centers for Disease Control and Prevention)

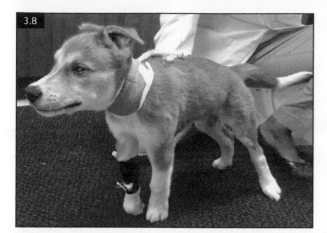

Fig. 3.8 Muscle rigidity in a dog with tetanus.

inoculation and are predominantly due to tetanospasmin toxin inhibition of gamma-aminobutyric acid (GABA) and glycine in the neurotransmitters of the brain and spinal cord. Animals with wound sites closer to the neurologic system (brain or spine) or with heavy spore contamination develop clinical signs more quickly and severely.

Geography
C. tetani is found worldwide.

Incidence and risk factors
The incidence of disease is low in dogs, and tetanus is very rare in cats. Young, large breed, athletic male dogs are most commonly affected because of the greater risk of puncture wounds. Affected cats tend to be young outdoor cats.[17]

Clinical signs
Affected dogs are typically alert, afebrile and in good body condition. Disease can be localized or generalized. A combination of spastic paralysis and voluntary muscle rigidity is the classic presentation (**Fig. 3.8**). Signs are often most prominent around the head (**Fig. 3.9**), and the generalized form is most often noted as erect ears, wrinkled forehead, lips drawn back in a grinning appearance (**Fig. 3.10**) and third eyelid prolapse with generalized muscle stiffness. Abnormal facial appearance or dysphagia may be most readily detected by owners. Lockjaw (inability to open the mouth) may also be present. A sawhorse appearance due to muscle tetany can be noted

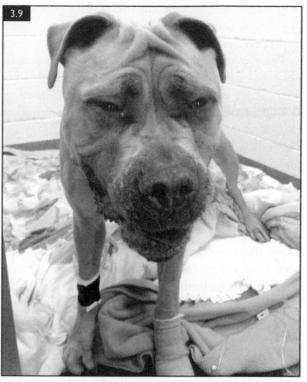

Fig. 3.9 Classic signs of tetanus spastic paralysis in a dog.

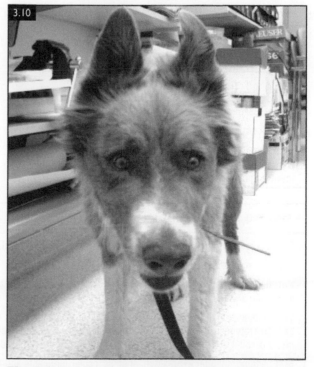

Fig. 3.10 "Grinning" appearance with canine tetanus.

(**Fig. 3.8**), and 50% of dogs have laryngeal spasm and hypersalivation.[18] Severe tetanus can cause hyperthermia.

Prior or existing wounds located on the feet or head, or caused by a foreign body, bite wound, post-operative site, grooming lesions (skin and nails) or tick bite may be noted.[18–20] Signs typically ascribed to clostridial infection (e.g. crepitus) are not often present and the affected wound area may not be obvious. One-third of dogs have no wound history[18, 20] or the wound may have healed over.

Neurologic signs can begin local to the wound site (localized tetanus) and then progress to the generalized form. Dogs are more likely to have head, facial and ocular involvement and generalized tetanus than cats. Cats are more likely to have localized tetanus confined to one limb, but this can progress to generalized.[17] There may be a recent history of lameness.

Diagnosis

Diagnosis of tetanus is through a combination of history, clinical signs, exclusion of differential diagnoses and supportive lab assessment. Hematology is typically unremarkable. Serology and culture are unrewarding or low-yield diagnostics. Isolation of *C. tetani* from tissue can be attempted but may not be successful. However, isolation of *C. tetani*, particularly with concurrent cytological evidence of gram-positive rods and/or spores (**Fig. 3.7**) is highly suggestive.

Therapy

A combination of supportive nursing care, wound management and specific, single-dose, IM human tetanus or IV equine antitoxin is indicated depending on the severity of clinical signs (*Table 3.5*). Antitoxin will reduce free toxin but will not reverse existing paralysis and clinical signs. Antitoxin administration is most helpful in reducing progression and worsening of clinical signs in severely affected patients, or those with suspected heavy wound contamination of spores.

Patients with generalized tetanus and hypoventilatory respiratory failure may require mechanical ventilation until control of the diaphragm and intercostal muscles is restored.

Antimicrobial therapy is indicated. Metronidazole (15 mg/kg q8–12h) is commonly used. Surgical invention and wound care may be required to assist in treatment of the infection and elimination of the anaerobic environment that supports *C. tetani* growth. Nursing care is important to provide comfort, reduce spasms and prevent complications (*Table 3.6*).

Prognosis/complications

Prognosis and treatment duration are based on severity of presenting clinical signs and ability of owners to commit to extended supportive care and cost. Patients with localized or generalized tetanus without complications have a good prognosis (50–80% survival) with appropriate therapy.[21] Improvement of clinical signs with therapy occurs within 1 week in dogs, but complete recovery can take 3–4 weeks.[21]

Table 3.5 **Treatment options for tetanus**	
Metronidazole	15 mg/kg IV or PO q8–12h
Tetanus equine antitoxin	100–1000 units/kg IV (preferred) or IM
Human tetanus immunoglobulin	500 units IM near wound site if wound noted

Table 3.6 **Management of tetanus**
Dim, darkened room to reduce the effect of light and noise stimulation
Sedation or anxiolytics to reduce stress and fear
Nutritional support in the form of nasal or esophageal tubes to support requirements during recovery and also reduce risk of aspiration and resultant pneumonia. Force feeding is not advised owing to high risk of aspiration
Muscle relaxants and anticonvulsants to reduce spasms and risk of hyperthermia. Suggested drugs include: acepromazine, benzodiazepines (diazepam or midazolam) or methocarbamol. Severely affected patients may require constant rate infusions of phenobarbital or propofol. Magnesium sulfate has also been used as an adjunctive treatment for severe muscle rigidity
Soft bedding, bladder expression, enemas, ocular lubricants and IV fluids (hydration and to remove effects of muscle damage), depending on patient need

Death is most commonly due to respiratory muscle paralysis, or secondary respiratory complications (aspiration pneumonia), multiple organ failure, disseminated intravascular coagulopathy (DIC), thromboembolism or cardiac arrhythmias.[18–20]

Prevention
Wound management
The key to prevention of tetanus is prompt identification of wounds and subsequent effective wound management to eliminate spore entry and reduce contamination. This is particularly important in dogs and cats that spend time outdoors or engage in high-risk activities for penetrating wounds (hunting, athletic events).

Vaccination
Although vaccination is the mainstay of tetanus prevention in some species (e.g. humans, horses), dogs and cats have low susceptibility to tetanus and vaccination is not indicated. However, in some parts of the world where dogs are deemed at high risk, the equine vaccine has been used in dogs.

Public health
Tetanus is not directly transmissible between humans and other animals.

CUTEREBRA MYIASIS
John Speciale

Definition
Cuterebra myiasis is the aberrant intracranial migration of a bot fly larva. The disease was first recognized as an acute focal vascular syndrome defined as feline ischemic encephalopathy. However, more recently, diverse pathologic mechanisms have been associated with intracranial or intraocular *Cuterebra* infection (**Fig. 3.11**).

Species affected
Cats, dogs and humans have all been infected with *Cuterebra* larvae, but only cats are frequently afflicted with intracranial invasion.[22]

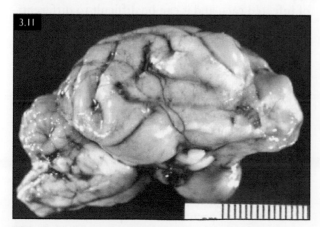

Fig. 3.11 Second-stage *Cuterebra* larva over the necrotic right olfactory bulb of a young cat. (Courtesy of Dr Alexander de Lahunta)

Etiology and pathogenesis
Adult *Cuterebra* flies emerge and breed in the late spring and survive for a few weeks. Females deposit eggs near rodent or rabbit burrows. Eggs stick to the fur of passing animals and are carried into the burrow. The eggs hatch and larvae enter the host and migrate to a subcutaneous site where they mature into second-stage larvae. They form a warble and grow into large third-stage larvae, which subsequently leave the host and pupate.

Although cats are an aberrant host for *Cuterebra* spp., the larvae often migrate successfully and benignly to a subcutaneous site. However, larval migration into the intracranial cavity or, much less often, into the spinal cord causes neurologic disease.

Clinical signs result from parasitic track lesions (**Fig. 3.12**), vasospasm (**Fig. 3.13**) and/or diffuse necrosis, presumably the result of the parasite's production and secretion of a neurotoxic or necrotizing substance (**Fig. 3.14**).

Geography
Cuterebra flies have only been identified in Central and North America.

Incidence and risk factors
The climate in the northeast leads to a predictable late summer or fall seasonal incidence. Seasonal occurrence may be less well defined in warmer areas

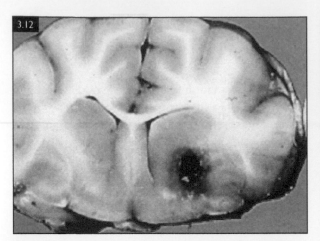

Fig. 3.12 Parasitic tract lesion in the basal ganglia of a cat. There is a cross-section of the larva within the tract. Note necrosis and edema of the adjacent brain parenchyma. (Courtesy of Dr Alexander de Lahunta)

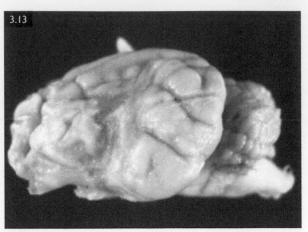

Fig. 3.13 Left cerebral atrophy in region of the left middle cerebral artery 2 months after acute onset of signs. Before identification of *Cuterebra* spp. the disease was defined as feline ischemic encephalopathy. (Courtesy of Dr Alexander de Lahunta)

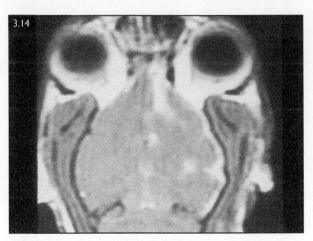

Fig. 3.14 T2-weighted MRI of a 2.5-year-old cat with signs consistent with *Cuterebra* infection. Not only is there hyperintensity extending from the left olfactory bulb into the thalamus, but there is also a notable diffuse hyperintensity over the ipsilateral meninges or brain surface. (Courtesy of Dr Alexander deLahunta)

of the western hemisphere. Cats that hunt outside (particularly in late summer or fall) are most likely to be exposed, infected and subsequently display signs consistent with cerebral migration.

Clinical signs

Onset of neurologic signs is peracute to acute. Clinical signs vary with the location of the parasite migration and the nature of the pathogenic process.[23] Signs caused by *Cuterebra* track lesions can vary over time, as different regions of the brain are affected and the immune response matures.

Hypo- or hyperthermia is common and the only physical abnormality other than neurologic deficits. Altered behavior is the most consistent sign. Depression to obtundation is noted most frequently, but some cats become abnormally aggressive. Seizures occur in approximately 25% of infected cats, and it can be difficult to differentiate altered behavior (i.e. primary lesion) from postictal changes.

Although signs may affect both sides of the brain, lateralization of signs is typical, with functional deficits more severe on one side. These may include: unidirectional circling, menace and/or visual deficits, hemi-attention and/or postural deficits.

Diagnosis

Definitive diagnosis of *Cuterebra* infestation requires necropsy, although recovery of *Cuterebra* larvae may not occur. Cerebrospinal fluid is likely to contain increased nucleated cells and protein but may be normal. Advanced imaging such as MRI can be helpful, but does not always demonstrate track lesions (**Fig. 3.15**).

Therapy

As with all neurologic diseases supportive treatment is important. Cats that have seizures should be treated with phenobarbital (3–5 mg/kg PO q12h). Treatment with an immunosuppressive dose of prednisone (2–3 mg/kg PO q24h initially and gradual tapering based on improvement) is justified. Treatment with ivermectin (400 μg/kg IM) has been recommended, following pre-treatment with diphenhydramine (4 mg/kg).

Prognosis/complication

Prognosis depends on the areas of the brain that are affected, but is considered fair to guarded with appropriate care. Sudden death may occur, whereas uncontrolled seizures, cost of care or intolerable behavior changes often lead to euthanasia.

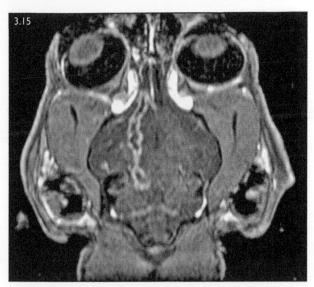

Fig. 3.15 T1-weighted contrast-enhanced image of a 2-year-old cat with an acute history of a right cerebral syndrome. The track lesion is similar to that in Fig. 3.14 but there is less diffuse involvement and the contrast enhancement demonstrates an associated inflammatory response. (Courtesy of Dr Andy Shores)

DISKOSPONDYLITIS
J Scott Weese

Definition

Diskospondylitis is an infectious and inflammatory disorder of the intervertebral disks and adjacent vertebrae. Local inflammation can result in varying degrees of local and systemic illness and neurologic abnormalities. Although disease can occur at any location in the spinal column, thoracic and lumbar disease are most common.

Species affected

Dogs are much more commonly affected than cats.

Etiology and pathogenesis

Bacteria are most often involved, particularly *Staphylococcus pseudintermedius*, *Streptococcus canis* and Enterobacteriaceae. *Brucella canis* (**Fig. 3.16**) is less commonly involved, although a range of other aerobic bacteria can occasionally cause disease. Fungal infections caused by opportunistic fungi such as *Aspergillus* spp. can occur.

The pathophysiology of disease relates to localization of opportunistic bacteria at the disk space, with development of a local infection that may extend to adjacent vertebrae. Slow blood flow in the area may facilitate establishment of the infection, and poor vascularity of the disk and adjacent bone can hamper the immune response and effectiveness of antimicrobial therapy. A cause is rarely identified but can include bacterial translocation (e.g. from the gastrointestinal tract or mouth), penetrating wound, foreign bodies and extension of local soft tissue infections. Postoperative infections may occur after spinal procedures.

Geography

There is no apparent geographic predisposition, although the relative role of certain pathogens (e.g. *B. canis*, fungi) varies geographically.

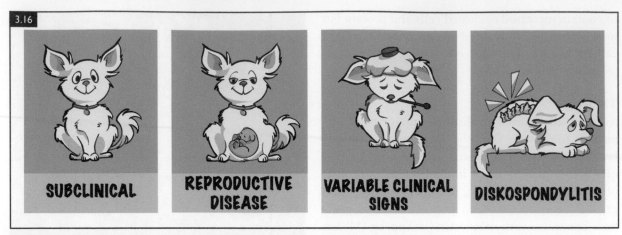

Fig. 3.16 Clinical presentations of *Brucella canis* infection in dogs: subclinical, reproductive disease (abortion), variable and/or vague clinical signs (lymphadenopathy, uveitis), diskospondylitis.

Incidence and risk factors

The incidence is poorly defined, as are risk factors. Events that predispose to bacterial translocation (e.g. dental disease, gastrointestinal disease) or immunosuppression likely play a role, but obvious inciting causes are not usually identified. Any age, breed and sex can be affected.

Clinical signs

Spinal pain is most commonly observed. Concurrent systemic signs such as fever may be present in a minority of cases. Neurological deficits may be present, and the severity and signs depend on the amount of nerve compression and the location. Ataxia and paresis are most common. Paralysis is rare. The degree of pain, ataxia and paresis, if present, should be carefully documented to aid in assessment of response to treatment.

Diagnosis

Diagnosis can be challenging, particularly early in disease and if advanced imaging is not possible. Consistent clinical signs are often used for a presumptive diagnosis, particularly because diskospondylitis is often the most treatable of the likely differential diagnoses.

Imaging

Imaging should be performed whenever possible (**Fig. 3.17**). Survey spinal radiographs can provide a definitive diagnosis but may have low sensitivity in the first few weeks of disease. Common abnormalities include irregularity of the endplates and narrowing of the intervertebral disk space. Evidence of osteomyelitis and bony proliferation can be observed in more advanced cases.

Myelography can be performed to evaluate spinal cord compression, particularly in acute cases or when the clinical relevance of radiographic abnormalities is in debate. However, CT or MRI is preferable to myelography and performing one of these is ideal in all cases.

Ultrasound-guided aspiration of the disk can be performed to obtain a sample for culture.

Brucella serology

This should be performed in all cases. Consideration should be given to performing testing before submission of cultures in high-risk cases, because of the biosafety risks associated with isolation of *Brucella* spp.

Culture

Aerobic culture and susceptibility testing should be performed on all cases. Specimens may include disk aspirates, blood and urine. Fungal culture is typically reserved for cases where there is cytologic evidence of fungal involvement or some other factor that suggests fungal disease.

Cytology

Cytologic examination of disk or local aspirates should be performed to guide empirical therapy (e.g. rods vs. cocci) and to identify rare infections caused by fungi or atypical pathogens such as *Actinomyces* or *Nocardia* spp.

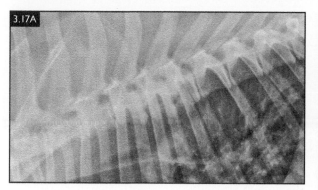

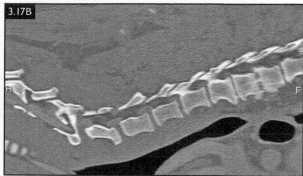

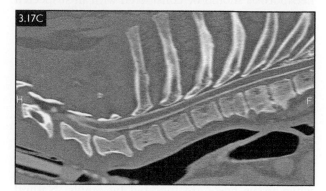

Fig. 3.17 Radiograph (A) and CT images (B, C) demonstrating a spinal lesion at T5–T6 consistent with diskospondylitis. (Courtesy of Atlantic Veterinary College)

Therapy

Empirical therapy should be started while awaiting culture results, unless clinical signs are mild and there is a desire to await *Brucella* serology results before culture sample collection. Amoxicillin/clavulanic acid or a first-generation cephalosporin (e.g. cephalexin) is commonly used as they are effective against staphylococci (excluding methicillin-resistant staphylococci) and have some activity against gram-negative organisms. Clindamycin is a good option if staphylococci are known or highly suspected because of its spectrum and good bone levels. Fluoroquinolones or third-generation cephalosporins can be effective but should be reserved for documented infections caused by gram-negative organisms. Some response to treatment is expected within the first few days. Lack of response should lead to reconsideration of the diagnosis and potentially a change in antimicrobial therapy if cultures were negative.

Duration of treatment is poorly defined. A minimum of 6–8 weeks should be considered, even if there is prompt and complete clinical response. Cases should be approached assuming the potential need for 1 year, or more, of treatment. Repeated imaging can be of use to determine therapy duration, but residual signs or recurrence can occur despite apparent resolution, even on CT or MRI.

Surgical intervention is typically reserved for serious cases with spinal cord compression or unstable vertebral body fracture.

Prognosis/complications

The prognosis is reasonable provided an adequate duration of treatment can be given and neurologic signs are not severe. Clinical signs usually improve within the first few days and neurologic deficits may improve over 2–4 months.

Public health and infection control

B. canis is a significant public health risk and diagnosis of this pathogen may result in an intervention by public health authorities. Exposure to urine from intact dogs is the greatest risk. It is prudent to handle diskospondylitis cases with contact precautions until *Brucella* serology is available, particularly in dogs from regions where the disease is endemic.

NEOSPORA CANINUM
Michelle Evason and Susan Taylor

Definition

Neospora caninum is a protozoal parasite that most often causes disease in puppies less than 6 months old. Classically, pelvic limb weakness progressing to rigid hindlimb hyperextension is noted. Prompt clinical recognition in young puppies is critical for treatment and improved prognosis. In older dogs, neosporosis should be considered with all suspected inflammatory CNS presentations (e.g. granulomatous meningoencephalitis).

Species affected

Dogs and wild canids are the main definitive hosts and shed oocysts in their feces.[24] Intermediate hosts include dogs, cattle, sheep, goats, horses, bison, water buffalo, white-tailed deer and foxes.[24] After ingestion of oocysts, tissue cysts can develop in intermediate hosts, with completion of the life cycle when tissue cysts are ingested by canids. Natural infection in cats has not been documented. *N. caninum* is a major cause of abortions in cattle, and dogs are the presumed source of infection.[25]

Etiology and pathogenesis

Dogs can be both definitive and intermediate hosts. Clinically important transmission of infection is thought to occur differently in puppies vs. adult dogs.

Puppies

Transplacental infection is considered the most common transmission route. This most often occurs when a bitch with persistent infection (tissue cysts) has reactivation of infection during pregnancy and transmits *N. caninum* to her pups. There may also be transmission through milk (lactation). Reactivation of the bitch's chronic infection and transplacental transmission often occur in successive litters.[24, 26]

Adult dogs

Ingestion of infected cattle (or other intermediate host) tissues containing cysts is considered the most common means of transmission. This may explain the higher prevalence in rural dogs and those on dairy farms (e.g. access to dead livestock).[27] Fecal transmission is less common in dogs.[24] Approximately 1 week after ingesting tissue cysts containing bradyzoites, dogs begin shedding varying numbers of oocysts in their feces.[28] Oocyst shedding may continue for months. Oocyst sporulation (resulting in infectivity) occurs 24–72 hours after oocysts are outside the body.[28]

In dogs with normal immune defenses clinical disease does not occur. Organisms become encysted as bradyzoites within tissue cysts and remain static, resulting in chronic (latent) infection. Immunosuppressed dogs may develop clinical disease due to bradyzoite activation and tachyzoite replication, followed by cell rupture and necrosis.[29] Widespread multi-organ dissemination of tachyzoites occurs in the acute phase. However, spread may also be restricted to the muscles or nervous tissues, where continued replication can lead to clinical disease.

Geography

Worldwide, typically maintained in the environment between dogs and cattle.

Risk factors

Labrador Retrievers are over-represented in reports of pediatric and adult-onset neosporosis.[26, 30] This may be related to a genetically based immune deficiency or susceptibility to infection.

Common clinical signs

Pediatric neosporosis (<6 months)

Puppies may be clinically normal at birth, then develop signs 3–16 weeks later. Occasionally multiple pups in a litter will be clinically affected.[24] The classic early sign in puppies is progressive weakness in the pelvic limbs, a crouched bunny-hopping gait, quadriceps muscle atrophy and loss of the patellar reflex. This rapidly progresses to rigid hyperextension of the pelvic limbs due to denervation atrophy and fibrous contracture of the quadriceps and gracilis muscles while the bones of the limb continue to grow (**Fig. 3.18**).

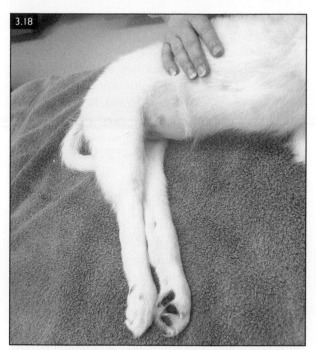

Fig. 3.18 Rigid hindlimb extension in a puppy with neosporosis. (Courtesy of Dr Susan Taylor)

Adult dogs

Affected dogs may be presented with progressive cerebellar dysfunction and ataxia, or with signs of progressive multifocal CNS disease including paresis, paralysis, ataxia, head tilt and/or seizures.[26, 30] Less commonly, infection can be widespread, resulting in myocarditis, hepatitis, dermatitis, ocular lesions, interstitial pneumonia and pancreatitis.[26, 30]

Diagnosis

Recognition of pediatric neosporosis based on typical early features is critically important for successful treatment. Serology is sometimes diagnostic, as is muscle biopsy; however, treatment is ideally initiated based on clinical suspicion before results of diagnostic testing.

Diagnosis is more difficult in adult dogs, where neosporosis is a differential diagnosis for a variety of infectious and non-infectious inflammatory disorders affecting the brain. Definitive diagnosis of neosporosis can be made through identification of organisms in affected muscle tissues (antemortem)

using immunohistochemical (IHC) staining, PCR on CSF and immunofluorescent assay (IFA).[26]

Laboratory abnormalities

The CBC and biochemistry may be normal, or non-specific for inflammation, muscle atrophy/damage and necrosis (high creatine kinase and aspartate transaminase).[26, 31]

Fecal testing is of limited use because it is rare to discover oocytes and, when present, they cannot be differentiated grossly from *Hammondia heydorni* oocytes.

Cytology may reveal tachyzoites in an aspirate and/or smear from body tissue or fluid. CSF analyses can be normal or reveal a mild-to-marked mixed mononuclear pleocytosis, with elevated protein content. A positive PCR CSF result, along with high titers of serum antibodies (IFA >1:800) is considered strongly suggestive of infection.[26]

Radiology/imaging

Radiology and ultrasound (abdominal and/or echocardiogram) will be normal in most dogs with neurologic and muscle disease. MRI in adult dogs may be consistent with cerebellar atrophy and inflammation within the brainstem or other regions within the brain.

Electromyographic results and nerve conduction velocities may be abnormal, particularly in pediatric neosporosis where radiculoneuritis, denervation and myositis are all present in the pelvic limbs.

Serology and PCR

Serological (IFA) testing can be helpful, and a titer greater than 1:800 in a dog with supportive clinical signs strongly suggests infection.[31] Unfortunately, many dogs without clinical disease can be seropositive with high titers (>1:800),[31] and some dogs with clinical disease may have negative titers. Therefore, it is advised to use serologic testing together with clinical signs. In the presence of signs suggesting neosporosis, a titer greater than 1:800 strongly supports diagnosis. A high titer (>1:800) on inflammatory CSF is also considered suggestive.

PCR can be similarly helpful; however, false negatives can occur. This diagnostic needs to be interpreted in light of clinical signs. PCR of the CSF was positive in four of five adult dogs with intracranial neosporosis in one study.[26]

Histopathology

Neospora caninum may be identified in muscle tissue or CNS using IHC staining. Muscle biopsy should be considered when there are negative or inconclusive results, particularly in puppies with suspected pediatric neosporosis.

Therapy

Supportive nursing care, together with prompt diagnosis and specific treatment, may improve prognosis and patient outcomes.

Clindamycin (10–15 mg/kg PO q12h for 8–12 weeks) is typically recommended,[30] although longer durations have also been used. Trimethoprim sulfonamide (15–20 mg/kg PO q12h) has also been used alone or concurrently with clindamycin for the same duration. Glucocorticoid therapy is not usually advised because disease rapidly progresses and disseminates with immune suppression.[24, 26, 30] There is no available therapy for dormant *N. caninum* bradyzoite tissue cysts, as drugs do not kill these.[31]

PSEUDORABIES
Andrew S Bowman

Pseudorabies, also known as Aujeszky's disease and "mad itch", is caused by suid alpha-herpesvirus-1. It is a viral disease of pigs that can spill over to infect many other animal species and rarely cause a highly fatal, neurologic disease in dogs and cats.[32] Feral or domestic swine are the reservoirs. Aberrant hosts typically become infected after ingestion of the virus during consumption of raw pork products.

Pseudorabies is commonly recognized by the onset of severe pruritus, usually of the head and neck, leading to self-mutilation (**Fig. 3.19**). Multiple cranial nerve deficits (e.g. hypersalivation, mydriasis, trismus, head tilt, pharyngeal paralysis) may develop rapidly. Anisocoria and dysphonia are common in affected cats.[33] Affected animals become progressively depressed, lethargic and weak, leading to recumbency, coma and death. Vomiting, ataxia, convulsions, fever, dyspnea and cardiac arrhythmias have also been

Prognosis/complications

Most puppies with pediatric neosporosis are euthanized because they develop rigid hyperextension of their pelvic limbs that does not resolve with treatment.[24, 26] However, with committed owners, early diagnosis and treatment initiated before fibrosis, prognosis for functional recovery can be good. Puppies and adult dogs with systemic neosporosis, cerebellar atrophy or multifocal CNS disease have a guarded prognosis for recovery.

Prevention

Efforts to decrease environmental (food and water) contamination with oocysts should be made on farms and livestock facilities.[25] Dogs should not be allowed to eat dead cattle or sheep. Meat/tissue along with offal and aborted material should be promptly disposed of.[25]

All infected dogs or puppies should be reported to the breeder, and responsible breeders should remove infected bitches from breeding. Breeders should promptly contact all owners of puppies from the litter so that they can be tested, monitored and perhaps treated.

reported. Direct fluorescent antibody testing on brain, PCR, virus isolation and histologic examination are used for confirmation of the diagnosis.

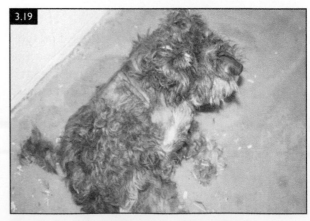

Fig. 3.19 A dog with pseudorabies and severe pruritus. (Courtesy of Dr Tony Forshey)

There is no effective treatment. Supportive care and heavy sedation or anesthesia can be used to minimize self-mutilation and control convulsions.

Pseudorabies can be prevented by avoiding direct contact with pigs and raw pork products.

RABIES
Jason W Stull and Susan Taylor

Definition

Rabies is an acute progressive neurologic disease that develops when the rabies virus enters the body through a wound (most commonly from a bite) or mucous membranes. The virus travels to the brain, resulting in encephalitis, associated behavioral and neuromuscular changes, and invariably death. All mammals are susceptible.

Etiology and pathogenesis

Rabies is an enveloped RNA virus from the family Rhabdoviridae and genus *Lyssavirus*. It can be divided into variants that correspond to specific regions or animal hosts (e.g. bat variant, which circulates primarily in bats). Viral variants can be transmitted to any susceptible host, although they are unlikely to continue to circulate in the non-adapted species. Disease almost always occurs following the bite of an infected animal with rabies virus in its saliva. Very rarely transmission may occur when the virus crosses mucosal surfaces or the placenta. Transmission cannot occur through intact skin or through contact with blood.

Following entry into an animal, the virus travels along the peripheral nerves to the CNS. The virus damages motor neurons, resulting in clinical disease. After CNS infection, the virus spreads further along peripheral nerves, making its way to the salivary glands and saliva. The incubation period is generally 3–12 weeks, but can range from several days to months, rarely exceeding 6 months.[34]

Geography

Rabies virus is present in much of the world, although there are some rabies-free countries (e.g. United Kingdom).

Incidence and risk factors

In most of the northern hemisphere rabies predominantly cycles in wildlife, whereas in the southern hemisphere feral dogs are the main source of transmission. Raccoons, skunks, foxes, coyotes and insectivorous bats are the wildlife vectors in various locations within North America. In Europe, bat and fox rabies predominate. Canine rabies is common in South America, Africa and Asia (**Fig. 3.20**).

Clinical signs

Rabies can cause a wide range of signs and should be considered in any animal with an acute history of altered mentation or lower motor neuron paralysis. Several phases are commonly described, although not all animals reveal signs of each phase. Rabies can mimic many different clinical conditions, sometimes resulting in vague disease that is not recognized as neurologic in origin until it is advanced. A 2- to 3-day prodromal phase is marked by anxiety, fever, pupillary dilation and behavioral change. Animals may lick or chew at the site of virus introduction. This may progress to a "furious phase" characterized by 1–7 days of markedly abnormal behavior, including restlessness, aggression, excitability, photophobia, hiding, hyperesthesia and psychotic behaviour (**Fig. 3.21**). Dogs may compulsively eat foreign objects and may attack their surroundings or moving objects. Incoordination, loss of balance, disorientation and seizures develop, followed by death. Some dogs develop a progressive lower motor neuron paralysis ("paralytic phase") (**Fig. 3.22**) characterized by weakness, loss of limb reflexes and weakness or paralysis of the pharyngeal, laryngeal and masticatory muscles, causing hypersalivation, a hoarse bark and a dropped jaw. Coma and respiratory paralysis follow.

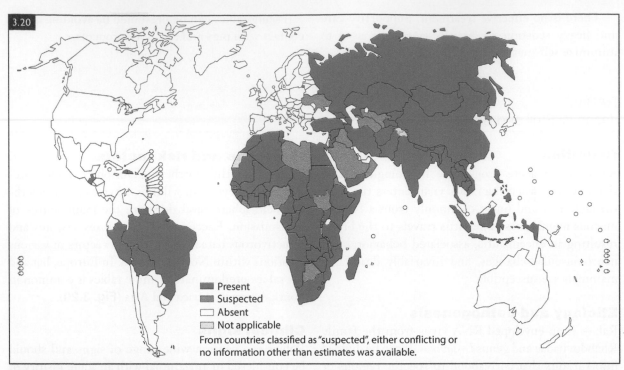

Fig. 3.20 International distribution of canine rabies. (Courtesy of the World Health Organization, http://www.who.int/rabies/Presence_dog_transmitted_human_Rabies_2014.png?ua=1)

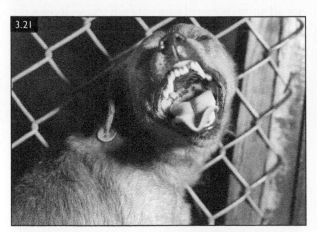

Fig. 3.21 Dog demonstrating aggressive behaviour resulting from rabies. (Courtesy of US Centers for Disease Control and Prevention)

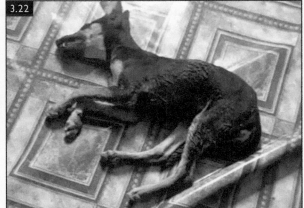

Fig. 3.22 A feral dog with end-stage rabies. (Courtesy of Dr Philip Mshelbwala)

Findings are progressive over days, with most infected dogs and cats succumbing to respiratory failure within 10 days of onset of signs.

Diagnosis

Diagnosis is based on suggestive clinical signs, although many neurologic diseases can produce similar signs. A history of exposure to the virus or a potential wildlife reservoir and lack of rabies vaccination provides an increased index of suspicion. Given the delay between exposure and clinical disease, bite wounds may no longer be observed. Once a high index of suspicion of rabies is present, euthanasia for rabies testing is warranted.

The highly sensitive and specific fluorescent antibody test performed on brain tissue is the international gold standard.[35] The head or body of an animal (deceased or euthanized) suspected of having rabies should be immediately cooled and maintained refrigerated (not frozen).

Therapy

Rabies in animals is not treatable. Once rabies is strongly suspected, euthanasia is warranted followed by submission of the brain for rabies testing.

Prognosis/complications

Rabies uniformly results in death in companion animals, within 1–10 days of clinical onset.

Prevention

Vaccination

Rabies in vaccinated dogs and cats is extremely rare.[36] Local regulations for vaccination should be followed, and often consist of a requirement to vaccinate all dogs and cats after 12 weeks of age, 1 year later, then every 3 years (or as indicated for the vaccine).[37] Due to antibody development, animals are considered vaccinated 28 days after first vaccination and immediately after subsequent vaccinations.

Reducing exposure risk

Exposure to wild animals should be limited, especially known rabies reservoir species. Dogs and cats entering rabies-free countries may be quarantined and/or require demonstration of proof of vaccination.

Post exposure

After exposure to a known rabid animal or a suspect rabid animal when confirmatory testing is not possible (e.g. fighting with a rabies reservoir species that was not caught for testing), local requirements must be followed but typically include prompt vaccination and often quarantine, with variation depending on previous vaccination status.[34] In unvaccinated animals, this usually involves euthanasia or 3–6 months of quarantine.

Public health and infection control

See *Table 3.7*. People bitten by animals should be instructed to wash the wound immediately and thoroughly with soap and water, and urgently seek medical advice regarding the need for rabies post-exposure prophylaxis (PEP: vaccine, rabies immunoglobulin), depending on the biting species, ability to quarantine the animal, rabies epidemiology in the area and the victim's previous rabies vaccination status.[38]

Local public or animal health authorities should be consulted regarding animals exposed to known or suspected rabid animals and bites to people. An apparently healthy dog or cat (regardless of rabies vaccination status) that bites a person should be monitored for 10 days following the bite; dogs and cats shed the virus for a few days before the onset of clinical signs and during illness. If no signs of illness occur in the animal, it was not shedding rabies at the time of the bite.[34] All bites should be reported to authorities as required by law.

Rabies virus is readily deactivated by ultraviolet light, heat, desiccation and disinfectants. Contaminated objects should be cleaned with soap and water, allowed to dry and disinfected with a 1:32 solution of household bleach. For other areas (e.g. animal fur), once dry (e.g. exposure to air for several hours) the virus is considered deactivated. The virus may remain viable for longer (days to weeks) when a body is refrigerated or frozen.[39]

Table 3.7 **Selected rabies resources**
US Centers for Disease Control and Prevention. Rabies. Available at: http://www.cdc.gov/rabies/index.html
Day MJ *et al.* (2016) WSAVA Guidelines for the vaccination of dogs and cats. *J Small Anim Pract* 57:E1–45. Available at: http://www.wsava.org/guidelines/vaccination-guidelines
National Association for State Public Health Veterinarians. Available at: http://nasphv.org/
OIE – World Organisation for Animal Health. Rabies. Available at: http://www.rr-asia.oie.int/disease-info/rabies/
RabiesAware.org. Rabies laws and vaccination in the US. Available at: http://www.rabiesaware.org/
World Health Organization. Rabies. Available at: http://www.who.int/rabies

TICK PARALYSIS
Michelle Evason

Definition

Tick paralysis presents as a flaccid (lower motor neuron) paralysis leading to respiratory compromise and death in dogs and cats if untreated. The condition is due to female tick bite and the resultant toxin secretion. The most commonly associated ticks in North America include *Dermacentor andersoni* (**Fig. 3.23**), *D. variabilis* and rarely *Ixodes scapularis*, whereas in Australia the causative tick is *Ixodes holocyclus* (**Fig. 3.24**). Therapy consists of prompt removal of the offending tick and supportive care.

Species affected

Domestic and wild dogs and cats, cattle, sheep, goats and humans.

Etiology and pathogenesis:

A neurotoxin produced in the salivary glands of the female tick has been identified as paralyzing to the host after 4–5 days of tick feeding.[40] It is thought that different tick bites (e.g. *Dermacentor* vs. *Ixodes* spp.) have varying toxicities,[40] which is why clinical signs and time of recovery from tick paralysis differ between Australia and North America. Clinical signs are related to the reduction of neurotransmitter release from the presynaptic nerve of the neuromuscular junction, resulting in decreased nerve conduction and flaccid paralysis.[40]

Geography

Worldwide, but more frequently reported in the Pacific Northwest of Canada and the USA, southwestern Canada and eastern Australia.[40, 41]

Incidence and risk factors

The incidence of clinical disease is unknown. Risk factors for dogs and cats are related to increased tick exposure through lifestyle (e.g. stray or feral) and higher tick population seasons.[41]

Clinical signs

Classically, signs include an acute ascending symmetric paralysis that progresses over hours to days, resulting in a flaccid weakness that begins in the hindlimbs.[40, 41] Weakness progresses to the forelimbs, and failure of respiratory muscles occurs. Less commonly, focal weakness has been observed.[40]

Dogs can develop direct cardiotoxicity and concurrent gastrointestinal signs related to megaesophagus (regurgitation), leading to pulmonary edema and aspiration pneumonia.

Cats may have primary respiratory compromise and gait abnormalities.[41]

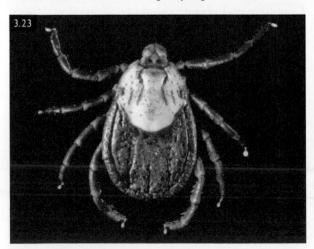

Fig. 3.23 Adult female *Dermacentor andersoni*. (Courtesy of Dr Christopher Paddock)

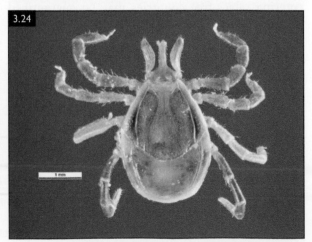

Fig. 3.24 *Ixodes holocyclus* adult female. (Courtesy of Walker, K (2006) Australian paralysis tick [*Ixodes holocyclus*]. Updated on 9/14/2006 1:57:55 PM Available online: PaDIL http://www.padil.gov.au)

Diagnosis

Diagnosis is based on clinical suspicion, history of exposure to ticks (or travel to a tick endemic region), or through locating an engorged tick. Shaving patients to remove hair can aid tick identification and improve prognosis (**Fig. 3.25**).[41]

Therapy

Therapy consists of prompt tick identification, removal and supportive care. This may consist of a quiet environment, anti-anxiolytics, and prudent risk–benefit assessment of administration of tick antitoxin based on initial clinical signs. Canine tick antitoxin serum and ventilatory support in cats with respiratory compromise improved outcome in an Australian study.[41] Intensive care and monitoring may be needed, particularly for patients with respiratory compromise.

Monitoring

Clinical improvement typically occurs 24 hours after tick removal with North American ticks. However, improvement can be delayed with *I. holocyclus* (Australia) and clinical signs may progress even after tick removal.

Prognosis/complications

The prognosis for dogs and cats given early therapy is excellent; however, those who present with severe

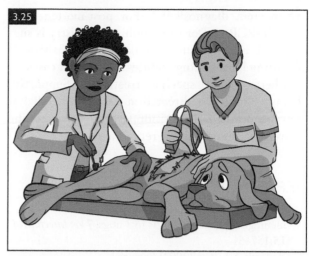

Fig. 3.25 Ascending symmetric lower motor neuron (flaccid) paralysis in a dog being examined for suspected tick paralysis.

complications or presentations (e.g. respiratory compromise, worsened paralysis and hypothermia) have a more guarded prognosis.[41] Disease can be fatal, particularly without treatment.[40, 41]

Prevention and infection control

Prevention is dependent on tick checks and effective tick prevention products applied consistently and correctly.

WEST NILE VIRUS AND EASTERN EQUINE ENCEPHALITIS VIRUS
Jason W Stull and M Casey Gaunt

West Nile virus (WNV) and eastern equine encephalitis virus (EEEV), belonging to the genera *Flavivirus* and *Alphavirus*, respectively, can cause acute encephalitis. Both viruses are maintained in bird–mosquito–bird cycles, with spillover into mammalian hosts via the bites of infected mosquitoes. Although exposure may be common in some regions,[42] clinical illness is extremely rare in dogs and has not been described in cats. However, WNV seroprevalence can be high in both dogs and cats.[42]

In clinically affected animals, the viruses spread to the nervous system, causing encephalitis or encephalomyelitis. Lethargy, mental dullness, anorexia, fever, ataxia, generalized muscle tremors, conscious proprioceptive deficits, seizures and flaccid paralysis can occur. Clinical cases of EEE have been restricted to young (<6 months old) dogs.[43, 44] Infected cats and dogs do not develop an adequate viremia to transmit the viruses to biting mosquitoes and are therefore dead-end hosts.

Antibodies to WNV infection are generally evident by 7 days following infection. Acute and convalescent serum samples should be tested using IgM enzyme-linked immunosorbent assay (ELISA) and virus neutralization assays. The use of rapid real-time reverse transcriptase (RT)-PCR assays on tissue biopsy samples or synovial fluid samples, along with IgM serology, has been recommended for antemortem diagnosis.[43, 45] For post-mortem testing, RT-PCR and/or immunohistochemistry is suggested. It is important to speak to public health staff regarding local testing abilities and suspect cases.

There is no specific treatment. Supportive therapy should be directed at maintaining hydration, perfusion and nutrition, as well as controlling neurologic signs. Antipyretics, anti-nausea agents and antiepileptic drugs should be administered as indicated.

Prognosis is difficult to estimate given the limited number of clinically infected dogs and cats identified; however, it appears poor. All reported animals naturally infected with resulting clinical disease have died. Preventing mosquito bites is paramount to WNV and EEEV prevention in all species.

REFERENCES

1 Cizinauskas, S *et al.* (2001) Streptococcal meningoencephalomyelitis in 3 dogs. *J Vet Intern Med* **15**:157–61.

2 Radaelli, ST *et al.* (2002) Bacterial meningoencephalomyelitis in dogs: a retrospective study of 23 cases (1990–1999). *J Vet Intern Med* **16**:159–63.

3 Martinez-Gutierrez, M *et al.* (2016) Diversity of susceptible hosts in canine distemper virus infection: a systematic review and data synthesis. *BMC Vet Res* **12**:78.

4 Sykes, J (2014) Canine distemper virus infection. In *Canine and Feline Infectious Disease*. J Sykes, ed. Elsevier, St. Louis, MO, pp.152–65.

5 Pesavento, PA *et al.* (2014) Common and emerging infectious diseases in the animal shelter. *Vet Pathol* **51**:478–91.

6 Sokolow, SH *et al.* (2005) Epidemiologic evaluation of diarrhea in dogs in an animal shelter. *Am J Vet Res* **66**:1018–24.

7 Amude, AM *et al.* (2007) Clinicopathological findings in dogs with distemper encephalomyelitis presented without characteristic signs of the disease. *Res Vet Sci* **82**:416–22.

8 Greene, CE (2012) Canine distemper. In *Infectious Diseases of the Dog and Cat*, 4th ed. CE Greene, ed. Elsevier, St. Louis, MO, pp.25–42.

9 Barsanti, J (2012) Botulism. In *Infectious Diseases of the Dog and Cat*, 4th ed. CE Greene, ed. Elsevier, St. Louis, MO, pp.447–60.

10 Penderis, J (2012) Tetanus and botulism. In *Small Animal Neurological Emergencies*. SR Platt, ed. CRC Press, London, pp.416–22.

11 Horowitz, BZ (2005) Botulinum toxin. *Crit Care Clin* **21**:825–39, viii.

12 Humeau, Y *et al.* (2000) How botulinum and tetanus neurotoxins block neurotransmitter release. *Biochimie* **82**:427–46.

13 Elad, D *et al.* (2004) Natural *Clostridium botulinum* type C toxicosis in a group of cats. *J Clin Microbiol* **42**:5406–8.

14 Fernandez, RA *et al.* (1999) Botulism: laboratory methods and epidemiology. *Anaerobe* 5:165–8.

15 Shapiro, RL *et al.* (1998) Botulism in the United States: a clinical and epidemiologic review. *Ann Intern Med* 129:221–8.

16 Rutter, CR *et al.* (2011) Outcome and medical management in dogs with lower motor neuron disease undergoing mechanical ventilation: 14 cases (2003–2009). *J Vet Emerg Crit Care* **21**:531–41.

17 Malik, R *et al.* (1989) Three cases of local tetanus. *J Small Anim Pract* **30**:469–73.

18 Burkitt, JM *et al.* (2007) Risk factors associated with outcome in dogs with tetanus: 38 cases (1987–2005). *J Am Vet Med Assoc* **230**:76–83.

19 Greene, CE (2012) Tetanus. In *Infectious Diseases of the Dog and Cat*, 4th ed. CE Greene, ed. Elsevier, St. Louis, MO, pp.423–31.

20 Sykes, J (2014) Tetanus and botulism. In *Canine and Feline Infectious Disease*. J Sykes, ed. Elsevier, St. Louis, MO, pp.520–30.

21 Bandt, C *et al.* (2007) Retrospective study of tetanus in 20 dogs: 1988–2004. *J Am Anim Hosp Assoc* **43**:143–8.

22 Bowman, DD *et al.* (2002) *Feline Clinical Parasitology*. Iowa State University Press, Ames, IA.

23 Glass, EN *et al.* (1998) Clinical and clinicopathologic features in 11 cats with *Cuterebra* larvae myiasis of the central nervous system. *J Vet Intern Med* **12**:365–8.

24 Dubey, JP *et al.* (2011) Neosporosis in animals – the last five years. *Vet Parasitol* **180**:90–108.

25 Reichel, MP *et al.* (2014) Control options for *Neospora caninum* – is there anything new or are we going backwards? *Parasitology* **141**:1455–70.

26 Garosi, L *et al.* (2010) Necrotizing cerebellitis and cerebellar atrophy caused by *Neospora caninum* infection: magnetic resonance imaging and

clinicopathologic findings in seven dogs. *J Vet Intern Med* **24**:571–8.

27 Dijkstra, T *et al.* (2002) Point source exposure of cattle to *Neospora caninum* consistent with periods of common housing and feeding and related to the introduction of a dog. *Vet Parasitol* **105**:89–98.

28 Gondim, LFP *et al.* (2005) Effects of host maturity and prior exposure history on the production of *Neospora caninum* oocysts by dogs. *Vet Parasitol* **134**:33–9.

29 Ordeix, L *et al.* (2002) Cutaneous neosporosis during treatment of pemphigus foliaceus in a dog. *J Am Animal Hosp Assoc* **38**:415–19.

30 Barber, JS *et al.* (1998) Naturally occurring vertical transmission of *Neospora caninum* in dogs. *Int J Parasitol* **28**:57–64.

31 Lavely, JA (2014) Pediatric seizure disorders in dogs and cats. *Vet Clin North Am* **44**:275–301.

32 Davison, AJ (2010) Herpesvirus systematics. *Vet Microbiol* **143**:52–69.

33 Henke, D *et al.* (2012) Pseudorabies. In *Infectious Diseases of the Dog and Cat*, 4th ed. CE Greene, ed. Elsevier, St. Louis, MO, pp.198–201.

34 Brown, CM *et al.* (2016) Compendium of animal rabies prevention and control. *J Am Vet Med Assoc* **248**:505–17.

35 Lembo, T *et al.* (2006) Evaluation of a direct, rapid immunohistochemical test for rabies diagnosis. *Emerg Infect Dis* **12**:310–13.

36 Murray, KO *et al.* (2009) Rabies in vaccinated dogs and cats in the United States, 1997–2001. *J Am Vet Med Assoc* **235**:691–5.

37 WSAVA publishes updated guidance on vaccination of dogs and cats: https://www.wsava.org/Guidelines/Vaccination-Guidelines

38 Rupprecht, CE *et al.* (2010) Use of a reduced (4-dose) vaccine schedule for postexposure prophylaxis to prevent human rabies: recommendations of the advisory committee on immunization practices. *MMWR Recomm Rep* **59**:1–9.

39 Lewis, VJ *et al.* (1974) Limitations of deteriorated tissue for rabies diagnosis. *Health Lab Sci* **11**:8–12.

40 Edlow, JA *et al.* (2008) Tick paralysis. *Infect Dis Clin North Am* **22**:397–413, vii.

41 Leister, E *et al.* (2018) Clinical presentations, treatments and risk factors for mortality in cats with tick paralysis caused by *Ixodes holocyclus*: 2077 cases (2008–2016). *J Feline Med Surg* **20**:465–78.

42 Kile, JC *et al.* (2005) Serologic survey of cats and dogs during an epidemic of West Nile virus infection in humans. *J Am Vet Med Assoc* **226**:1349–53.

43 Farrar, MD *et al.* (2005) Eastern equine encephalitis in dogs. *J Vet Diagn Invest* **17**:614–17.

44 Oliver, J *et al.* (2016) Geography and timing of cases of eastern equine encephalitis in New York State from 1992 to 2012. *Vector Borne Zoon Dis (Larchmont, NY)* **16**:283–9.

45 Cannon, AB *et al.* (2006) Acute encephalitis, polyarthritis, and myocarditis associated with West Nile virus infection in a dog. *J Vet Intern Med* **20**:1219–23.

BACTERIAL CYSTITIS
Michelle Evason and J Scott Weese

Definition

Bacterial cystitis is a common problem that occurs when bacteria proliferate and cause inflammation in the lower urinary tract. There are two main classifications. "Sporadic cystitis" is most common. "Recurrent or refractory cystitis" is when patients have had three or more episodes of bacterial cystitis in a year. Bacterial cystitis must be differentiated from subclinical bacteriuria (where bacteria are present in urine in the absence of clinical signs) and infections of other parts of the genitourinary tract (e.g. pyelonephritis, prostatitis) (**Fig. 4.1**).

Species affected

Dogs and cats, with dogs more often affected.

Etiology and pathogenesis

Although urine has often been considered to be sterile, it is increasingly evident that bacterial colonization or contamination occurs frequently in healthy animals. Evidence of a "urine microbiome" exists and subclinical bacteriuria is commonly encountered. Bacterial cystitis is defined as inflammation occurring in response to the presence of bacteria in the bladder, and occurs through a combination of host and pathogen (e.g. bacterial numbers, virulence factors) properties.

Gram-negative bacteria, particularly Enterobacteriaceae (e.g. *Escherichia coli*, *Klebsiella* spp.) are most commonly involved, followed by staphylococci (e.g. *S. pseudintermedius*, *S. aureus*, *S. felis*), streptococci, *Proteus* spp. and enterococci.[1-3]

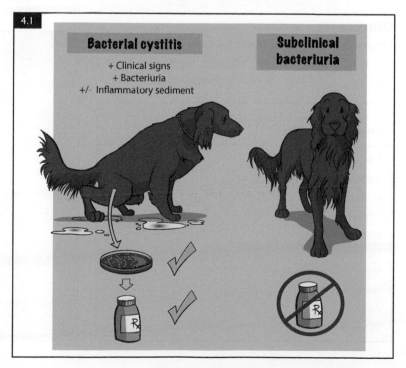

Fig. 4.1 Comparison of bacterial cystitis and subclinical bacteriuria.

Incidence and risk factors

Lower urinary tract disease (LUTD) is a leading cause of veterinary visits and antimicrobial use in dogs and cats. Sporadic cystitis may not be associated with an identifiable risk factor but is common in dogs, particularly females. Recurrent or refractory cases are almost always associated with some underlying anatomical, functional or immunological risk factors (*Table 4.1*, **Fig. 4.2**), although the underlying factor is not always apparent. Cats are less likely to develop bacterial cystitis than dogs, and LUTD, particularly in a young cat, is much more likely to be feline idiopathic cystitis (FIC).

Subclinical bacteriuria is relatively common in some populations, particularly older cats, obese individuals, and patients with endocrine abnormalities (e.g. diabetes mellitus, hypothyroidism) or renal compromise.[4-6] However, evidence that this corresponds to a risk of bacterial cystitis is lacking.

Clinical signs

Clinical signs are related to inflammation of the lower urinary tract and may include straining or difficulty with urination, painful urination, blood in urine (**Fig. 4.3**), and increased urgency and frequency of small amounts of urine. Cats may urinate outside the litter box.

Diagnosis

Diagnosis is often based on the presence of clinical signs of LUTD, but this is not definitive, particularly in cats with FIC. Urinalysis should be performed in all cases.

Urinalysis

This may show dilute to concentrated urine, bacteriuria, mild-to-moderate proteinuria, glucosuria, pyuria and haematuria, and can include casts. Urease-producing bacteria (e.g. *Staphylococcus* spp., *Proteus* spp., *Corynebacterium urealyticum*) typically produce an alkaline pH and concurrent struvite crystalluria. Cytology is a very useful but

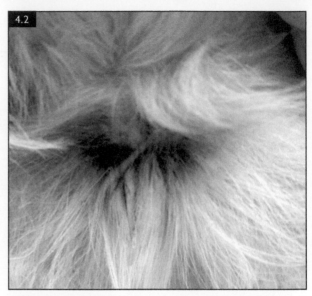

Fig. 4.2 Vulvar staining on a female English Setter with recurrent cystitis likely related to urinary incontinence.

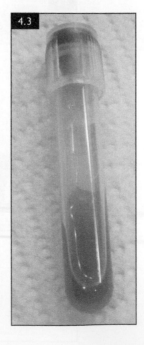

Fig. 4.3 Grossly abnormal urine collected from a female English Setter with bacterial cystitis.

Table 4.1 **Potential risk factors for recurrent or refractory cystitis**
Ectopic ureter
Mesonephric duct abnormalities
Abnormal vulvar conformation
Obesity
Bladder wall mass
Rectal fistula
Urinary incontinence
Urine retention
Endocrinopathy
Polypoid cystitis

overlooked tool. Pyruria, hematuria and bacteria are typically observed (**Fig. 4.4**).

Bacterial culture

Urine culture is always useful and should be done in all cases of recurrent or refractory disease. Cystocentesis should be performed for collection of culture specimens unless samples can be collected cleanly, kept refrigerated, be processed by the laboratory within a few hours and be interpreted with a cutoff of ≥100,000 colony-forming units (CFU)/mL.[7] Interpretation of susceptibility testing should be done using urine breakpoints, when they are available. With drugs that are concentrated in urine (e.g. penicillins, cephalosporins, fluoroquinolones), serum breakpoints may underestimate the potential efficacy, and drugs that are reported as intermediate or even resistant may sometimes be effective for cystitis.

Diagnostic imaging

Radiographs are typically normal with bacterial cystitis, except in the case of a recurrent (complicated) urinary tract infection (UTI) where an underlying urolith or renolith may be noted (**Fig. 4.5**). Emphysematous cystitis is indicated by radiolucency within the bladder wall or associated with the bladder lumen (**Fig. 4.6**).

Contrast radiography may be of benefit to identify abnormalities predisposing to a recurrent (complicated) UTI (**Fig. 4.7**). Examples of these include bladder diverticuli, neoplasia, cysts or, more commonly, urate calculi.

Cystoscopy

Cystoscopy can be extremely helpful in identifying the cause of recurrent disease (**Figs. 4.8, 4.9**), after appropriate diagnostics such as CBC, serum chemistry and endocrine testing have been completed. Biopsies and specimens for culture may also be obtained.

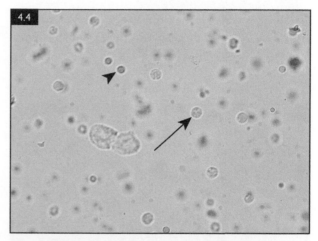

Fig. 4.4 Urine cytology from a dog with bacterial cystitis. Note the white blood cells (arrow) and red blood cells (arrowhead). (Courtesy of Dorothee Bienzle)

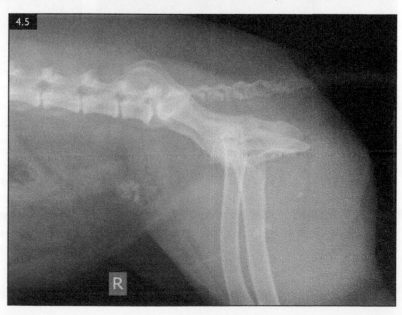

Fig. 4.5 Lateral abdominal radiograph of a dog with struvite urolithiasis. Note the numerous smooth radiodense uroliths in the bladder and urethra. (Courtesy of Atlantic Veterinary College)

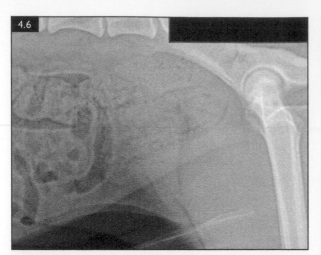

Fig. 4.6 Lateral radiograph showing emphysematous cystitis. (Courtesy of Jinelle Webb)

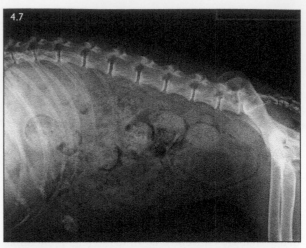

Fig. 4.7 Lateral radiograph showing emphysematous cystitis due to *E. coli* infection in a diabetic dog. (Courtesy of Holland Street Veterinary Clinic)

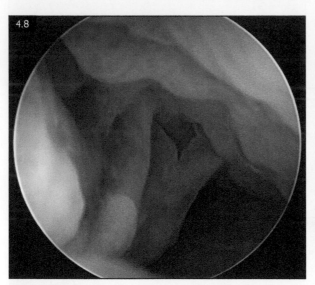

Fig. 4.8 Cystoscopic image of the bladder of a dog with cystitis. The mucosa is hyperemic but no other overt abnormalities are noted. (Courtesy of Alice Defarges)

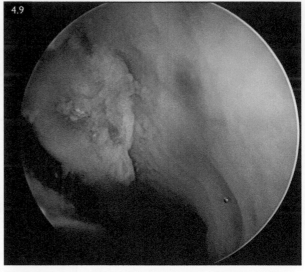

Fig. 4.9 Cystoscopic image of a transitional cell carcinoma. Note the mass and the irregular mucosa, along with patches of mucosal hyperemia adjacent to the mass. (Courtesy of Alice Defarges)

Therapy

Common treatment options are presented in *Table 4.2*.[8] Short (3–5 days) treatment durations are recommended for sporadic cystitis. For recurrent or refractory cases, duration depends on the underlying etiology. Short (3–5 days) or longer durations (10–14 days) may be indicated depending on the disease process.

Prevention

Prevention of cystitis involves identification and control of underlying risk factors, which is possible in some cases but not others. Investigation of risk factors is indicated in all recurrent cases to determine whether prevention is possible.

Table 4.2 **Antimicrobial options for bacterial cystitis**

TYPE	DRUG	DOSE	COMMENTS
First line	Amoxicillin	11–15 mg/kg PO q12h	Good routine option for cystitis. Urine breakpoints should be used for susceptibility testing
	Amoxicillin/clavulanic acid	12.5–25 mg/kg PO q12h (dose based on combination of amoxicillin + clavulanic acid)	Not clear whether it is better than amoxicillin alone for sporadic bacterial cystitis. Urine breakpoints should be used
	Trimethoprim sulfadiazine/ trimethoprim sulfamethoxazole/ ormetoprim sulfadimethoxine	15–30 mg/kg PO q12h\n\nNote: dosing is based on total trimethoprim + sulfa concentration	Adverse effects are of lesser concern with typical short durations. Avoid in dogs that may be sensitive to KCS, hepatopathy, hypersensitivity and skin eruptions
Second line	Cefovecin	8 mg/kg single SC injection. Can be repeated once after 7–14 days	Duration and spectrum are greater than are typically needed. Only use when oral treatment is not possible. Ineffective against enterococci
	Cefpodoxime proxetil	Dogs: 5–10 mg/kg q24h PO\nCats: no dose established	Ineffective against enterococci
	Doxycycline	5 mg/kg PO q12h	Not for routine use but potentially useful with multidrug-resistant bacteria
	Enrofloxacin	5 mg/kg PO q24h (cats)\n5–20 mg/kg q24h (dogs)	Reserve for documented resistant cystitis. Do not exceed 5 mg/kg/day of enrofloxacin in cats
	Fosfomycin	40 mg/kg PO (with food) q12h	Should be reserved for multidrug-resistant infections. Do not use in cats
	Marbofloxacin	2.7–5.5 mg/kg PO q24h	Reserve for documented resistant cystitis
	Nitrofurantoin	4.4–5 mg/kg PO q8h	Useful for many multidrug-resistant pathogens
	Orbifloxacin	Tablets: 2.5–7.5 mg/kg PO once daily\nSuspension (cats): 7.5 mg/kg once daily	Reserve for documented resistant cystitis
	Pradofloxacin	Dogs: 3–5 mg/kg PO once daily\nCats: 3–5 mg/kg once daily (tablets) or 5–7.5 mg/kg once daily (suspension)	Reserve for documented resistant cystitis

Abbreviations: KCS, keratoconjunctivitis sicca

BRUCELLOSIS (*BRUCELLA CANIS*)
Michelle Evason

Definition
Brucella canis is a gram-negative bacterium that primarily causes reproductive disease in dogs, but is also an important cause of diskospondylitis. Subclinical (and chronic) infections are common, and evidence of infertility or abortion in breeding facilities should prompt testing. Disease eradication is challenging because of poor (or lack of) response to antimicrobial therapy. *B. canis* is zoonotic, and human risk is typically through contact with infected breeding dogs.

Species affected
Dogs and wild canids are primarily affected.

Etiology and pathogenesis

Brucella canis is transmitted through direct (e.g. dog to dog) oral, nasal or venereal exposure to infected body fluids such as urine, vaginal discharge, aborted fetus, semen and less frequently saliva, milk or nasal or conjunctival discharge. In crowded kennels, inhalation and fomite (e.g. contaminated water bowl, food, soil or bedding) transmission are important routes of infection.[9] Recurrent (or continuous) bacteremia can occur for years after infection. Shedding occurs readily, increasing risk of contagion.

Geography

The bacterium can be found worldwide, although the prevalence varies by region. The southern USA, Mexico, South and Central America, China and Japan are higher-risk areas.[10, 11] Given the increased importation of breeding dogs and semen for artificial insemination (AI), this is regarded as a global concern.[12]

Incidence and risk factors

Seroprevalence rates vary depending on the sampled population (e.g. stray, shelter, pet dog, breeding facility) and region.[9, 10] Underdiagnosis and underreporting are concerns.

Risk factors (seropositive status and clinical disease) include history of being a stray, feral or breeding dog, or living in a breeding facility or kennel. Dogs with diskospondylitis are most commonly intact males, and less commonly spayed females.[13]

Clinical signs

(See **Fig. 3.16**, page 110.)

Infected dogs may have no clinical signs or a wide range of reproductive disorders.[14] Overt clinical signs include abortion, weak pups that die shortly postbirth, orchitis, prostatitis, infertility (bitch or stud) and placentitis. Late term pregnancy loss (weeks 7–9) is the hallmark of brucellosis. Diskospondylitis, uveitis, lymphadenopathy, splenomegaly and dermatitis can also occur. Spinal pain is usually present with diskospondylitis.[13]

Diagnosis

Diagnosis can be challenging. Repeated testing (or a combination of diagnostic assays) to ensure presence or confirmation of infection and avoid false positives is required. In breeding facilities, testing multiple dogs is advised to improve successful diagnoses. In many areas *B. canis* is reportable to local or national public health organizations, so confirmatory testing may be directed by public health or animal health personnel.

Typically, diagnosis is confirmed through consistent clinical signs, together with PCR and serology (rapid slide agglutination test [RSAT], enzyme-linked immunosorbent assay [ELISA], immunofluorescent assay [IFA]), or through positive blood or urine culture. In some countries testing of semen is required before importation.

Laboratory assessment is frequently normal. Abnormalities may include neutrophilia, hypoalbuminemia and hyperglobulinemia. Urinalysis may be normal despite urinary shedding of the bacterium.

Cytology of the semen, liver or spleen may show inflammation or organisms. Ejaculate abnormalities may be noted, such as low sperm counts, poor motility or the absence of sperm in samples.

Culture of urine and other fluids has low sensitivity. However, blood culture is more likely to be successful early in infection (e.g. 8 weeks) and is regarded as the gold standard of diagnosis. Prior antibiotic therapy can interfere with culture results,[9] and negative culture does not rule out infection. Culture should be performed only by laboratories with enhanced biosafety practices required for *Brucella* isolation.

Imaging is not specific for brucellosis. Diskospondylitis may be noted on plain radiographs; however, CT and MRI are more sensitive. Abdominal or testicular ultrasonographic findings may vary widely or appear normal. Splenic, liver or lymph node enlargement may be noted, in addition to prostatic or testicular abnormalities.

Serologic testing may be used to screen dogs as part of breeder and kennel management, for diagnosis of disease and for monitoring response to treatment. Seroconversion can be noted 1–4 weeks post-infection. Both false-positive (typically due to cross-reaction with other bacteria) and false-negative results are a concern with currently available assays. False negatives may occur with early infection and lack of (or limited) antibody response. Confirmation of positive results is critical, particularly before instituting any kennel culling or changes in breeding programs.

Screening tests include the quick and readily available RSAT and the 2-mercaptoethanol modified (ME) RSAT. The tube agglutination test (TAT) can provide quantitative antibody results. Agar gel immunodiffusion (AGID) is frequently used to confirm positive RSAT, ME-RSAT or TAT results. Indirect IFA and ELISA tests are also available; however, false negatives are a concern with IFA and the ELISA is considered more specific.[14] Positive screening test results (RSAT or ME-RSAT) are ideally confirmed with blood culture, AGID or a validated PCR or ELISA.[9]

PCR for *B. canis* DNA can be performed on semen, urine or blood, and will detect either live or dead organisms.

Therapy

Therapy rarely results in complete elimination of the organism. Antimicrobial therapy is advised in conjunction with neutering. Doxycycline (10–15 mg/kg q12h) for 1–2 months, together with an aminoglycoside (streptomycin 20 mg/kg IM q24h) for 1–2 weeks, is thought to be most successful, although clear data are lacking. Anecdotally, enrofloxacin has been used to maintain fertility; however, dogs continued to shed *B. canis*.[15] Additional therapy (e.g. analgesia, level of nursing care) will vary depending on degree of debilitation.

After therapy, retesting is recommended until a negative test result has been achieved.[9] After this time, reassessment with serology every 4–6 months to monitor for relapse should occur. Antimicrobial therapy can reduce antibody titers and improve serologic results; however, relapses are common.

Prognosis/complications

Prognosis is considered guarded and eradication of disease is extremely difficult. Dogs with diskospondylitis can make a complete clinical recovery but remain seropositive, and are considered infected for life. Owners must be counseled regarding zoonotic concerns, and breeders must understand the risk of continued exposure in their breeding population. Recovery from clinical brucellosis does not protect from future infections.

Prevention

Prevention through monitoring, quarantine and elimination of infected dogs is the most effective strategy. A minimum of annual testing of breeding dogs and quarantine pending assessment of all new dogs before kennel entry is advised. At the optimum, two negative screening tests (30 days apart) would occur before admission. This translates into an 8- to 12-week isolation period.[9] For breeding facilities, testing 3–4 weeks before breeding or AI is advised.

Rehoming of dogs with known *B. canis* or from kennels where *B. canis* status is unknown is not recommended, unless confirmation of negative status (prior to new ownership and repeated 6–8 weeks later) can be performed.

CANINE TRANSMISSIBLE VENEREAL TUMOR
J Paul Woods and Michelle Evason

Definition

Canine transmissible venereal tumor (CTVT) is a transmissible round cell neoplasm usually spread by coitus. It is less commonly spread by licking, biting and sniffing tumor-affected areas.[16]

Etiology and pathogenesis

CTVTs are infectious, clonally transmissible, round cell neoplasms usually spread as an allograft of cancer cells through breeding, and less commonly by licking, biting and sniffing tumor-affected areas. Transmission occurs via exfoliation and implantation of viable tumor cells on to abraded genital mucosa.[17] Lesions generally appear within 2–6 months of mating, and may grow slowly (over years), unpredictably or invasively, eventually becoming malignant and metastatic. The most common sites of infection are the external genitalia, but others include the nasal and oral cavities, subcutaneous tissues and eyes.

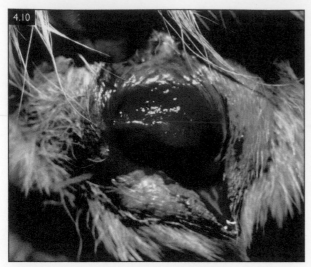

Fig. 4.10 Transmissible venereal tumor in the vagina. (Courtesy of Claudia Barton)

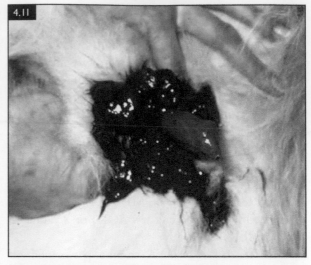

Fig. 4.11 Transmissible venereal tumor affecting the caudal aspect of the penis. (Courtesy of Claudia Barton)

Lesions are typically localized; however, metastasis can occur in 5–17% of cases. Common metastasis sites include draining regional lymph nodes (e.g. inguinal, iliac, tonsils), subcutaneous tissue, skin, eyes, oral mucosa, liver, spleen, peritoneum, hypophysis, brain and bone marrow.

Incidence and risk factors

CTVT has a worldwide distribution with its highest prevalence in tropical and subtropical areas. In enzootic areas, where breeding is poorly controlled and there are high numbers of free-roaming, sexually active dogs, CTVT is the most common canine tumor.

Because CTVT is primarily spread by coitus, free roaming, sexually intact mature dogs are at greatest risk. There is no sex predilection (except entire vs. neutered) and no heritable breed-related predisposition. In endemic areas, CTVT is most common (80% of cases) in dogs 2–5 years of age.

Clinical signs

In most cases neoplastic foci can be detected on the genitalia. The tumor is cauliflower like, pedunculated, nodular, papillary or multilobulated, ranging in size from small nodules (1–3 mm) to large masses (10–15 cm). The mass is firm but friable; the surface is often ulcerated and inflamed and may be hemorrhagic and infected. The tumor may occur deep in the prepuce or vagina and be difficult to see, so that bleeding may be misdiagnosed as estrus, urethritis, cystitis or prostatitis. In female dogs, the lesions are usually located in the posterior vestibule or vagina (**Fig. 4.10**). In male dogs, lesions are usually on the caudal part of the penis, requiring caudal retraction of the penile sheath for visualization (**Fig. 4.11**). The tumor often oozes a serosanguineous or hemorrhagic fluid. CTVT may also develop at extragenital sites such as skin, subcutis, oral and nasal cavities, eyes and anus, although most are secondary to genital lesions.

Metastasis occurs occasionally to draining regional lymph nodes, subcutaneous tissue, skin, eyes, oral mucosa, liver, spleen, peritoneum, hypophysis, brain and bone marrow. Because CTVT is also transmitted by licking, sniffing and biting, many cases of reported metastases may actually be spread by mechanical extension or auto- or hetero-transplantation.

Extragenital lesions can cause sneezing, epistaxis, epiphora, halitosis, tooth loss, exophthalmos, skin masses, facial deformation, regional lymph node enlargement, neurologic deficits and behavioral changes.

Diagnosis

Diagnosis of CTVT is based on environmental history, signalment, history, clinical signs, physical

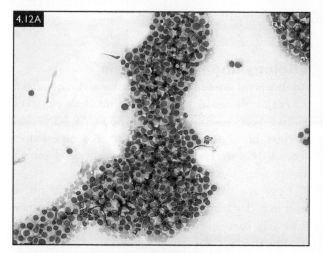
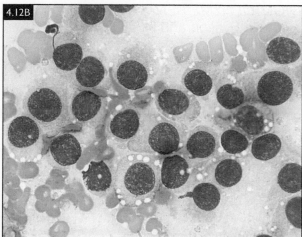

Fig. 4.12 Low (A) and high (B) magnification of transmissible venereal tumor cytology. (Courtesy of Claudia Barton)

findings, cytologic examination of cells obtained by swabs, fine-needle aspiration (FNA) or imprint of the tumors, and/or histologic examination of a biopsy from the mass.

Characteristic cytology typically confirms the diagnosis. Exfoliative cytology demonstrates uniform, discrete, round-to-polyhedral-shaped cells with moderately abundant pale blue cytoplasm and an eccentrically located nucleus, with occasional binucleation and mitotic figures (**Fig. 4.12**). Single or multiple nucleoli are often observed, surrounded by clumped chromatin. The most characteristic feature is the presence of numerous, discrete, clear cytoplasmic vacuoles.

Histopathology can show compact masses of round or polyhedral cells with slightly granular, vacuolated, eosinophilic cytoplasm. Neoplastic cells are arranged in a diffuse pattern and supported by thin trabeculae of fibrovascular tissue.

Specific molecular techniques (e.g. *in situ* PCR of the rearranged *LINE-c-myc* gene sequence) can confirm the diagnosis but are rarely needed.

Therapy

In most cases CTVT remains localized and rarely becomes disseminated in an immunocompetent host.

Chemotherapy is the treatment of choice. Single agent vincristine (0.5–0.7 mg/m² or 0.025 mg/kg IV) once weekly for 3–6 treatments (1 treatment past clinical remission) can result in complete and durable response in most cases (90–95%). Resistant cases can be treated with doxorubicin (25–30 mg/m² IV q21 days for 3 treatments). Other protocols have employed cyclophosphamide, vinblastine, methotrexate, L-asparaginase and prednisolone.

Surgical excision (cryosurgery) and radiation therapy can be effective, particularly for chemoresistant cases.

In some cases, lesions can spontaneously regress. However, spontaneous regression is uncommon and has been associated with immune responses against the tumor.

Prognosis

Prognosis for complete remission with chemotherapy (vincristine) or radiation is excellent. Spontaneous regression usually starts within 3–6 months after implantation of cancer cells, and prognosis is good in these cases. However, self-regression is unlikely if tumors are present for over 9 months.

Prevention

In regions free of CTVT occasional cases occur following travel of dogs to or from endemic areas. Therefore, veterinarians may act as the first line of defense against the introduction of CTVT into nonendemic areas.

DIOCTOPHYME RENALE (GIANT KIDNEY WORM)
Michelle Evason and Jinelle A Webb

Definition
Dioctophyme renale is a large nematode (30–60 cm) that may infect and destroy the kidneys of dogs and rarely cats. Mild dysuria with hematuria can be present, although in most animals infection is discovered incidentally during abdominal surgical procedures.

Species affected
Dogs, foxes, mink, ferrets, otters and other fish-eating carnivores can be infected. It is rarely reported in cats, pigs, horses and humans.

Etiology and pathogenesis
Adult worms are red–purple in color and range from 30 cm to 60 cm in length. The life cycle can take up to 2 years to complete, and the prepatent period is thought to be 155 days. Winter temperatures (i.e. <10°C) are less favorable for egg development and prolong the life cycle.

Eggs are passed in the urine of the definitive host (e.g. dog), ingested by the annelid intermediate host (e.g. earthworm) and may develop into third- or fourth-stage larvae (**Fig. 4.13**). Alternatively,

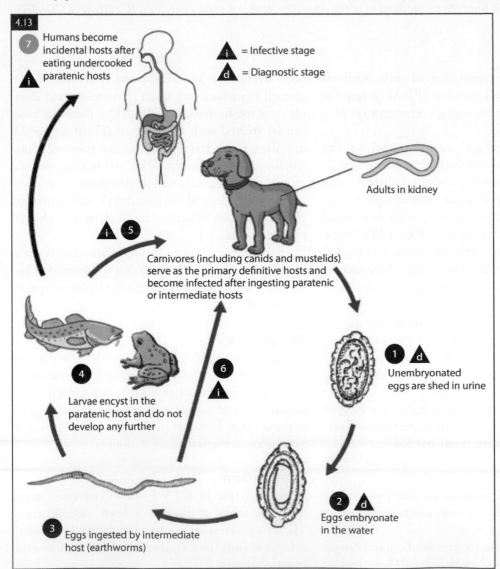

4.13

7 Humans become incidental hosts after eating undercooked paratenic hosts

i = Infective stage
d = Diagnostic stage

Adults in kidney

5 Carnivores (including canids and mustelids) serve as the primary definitive hosts and become infected after ingesting paratenic or intermediate hosts

1 **d** Unembryonated eggs are shed in urine

4 Larvae encyst in the paratenic host and do not develop any further

6 **i**

2 **d** Eggs embryonate in the water

3 Eggs ingested by intermediate host (earthworms)

Fig. 4.13 Life cycle of *Dioctophyme renale*. (Courtesy of Centers for Disease Control and Prevention)

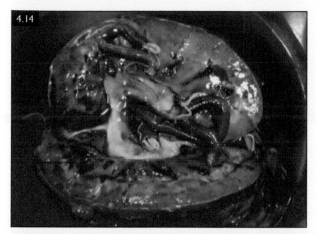

Fig. 4.14 *Dioctophyme renale* in the kidney of a dog after nephrectomy. (Courtesy of Dinaz Nagawalla)

frogs or fish (paratenic hosts) may ingest annelids, and larvae can encyst and develop into the third or fourth stage within these hosts. After the dog (or another definitive host) consumes infected fish, frogs or annelids, the larvae leave the intestinal tract and migrate to the kidney (**Fig. 4.14**). Maturation occurs, and the adult worms gradually destroy the kidney parenchyma. The right kidney is more likely to be affected than the left, possibly owing to its proximity to the duodenum.[18] The affected kidney may become a distended sac containing one to four adult worms. Rarely, the sac ruptures and worms can be found in the abdominal cavity with (or without) concurrent peritonitis. Worms may also be found in the bladder, entwined around a liver lobe or encysted within the abdominal cavity.[18–20]

Geography
This parasite can be found throughout North and South America and Asia.[18–20]

Prevalence, incidence and risk factors
Prevalence and incidence are largely unknown. Urinary prevalence and seroprevalence have been reported as 14% and 16%, respectively, in apparently healthy dogs in one endemic region.[18] However, the incidence of active infestation appears to be very low in most regions.

Consuming a diet high in raw fish, indiscriminate eating and ingestion of annelids, fish or frogs, outdoor lifestyle (e.g. stray, feral, hunting dogs), and living near rivers, lakes and streams are risk factors.[18, 21] Bitches were more likely to be affected in one study.[18]

Clinical signs
Most infected dogs have no clinical signs. Those with more advanced disease may display lower urinary tract signs (e.g. dysuria, hematuria, pollakiuria), lumbar pain, weight loss, palpable renomegaly, fever or signs consistent with renal failure.[19–21]

Diagnosis
Diagnosis is usually based on incidental identification of eggs in the urine or adult worms during exploratory laparotomy.

Hematology and biochemistry
The CBC and serum biochemistry are usually normal, or may be consistent with inflammation (e.g. neutrophilia with left shift, lymphopenia, eosinophilia).[19, 22] Findings consistent with renal disease (e.g. elevated urea or creatinine) are rare because of compensation by the other kidney;[22] however, those may be noted with advanced disease.

Urinalysis may reveal eggs and inflammation, e.g. hematuria, proteinuria.[22]

Cytology
Urine sediment cytology may show ovoid (lemon-shaped) eggs with a thick pitted shell (**Fig. 4.15**).

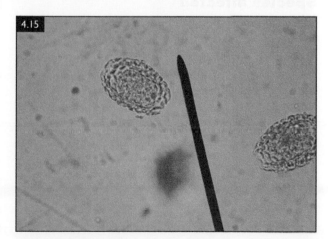

Fig. 4.15 *Dioctophyme renale*. Note the characteristic pitted and sculped shell. (Courtesy of Froggerlaura at English Wikipedia)

Eggs appear only when a gravid female worm is present. A negative finding does not rule out infection.

Imaging

Radiographs may be normal or show an enlarged kidney. Abdominal ultrasound may reveal a cyst-like ring- or band (worm)-filled structure within the kidney(s), loss (partial or complete) of normal kidney architecture or a cyst-filled sac within the peritoneal cavity.[19, 20, 22] CT (plain and contrast) has been used successfully to identify worms in the kidney and abdomen and determine the extent of renal destruction.[20] A skilled interpreter is required to avoid false-positive findings (e.g. confusion with intestinal loops or rings).

Serological testing

Serology (indirect enzyme-linked immunosorbent assay [ELISA]) may be useful in diagnosis, particularly for dogs that are infected with immature forms, male worms or have ectopic (outside the kidney) infection.[18, 23]

Therapy

Therapy consists of surgical removal of worms and frequently the affected kidney.[19, 22] A pyelogram may aid assessment of kidney function before consideration of removal. Removal of worms found within the abdomen is advised in cases of peritonitis.

Prognosis/complications

Prognosis can be excellent with early identification of infection and surgical removal. Clinical improvement is typically noted within a few days of therapy, and the unaffected (usually left) kidney is able to compensate without impact on clinical or laboratory function.[19, 22]

Prevention

Reduction of raw fish in the diet may reduce the incidence of infection.

FUNGAL URINARY TRACT INFECTION
Michelle Evason

Definition

Fungal infections rarely occur in the upper or lower urinary tracts.

Species affected

Dogs and cats.

Etiology and pathogenesis

Candida spp. are most often involved. Infection can occur via ascending infection or hematogenously. Subclinical infections may occur. As with bacteria, the presence of fungi in a urine sample does not, by itself, indicate the presence of disease or necessitate therapy.

Incidence and risk factors

Infections are rare and poorly described. They are typically associated with a breakdown in normal host defense mechanisms or concurrent immuno-suppression (e.g. corticosteroid therapy). Infections are most commonly reported in complex cases, often with indwelling devices (e.g. subcutaneous urethral bypass) and long-term or recurrent antimicrobial exposure.

Clinical signs

Clinical signs are indistinguishable from bacterial cystitis, and attributable to lower urinary tract inflammation (e.g. dysuria) or pyelonephritis (e.g. acute kidney injury).

Diagnosis

Fungi are usually apparent cytologically (**Fig. 4.16**). Fungal culture should be performed when cytology is indicative of fungal infection.

Therapy

Treatment can be challenging because of the complex nature of most cases and the common presence of an indwelling device. Removal or replacement of any devices is ideal.

Fungal susceptibility testing results can guide treatment, when available. Not all available antifungals are excreted in urine. Fluconazole is the drug of choice, but amphotericin B can also be used (*Table 4.3*). Drugs such as itraconazole that are not highly excreted in urine should not be used for cystitis; however, they can be used for pyelonephritis because tissue, not urine, drug levels are important for this location. This strategy (e.g. using itraconazole) is typically reserved for cases when fluconazole cannot be used.

Prevention

Prevention is difficult as this is an uncommon infection, typically occurring in high-risk patients. Managing underlying comorbidities and good maintenance of indwelling devices are the main preventive measures.

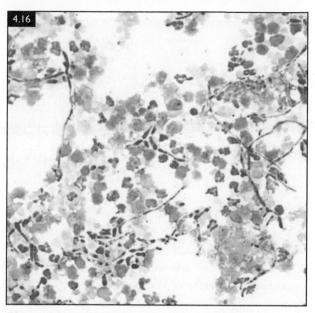

Fig. 4.16 Funguria in a cat with *Candida* urinary tract infection. (Courtesy of Allyson Berent)

Table 4.3 **Antifungal therapy for urinary tract infections**

DRUG	DOSE	COMMENT
Fluconazole	5–10 mg/kg PO q24h	Drug of choice
Amphotericin B (lipid complex)	Dogs: 1–3.3 mg/kg IV over 2 h q48h to total cumulative dose of 24–30 mg/kg	Reasonable option for upper and lower urinary tract infections, but greater risk of adverse effects
	Cats: 1 mg/kg IV over 2 h q48h to total cumulative dose of 12 mg/kg	
Flucytosine	25–50 mg/kg PO q6h or 50–65 mg/kg PO q8h	Rarely used. A potential option for resistant pyelonephritis when renal function is still acceptable
Itraconazole	Dogs: 5–10 mg/kg PO q12h	Low and variable urine levels. Not appropriate for cystitis
	Cats: 5 mg/kg PO q24h	

LEPTOSPIROSIS
Jinelle A Webb

Definition

Leptospirosis is a bacterial infection that often results in kidney or liver disease, sometimes with compromise of other body systems. It is considered a re-emerging disease in many regions and can involve a variety of different serovars.

Species affected

Dogs (common) and cats (rare)

Etiology and pathogenesis

Leptospira spp. is a genus of highly motile obligate aerobic spirochetes (**Fig. 4.17**). Common pathogenic serovars and their main reservoir hosts are listed in *Table 4.4*. The bacteria are maintained within the renal tubules of reservoir hosts, which are predominantly wildlife but may include dogs (serovar Canicola) and cats (geographical variability in serovars).[24–26] Once excreted, the leptospires can

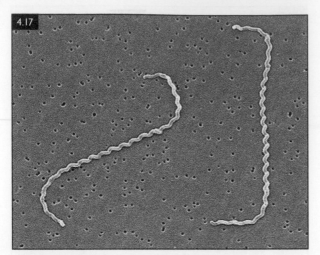

Fig. 4.17 Electron microscopy of *Leptospira* organisms. (Courtesy of Matthew Krecic).

remain viable for months in moist environments but die very quickly in dry environments. The highest incidence of leptospirosis in dogs occurs in October through December in northern temperate zones.[27–29]

Direct routes of infection are through abraded skin and intact mucous membranes. Indirect infection is through fomites such as drinking water bowls, food itself or food bowls, soil or bedding. The leptospiremic phase lasts approximately 7 days.

The pathogenicity of leptospires is because of their rapid multiplication within the blood and organs, which can result in kidney and/or liver disease, coagulopathy and vasculitis. Coagulopathy and vasculitis involving the lungs can lead to leptospiral pulmonary hemorrhage syndrome (**Fig. 4.18**), which appears to be more prevalent in Europe.[30]

Geography
Worldwide, with regional variation in incidence and serovars based on climate and reservoir host populations.

Incidence and risk factors
Incidence is regionally variable for dogs, and the disease is rare in cats. Risk increases with: exposure to wildlife; proximity to urban centers; outdoor activity; exposure to water/areas of flooding especially after periods of higher rainfall; lower socioeconomic areas; living within 2.5 km of a university, college, park or forest; being aged 4–10 years; kenneled or shelter; and lack of *Leptospira* vaccination.[24, 26, 29, 31, 32]

Clinical signs
The type and severity of clinical signs vary with the virulence of the organism, the infecting serovar,

Table 4.4 **Common reservoir hosts for different *Leptospira* serovars**

| SEROVAR | RESERVOIR HOSTS | |
	PRIMARY	SECONDARY
Australis	Rat, mouse	Bandicoot
Autumnalis	Mouse	Rat, raccoon, opossum, bandicoot
Batavia	Dog, rat, mouse	Hedgehog, vole, armadillo, shrew, bandicoot
Bratislava	Rat, pig, horse?	Mouse, raccoon, opossum, hedgehog, vole, fox, skunk, bandicoot
Canicola	Dog	Rat, raccoon, hedgehog, armadillo, vole, skunk, bandicoot
Grippotyphosa	Raccoon, vole, skunk, opossum	Mouse, rat, fox, squirrel, bobcat, shrew, hedgehog, weasel, mole, muskrat, bandicoot
Hardjo	Cow	Wild bovidae
Icterohaemorrhagiae	Rat	Mouse, raccoon, opossum, hedgehog, fox, skunk, muskrat
Pomona	Cow, pig, skunk, opossum	Mouse, raccoon, hedgehog, wolf, fox, woodchuck, vole, sea lion
Zanoni	Rat, mouse	Bandicoot

Source: Adapted from Greene, CE *et al.* (2012) Leptospirosis. In *Infectious Diseases of the Dog and Cat*, 4th ed. CE Green, ed. Elsevier, St. Louis, MO, pp.431–47.

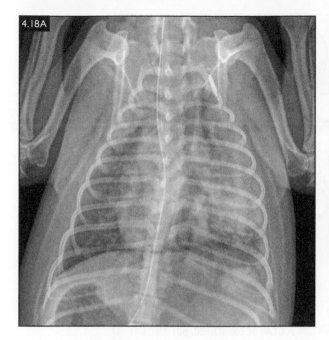

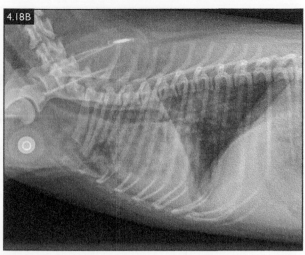

Fig. 4.18 Dorsoventral (A) and lateral (B) radiographs showing pulmonary leptospirosis in a dog.

host factors and the affected target organs. Most commonly, clinical signs are related to acute kidney disease, and therefore include polyuria/polydipsia or oliguria/anuria, vomiting, inappetence to anorexia, and lethargy. Acute liver disease may co-develop with acute kidney disease, sometimes resulting in jaundice. Less common are dyspnea, generalized or abdominal pain, and reluctance to move. Subclinical infections and chronic infections are also possible. Clinical signs may be vague early in the course of disease, with fever of unknown origin or depression being initially identified problems.

Diagnosis

Diagnosis of leptospirosis is typically confirmed with PCR or serology (**Fig. 4.19**, *Tables 4.5, 4.6*). PCR testing should be considered for patients that have not received an antimicrobial agent. Serological testing can be submitted simultaneously with PCR testing, when PCR testing is negative, or can be the sole test if a dog has received antimicrobial therapy. Serology test options include the patient-side (Witness™) IgM antibody test and IgG enzyme-linked immunosorbent assay (ELISA) testing for unvaccinated dogs, and acute and convalescent microscopic agglutination test (MAT) testing for

vaccinated dogs with a negative PCR test or those that have already received an antimicrobial. The Witness™ IgM antibody test can be used in dogs that have been vaccinated more than 3 months previously.

Laboratory abnormalities

Laboratory abnormalities vary with the infecting serovar, its virulence and the organs affected; they may include any or all of anemia, neutrophilia, lymphopenia, thrombocytopenia, hypoalbuminemia, azotemia, elevations in alanine aminotransferase (ALT), alkaline phosphatase (ALP) bilirubin, phosphorus or creatine kinase (CK), hyponatremia, hypochloremia, hypokalemia or hyperkalemia.

Urinalysis abnormalities commonly include hyposthenuria, mild-to-moderate proteinuria, glucosuria, pyuria, bilirubinuria and the presence of casts. Prolongation of prothrombin/partial thromboplastin time (PT/PTT), shortened PT and increased fibrinogen, D-dimer, fibrin degradation products (FDPs) and antithrombin may be present.

Imaging

Thoracic radiographic findings vary and are not specific to leptospirosis. Lung patterns may include

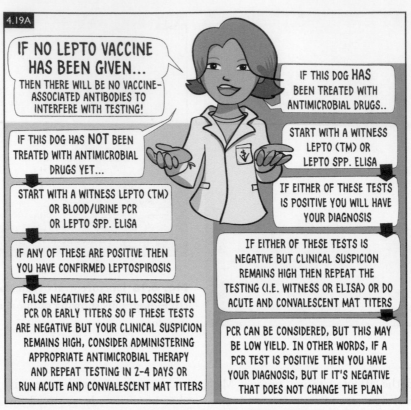

Fig. 4.19A Diagnosis of leptospirosis: dog not vaccinated against leptospirosis.

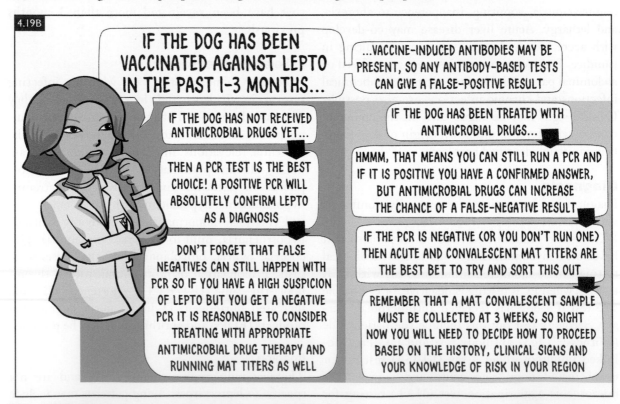

Fig. 4.19B Diagnosis of leptospirosis: dog vaccinated in the past 1–3 months against leptospirosis.

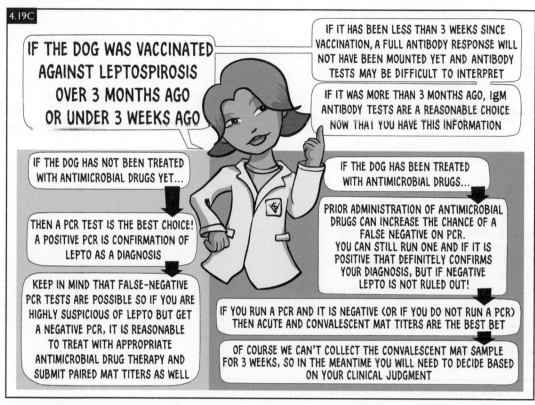

Fig. 4.19C Diagnosis of leptospirosis: dog vaccinated (<3 weeks or >3 months ago) against leptospirosis.

Table 4.5 **Comparison of testing options for leptospirosis**

	PCR	ELISA	ELISA	MAT
Target	Antigen (organism)	IgM antibodies	IgG antibodies	IgG and IgM antibodies
Qualitative or quantitative	Negative or positive only	Negative or positive only	Negative or positive only	Provides titers
Affected by antimicrobial use	Yes	No	No	No
Affected by vaccination	No	For 1–3 months	For months to years	For months to years
Turnaround time	~24 hours	30 minutes	~24 hours	7–35 days
Performance early in course of disease (i.e. with acute disease)	Fair, some false-negative results	Fair to good, may need repeat test (false negative)	Fair to poor	Fair, often need convalescent titer
Cost	$$–$$$	$	$$	$$$

Abbreviations: ELISA, enzyme-linked immunosorbent assay; Ig, immunoglobulin; MAT, microscopic agglutination test

Table 4.6 **Diagnostic options for leptospirosis**

Dog that has NOT received antimicrobials and is NOT vaccinated:
- Start with Witness Lepto™ in clinic, if available
- Otherwise *Leptospira* spp. ELISA and blood/urine PCR
  - If positive on any, treat as leptospirosis
  - If negative and clinical suspicion remains high, repeat testing in 2–4 days or do MAT; administer appropriate antimicrobials in case of a false negative

(Continued)

Table 4.6 **(Continued)**

Dog that has NOT received antimicrobials and HAS BEEN vaccinated in the previous 1–3 months:
- *Leptospira* spp. blood/urine PCR
  - If positive you have your diagnosis
  - If negative and clinical suspicion remains high, do MAT titers and administer appropriate antimicrobials in case of false-negative PCR

Dog that has received antimicrobials and is NOT vaccinated:
- Start with Witness Lepto™ in clinic, if available
- Otherwise *Leptospira* spp. ELISA
  - If positive on any, you have your diagnosis
  - If negative and clinical suspicion remains high, repeat testing or do MAT titers
- PCR can be considered but is low yield
  - If positive, you have a diagnosis

Dog that has received antimicrobials and HAS BEEN vaccinated in the previous 1–3 months:
- Acute and convalescent MAT titers
- Blood/urine PCR can be considered but is low yield
  - If positive, you have a diagnosis
- If clinical suspicion is reasonable, treat as leptospirosis while awaiting MAT results

Dog that has received antimicrobials and HAS BEEN vaccinated but not in the previous 1–3 months:
- Start with Witness Lepto™ in clinic, if available
- Otherwise acute and convalescent MAT titers
- PCR can be considered but is low yield
  - If positive, you have a diagnosis

Abbreviations: ELISA, enzyme-linked immunosorbent assay; MAT, microscopic agglutination test

nodular, diffuse, interstitial or alveolar (**Fig. 4.18**). In severely dyspneic dogs, lung changes may resemble those of bacterial pneumonia, blastomycosis or metastatic neoplasia.[26, 30]

Abdominal ultrasonographic findings are not specific to leptospirosis. Findings associated with the kidneys may include renomegaly, hyperechoic cortices, pyelectasia, prominent corticomedullary bands and perirenal effusion.

PCR

Leptospires can be detected in urine or blood by PCR, although urine testing gives a higher yield. Paired blood and urine samples are recommended to increase sensitivity. The rate of false-negative results is high, especially with previous antibiotic use.

Serology

Paired titers (acute and convalescent) obtained via the MAT are commonly used diagnostic tests for leptospirosis. Measurement of both acute and convalescent titers (i.e. paired sampling) is important,

especially in vaccinated animals, because post-vaccinal titers can be quite high (>1:6,400) and persist for months.[33, 34] A single high titer in an unvaccinated animal is suggestive but not diagnostic. A negative acute titer may be noted within the first week of illness. The serovar with the highest titer cannot be assumed to be the infecting serovar, and it is typical to see an increase in several serovars, even in non-vaccinated dogs.

An in-clinic antibody ELISA is available that detects IgM, which is formed early in the course of infection.[35, 36] The results are qualitative (positive or negative) and the infecting serovar is not identified. This test can be used in vaccinated animals, unless the vaccine was administered within the previous 2–3 months, in which case a false positive is possible. If a negative test is received and clinical suspicion remains high, the test should be repeated in 3–5 days in case the animal seroconverts in this time. The Witness™ test appeared to perform better than the ELISA early in the course of infection.[36] A positive test in an unvaccinated animal is strongly supportive of a diagnosis of leptospirosis. As IgM levels drop within weeks of infection, this test is not likely to be useful in uncommon cases of chronic leptospirosis.

An ELISA is also available that detects the lipoprotein LipL32, the most abundant lipoprotein on the surface of pathogenic leptospires. The results are qualitative (positive or negative) and the infecting serovar is not identified. Vaccinated animals are very likely to have a positive ELISA test, limiting the utility of this test in vaccinated animals. If a negative test is received and clinical suspicion remains high, the test should be repeated in 1 week in case the animal seroconverts in this time. A positive test in an unvaccinated animal is strongly supportive of a diagnosis of leptospirosis.

Therapy

An appropriate antimicrobial should be started after obtaining specimens for PCR testing but as soon as leptospirosis is suspected. This is to increase the chance of patient recovery and reduce zoonotic concerns. Currently, doxycycline or penicillin is recommended, with doxycycline (5 mg/kg PO q12h) most commonly used.[24, 26] In patients that cannot tolerate an oral antimicrobial because of ongoing anorexia or vomiting, an intravenously administered penicillin such as ampicillin (22 mg/kg IV q8h or 20 mg/kg IV q6h, reducing the dose for dogs with severe azotemia) may be needed. Once formerly anorexic dogs begin eating, and vomiting ceases, they can be transitioned to oral doxycycline. All infected dogs should receive the appropriate dose of doxycycline for 2 weeks to prevent chronic renal colonization and persistent leptospiruria.[24, 26]

Prognosis/complications

Most dogs have a good prognosis with appropriate, timely therapy. Survival rates for dogs with acute kidney disease are approximately 80%.[24] Kidney function may not return to normal for some dogs. These cases can be successfully managed in a similar way to dogs with chronic kidney disease. Complications associated with acute leptospirosis resulting in poor prognosis include anuric kidney disease, disseminated intravascular coagulation and pulmonary hemorrhage resulting in respiratory failure.

Prevention

Avoiding contaminated environments is the most effective way to reduce the risk of leptospirosis. However, with increased urbanization of the environment and encroachment into areas with abundant wildlife, avoiding contaminated areas is challenging. Avoiding areas with a high density of wildlife and slow-moving water is recommended. Suburban and urban small breed dogs are at risk because of sufficient contact with small water sources (e.g. puddles) and the potential high density of wild animals (e.g. raccoons) in some urban areas, especially parks.

Annual vaccination is effective at reducing the incidence and severity of clinical leptospirosis, and may reduce leptospiruria, thereby reducing contamination of the environment.[37] Vaccines available in North America currently contain four serovars (Grippotyphosa, Canicola, Icterohaemorrhagiae and Pomona), and are referred to as quadrivalent vaccines. Bivalent vaccines are more typical in Europe, containing two serovars (Canicola and Icterohaemorrhagiae), although there is a movement toward the use of quadrivalent vaccines.

Recovery from clinical leptospirosis does not protect against future infections; therefore, vaccinate upon recovery to lessen the risk of future infections. Vaccination should be considered for all dogs in endemic regions.

Public health and infection control

Although *Leptospira* spp. can be transmitted from infected dogs to humans, this has been only rarely reported.[24, 38] Infectious disease precautions should be taken with known or suspected leptospirosis cases, including clearly identifying all possible cases, avoiding contact with urine, taking care when moving the patient within the hospital, and limiting where the patient is permitted to urinate (**Fig. 4.20**).

Leptospires are easily killed with routine disinfectants and through desiccation. As dogs are unlikely to shed bacteria in their urine after 48 hours of antimicrobial use, treated animals

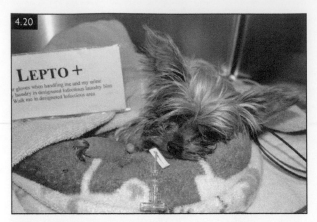

Fig. 4.20 Example of infection control signage for leptospirosis cases.

are often considered non-infectious by this time. Bathing the animal before ending enhanced infection control practices is reasonable in case there are viable leptospires living on the haircoat from urine contamination. However, it has been suggested that more study is needed to determine an accurate duration of leptospiruria after initiation of appropriate antimicrobial therapy.[26]

Clients should be instructed to avoid contact with their dog's urine for cases discharged from hospital before 48 hours of antimicrobial use. In addition, they should be counseled on the zoonotic potential of *Leptospira* spp. Although the risk of contracting the infection from their own pet is minimal, there is potential for exposure of both the human family and other pets in the shared environment. Recent consensus panels in the USA and Europe recommend a 2-week course of doxycycline for any dogs living in a household where a pet has been diagnosed with leptospirosis.[24, 26] This is probably more relevant for treatment of infection acquired from the same environment as the infected patient, rather than prevention of dog-to-dog transmission.

PROSTATITIS
Michelle Evason

Definition
Prostatitis is an infection of the prostate. It is almost always bacterial in origin and can be a difficult disease to manage.

Species affected
Dogs. Cats are rarely affected.

Etiology and pathogenesis
Prostatitis almost exclusively occurs in intact males and is typically associated with ascending infection from the urinary tract. Gram-negative bacteria such as *Escherichia coli* are most commonly involved, but streptococci and staphylococci can also cause disease.

Incidence and risk factors
The incidence is not well defined and varies regionally, in large part based on the prevalence of intact males. Intact status is the main risk factor. Prostatitis (acute or chronic) should be considered likely in any intact male dog with cystitis.

Clinical signs
Physical examination may be unremarkable, depending on the degree of systemic inflammation, prostatic enlargement and associated bacterial cystitis. Fever, weight loss, lethargy, purulent genital discharge and loss of appetite may be present. Signs of lower urinary tract disease may be noted, depending on the presence of concurrent cystitis and/or dysuria caused by an enlarged or abscessed prostate. A stiff gait may be observed. Sepsis is rare but can occur. Chronic cases may have mild to no clinical signs.

An enlarged and painful prostate may be palpable per rectum, but palpation cannot rule out prostatic disease because a palpably enlarged prostate is not always present. Care must be taken during palpation when a prostatic abscess is suspected to avoid rupture.

Diagnosis
Palpation of the prostate per rectum, CBC, serum biochemical profile, urinalysis and urine culture should be performed in all suspected cases. Hematologic evidence of acute or chronic infection may be present.

Diagnostic imaging

Ultrasonographic imaging is indicated to assess the size and structure of the prostate. In addition to detection of an enlarged prostate, it may help differentiate abscessation from neoplasia.

Dogs with prostatitis typically have normal radiographs; however, prostatic abscesses can cause prostatomegaly. Prostatic mineralization in a neutered dog should prompt further diagnostics to determine whether neoplasia is present.

Prostatic fluid evaluation

The third fraction of the ejaculate, fluid collected by urethral catheterization or fluid collected by fine-needle aspiration should be obtained. Suppurative inflammation is typically identified (**Fig. 4.21**). Culture of this fluid should also be performed. If discordant results are obtained from urine and prostatic fluid culture, prostatic fluid should be considered the relevant result unless contamination is suspected.

Brucella canis serology

This should be considered in all cases, particularly in dogs from endemic regions and when the animal will be used for breeding.

Therapy

Therapy involves selection of an appropriate antimicrobial with adequate penetration into the prostate and excellent gram-negative spectrum. Fluoroquinolones are the most common empirical choices, although trimethoprim sulfonamides are also reasonable. Changes can be made on the basis of culture results, but only drugs that cross the blood–prostate barrier well should be considered (e.g. fluoroquinolones, trimethoprim, clindamycin, macrolides). Four weeks of treatment is recommended for acute prostatitis, with 4–6 weeks for chronic cases.

Prostatic abscesses require surgical treatment, although careful ultrasound-guided drainage, together with antimicrobial therapy, may be performed for small abscesses (<2.5 cm). Castration is advised for all dogs with prostatitis. Other medical approaches such as finasteride, androgen receptor antagonists or gonadotropin-releasing hormone (GnRH) agonists can be considered, but are less useful in cases that are complicated by prostatic cysts or abscesses.

Prognosis

Prognosis is worsened by the presence of abscesses, neoplasia or cysts, and client unwillingness to castrate. Clinical cure is possible, particularly in acute cases.

Prevention

Neutering is the most effective preventive measure. Beyond that, addressing any comorbidities that predispose to bacterial cystitis would probably reduce the risk of prostatitis.

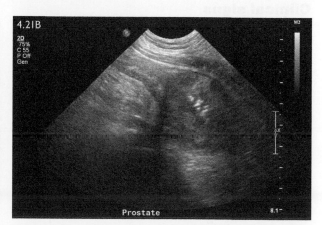

Fig. 4.21A, B Ultrasound examination of a male Labrador Retriever with a hypoechoic and enlarged prostate, with a small nodule and concurrent mineralization indicative of prostatitis and neoplasia. (Courtesy of Atlantic Veterinary College)

PYELONEPHRITIS
Michelle Evason

Definition
Pyelonephritis is a bacterial infection of the kidneys (renal pelvis and parenchyma).

Species affected
Dogs and cats.

Etiology and pathogenesis
Pyelonephritis is most often due to *Escherichia coli*,[39] likely due to the presence of bacterial adhesins that stick to the renal tubules, and also specific virulence factors. Other Enterobacteriaceae (e.g. *Enterobacter* spp.) may also be involved. Infection of the renal parenchyma can occur through ascending or hematogenous routes. The relative importance of each is unclear.

Incidence and risk factors
The incidence of pyelonephritis is unclear because definitive diagnosis can be a challenge.[39] It is potentially overdiagnosed but, because of the potential severity, it must be considered in animals with acute kidney injury. Risk factors are not well understood. Concurrent inflammatory and infectious diseases such as hepatitis, pancreatitis and pyometra were common in one case series.[39]

Clinical signs
Non-specific signs predominate, such as fever, anorexia, lethargy, vomiting, abdominal pain, diarrhea and dehydration.[39] These can be from pyelonephritis or underlying diseases. Cystitis is not necessarily present concurrently so there may be no outward evidence of urinary tract disease. Fever is potentially the most important clinical sign.[39]

Diagnosis
Diagnosis can be a challenge because a gold standard test is lacking, signs can be vague and non-specific, and it is difficult to rule out pyelonephritis. This likely leads to overdiagnosis, particularly in patient populations where renal disease and subclinical bacteriuria are common (e.g. geriatric cats).

Urinalysis
Pyuria, hematuria, bacteriuria and a reduced urine specific gravity are present in the majority of cases.[39]

Hematology
Azotemia and an inflammatory leukogram are common, but not always present.[39] Other changes may occur as a result of renal failure, such as hyponatremia, hypochloremia and alterations in serum potassium.

Culture
Culture is a critical part of both diagnosis and treatment selection. Cystocentesis samples should be collected, whenever possible.[8] Blood cultures may also be performed, particularly when fever is present, but they are of low yield. Pyelocentesis is often overlooked as a diagnostic test, and it can be particularly useful for confirmation of pyelonephritis.

Diagnostic imaging
Pyelectasia and hydroureter are the most common abnormalities (**Figs. 4.22, 4.23**).[39] However, these can be found in patients with other diseases or as a consequence of intravenous fluid therapy.[40]

Therapy
Therapy should begin once pyelonephritis is suspected and before culture and susceptibility results

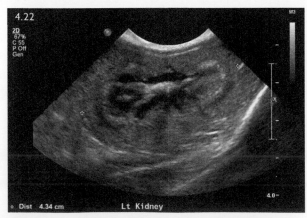

Fig. 4.22 Ultrasound examination of a female cat with an enlarged left kidney and left renal pelvis dilation secondary to *E. coli* pyelonephritis. (Courtesy of Atlantic Veterinary College)

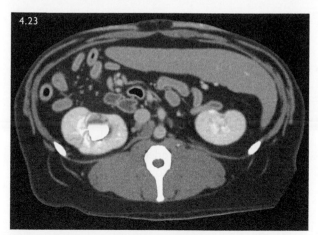

Fig. 4.23 CT image of a young female dog with ectopic ureters and concurrent *E. coli* pyelonephritis, revealing bilateral dilation of the renal pelves and ureters. (Courtesy of Atlantic Veterinary College)

are obtained. Unless there is reason to suspect otherwise (e.g. known infection at another body site), empirical treatment should target *E. coli*.[8] Efficacy is dependent on serum, not urine, antimicrobial levels, so some drugs that are useful for *E. coli* cystitis because of their ability to concentrate in the urine (e.g. amoxicillin ± clavulanic acid) should not be used for pyelonephritis. A fluoroquinolone is the most logical choice in most situations, for a duration of 10–14 days. Supportive care is dependent on the presence and severity of renal failure, as well as any comorbidities.

Prevention

Prevention is difficult and involves control of comorbidities and factors that might increase the risk of ascending infection or bacterial translocation.

PYOMETRA
Michelle Evason

Definition

Pyometra is a bacterial infection of the uterus, a condition that can be life threatening.

Species affected

Dogs and cats. Dogs are much more commonly affected.

Etiology and pathogenesis

Pyometra is thought to occur secondary to cystic endometrial hyperplasia, subsequent to a rise in serum progesterone levels. Ascending infection then occurs, most often with *Escherichia coli*. Other bacteria, including various gram-negative organisms, streptococci, staphylococci and anaerobes, are less commonly involved.

Geography

Pyometra occurs worldwide.

Risk factors

Pyometra typically occurs in middle-aged to older intact female dogs and cats. By 10 years of age, pyometra will have developed in roughly 25% of intact bitches.[41]

Clinical signs

Pyometra may be acute or chronic. Fever, dehydration, depression, anorexia, and abdominal or generalized pain may be present. In open-cervix pyometra purulent vaginal discharge may be noted, although this is absent in closed-cervix pyometra cases. Sepsis or shock may be present concurrently. Uterine rupture may occur in severe cases, resulting in severe septic peritonitis. Care must be taken during abdominal palpation to avoid uterine rupture.

Diagnosis
Hematology
The CBC results are variable and may range from normal to evidence of severe or chronic infection. Serum biochemical changes tend to be non-specific.

Diagnostic imaging
Imaging is critical for diagnosis. Ultrasound is more sensitive than radiographs but either is acceptable. An enlarged, fluid-filled uterus with a thickened wall is evident.

Bacterial culture

Culture specimens should be obtained from patients with open pyometra. Fine-needle aspiration of the uterus is not advised in pets with suspect pyometra. Blood cultures may also be considered for patients with sepsis.

Urinalysis

Concurrent cystitis may occur and, if present, this should be managed as for bacterial cystitis. Cystocentesis is not recommended because of the potential for uterine rupture. Urine cultures do not necessarily indicate or reflect the cause of pyometra.

Therapy

Supportive care may be required depending on the degree of systemic disease and whether evidence of sepsis is present. Prompt surgical removal of the uterus is indicated. Care must be taken during surgery owing to the high risk of uterine rupture and consequent peritonitis.

Prompt broad-spectrum antimicrobial therapy (e.g. ampicillin and a fluoroquinolone) is indicated in patients with systemic signs of disease. In stable patients, perioperative antimicrobials (preoperative, ± 24 h postoperative) are adequate because the source of infection has been removed.

Medical therapy, such as with prostaglandin $F_{2\alpha}$, can be tried in open-cervix pyometra when patients are otherwise healthy. Antimicrobial choices should be based on culture of uterine discharge.

Prevention

Spaying is the most effective preventive measure.

REFERENCES

1 Kroemer, S et al. (2014) Antibiotic susceptibility of bacteria isolated from infections in cats and dogs throughout Europe (2002–2009). *Comp Immun Microbiol Infect Dis* **37**:97–108.

2 Boothe, D et al. (2012) Antimicrobial resistance and pharmacodynamics of canine and feline pathogenic *E. coli* in the United States. *J Am Anim Hosp Assoc* **48**:379–89.

3 Ball, KR et al. (2008) Antimicrobial resistance and prevalence of canine uropathogens at the Western College of Veterinary Medicine Veterinary Teaching Hospital, 2002–2007. *Can Vet J* **49**:985–90.

4 Mayer-Roenne, B et al. (2007) Urinary tract infections in cats with hyperthyroidism, diabetes mellitus and chronic kidney disease. *J Feline Med Surg* **9**:124–32.

5 Forrester, SD et al. (1999) Retrospective evaluation of urinary tract infection in 42 dogs with hyperadrenocorticism or diabetes mellitus or both. *J Vet Intern Med* **13**:557–60.

6 McGhie, JA et al. (2014) Prevalence of bacteriuria in dogs without clinical signs of urinary tract infection presenting for elective surgical procedures. *Aust Vet J* **92**:33–7.

7 Sorensen, TM et al. (2016) Evaluation of different sampling methods and criteria for diagnosing canine urinary tract infection by quantitative bacterial culture. *Vet J* **216**:168–73.

8 Weese, JS et al. (2011) Antimicrobial use guidelines for treatment of urinary tract infections in dogs and cats: antimicrobial guidlines working group of the International Society for Companion Animal Infectious Diseases. *Vet Med Int* **4**:1–9.

9 Makloski, CL (2011) Canine brucellosis management. *Vet Clin North Am Small Anim Pract* **41**:1209–19.

10 Flores-Castro, R et al. (1977) Canine brucellosis: bacteriological and serological investigation of naturally infected dogs in Mexico City. *J Clin Microbiol* **6**:591–7.

11 Kauffman, LK et al. (2014) Early detection of *Brucella canis* via quantitative polymerase chain reaction analysis. *Zoonoses Publ Health* **61**:48–54.

12 Brower, A et al. (2007) Investigation of the spread of *Brucella canis* via the U.S. interstate dog trade. *Int J Infect Dis* **11**:454–8.

13 Kerwin, SC et al. (1992) Diskospondylitis associated with *Brucella canis* infection in dogs: 14 cases (1980–1991). *J Am Vet Med Assoc* **201**:1253–7.

14 Hollett, RB (2006) Canine brucellosis: outbreaks and compliance. *Theriogenology* **66**:575–87.

15 Wanke, MM et al. (2006) Use of enrofloxacin in the treatment of canine brucellosis in a dog kennel (clinical trial). *Theriogenology* **66**:1573–8.

16 Ganguly, B et al. (2016) Canine transmissible venereal tumour: a review. *Vet Comp Oncol* **14**:1–12.

17 Ostrander, EA et al. (2016) Transmissible tumors: Breaking the cancer paradigm. *Trends Genet* **32**:1–15.

18 Pedrassani, D et al. (2017) *Dioctophyma renale*: prevalence and risk factors of parasitism in dogs of São Cristóvão district, Três Barras county, Santa Catarina State, Brazil. *Braz J Vet Parasitol* **26**:39–46.

19 Ferreira, VL *et al.* (2010) *Dioctophyme renale* in a dog: clinical diagnosis and surgical treatment. *Vet Parasitol* **168**:151–5.

20 Rahal, SC *et al.* (2014) Ultrasonographic, computed tomographic, and operative findings in dogs infested with giant kidney worms (*Dioctophyme renale*). *J Am Vet Med Assoc* **244**:555–8.

21 Nakagawa, TLDR *et al.* (2007) Giant kidney worm (*Dioctophyma renale*) infections in dogs from Northern Paraná, Brazil. *Vet Parasitol* **145**:366–70.

22 Mesquita, LR *et al.* (2014) Pre- and post-operative evaluations of eight dogs following right nephrectomy due to *Dioctophyma renale*. *Vet Q* **34**:167–71.

23 Pedrassani, D *et al.* (2015) Improvement of an enzyme immunosorbent assay for detecting antibodies against *Dioctophyma renale*. *Vet Parasitol* **212**:435–8.

24 Sykes, JE *et al.* (2011) 2010 ACVIM small animal consensus statement on leptospirosis: diagnosis, epidemiology, treatment, and prevention. *J Vet Intern Med* **25**:1–13.

25 Hartmann, K *et al.* (2013) *Leptospira* species infection in cats: ABCD guidelines on prevention and management. *J Feline Med Surg* **15**:576–81.

26 Schuller, S *et al.* (2015) European consensus statement on leptospirosis in dogs and cats. *J Small Anim Pract* **56**:159–79.

27 Alton, GD *et al.* (2009) Increase in seroprevalence of canine leptospirosis and its risk factors, Ontario 1998–2006. *Can J Vet Res* **73**:167–75.

28 Gautam, R *et al.* (2010) Spatial and spatio-temporal clustering of overall and serovar-specific *Leptospira* microscopic agglutination test (MAT) seropositivity among dogs in the United States from 2000 through 2007. *Prev Vet Med* **96**:122–31.

29 Lee, HS *et al.* (2014) Signalment changes in canine leptospirosis between 1970 and 2009. *J Vet Intern Med* **28**:294–9.

30 Kohn, B *et al.* (2010) Pulmonary abnormalities in dogs with leptospirosis. *J Vet Intern Med* **24**:1277–82.

31 Raghavan, RK *et al.* (2012) Evaluations of hydrologic risk factors for canine leptospirosis: 94 cases (2002–2009). *Prev Vet Med* **107**:1–5.

32 Raghavan, RK *et al.* (2012) Neighborhood-level socioeconomic and urban land use risk factors of canine leptospirosis: 94 cases (2002–2009). *Prev Vet Med* **106**:324–31.

33 Barr, SC *et al.* (2005) Serologic responses of dogs given a commercial vaccine against *Leptospira interrogans* serovar Pomona and *Leptospira kirschneri* serovar Grippotyphosa. *Am J Vet Res* **66**:1780–4.

34 Martin, LE *et al.* (2014) Vaccine-associated *Leptospira* antibodies in client-owned dogs. *J Vet Intern Med* **28**:789–92.

35 Lizer, J *et al.* (2017) Evaluation of a rapid IgM detection test for diagnosis of acute leptospirosis in dogs. *Vet Rec* **180**:517.

36 Lizer, J *et al.* (2018) Evaluation of 3 serological tests for early detection of *Leptospira*-specific antibodies in experimentally infected dogs. *J Vet Intern Med* **32**:201–7.

37 Andre-Fontaine, G *et al.* (2003) Comparison of the efficacy of three commercial bacterins in preventing canine leptospirosis. *Vet Rec* **153**:165–9.

38 Vincent, C *et al.* (2007) La leptospirose: Cas de transmission d'un chien a un humain. *Reseau d'Alerte et d'Information Zoosanitaire (RAIZO) Bulletin Zoosanitaire* [no. 51], Quebec City, QC.

39 Bouillon, J *et al.* (2018) Pyelonephritis in dogs: Retrospective study of 47 histologically diagnosed cases (2005–2015). *J Vet Intern Med* **32**:249–59.

40 D'Anjou, MA, *et al.* (2011) Clinical significance of renal pelvic dilatation on ultrasound in dogs and cats. *Vet Radiol Ultrasound* **52**:88–94.

41 Egenvall, A *et al.* (2001) Breed risk of pyometra in insured dogs in Sweden. *J Vet Intern Med* **15**:530–8.

SKIN AND SOFT TISSUE DISEASES

CHEYLETIELLA SPP. (CHEYLETIELLOSIS)
Michelle Evason and Anette Loeffler

Definition

Cheyletiellosis, or "walking dandruff", is a highly contagious skin surface mite infestation that predominantly affects dogs and cats.

Etiology and pathogenesis

The three main *Cheyletiella* spp. are *C. yasguri* (dogs), *C. blakei* (cats) and *C. parasitivorax* (rabbits, dogs and cats). All species are easily spread by direct contact with infected animals, subclinical carriers or through contact with contaminated materials (e.g. grooming equipment, bedding, leashes). Fleas, lice and flies may also carry the mite, and serve as a source of infection.[1]

Mites live in pseudotunnels in epidermal debris, and do not burrow. They actively move about on the hair, which has resulted in the name "walking dandruff". Eggs are attached to the hair shaft, and an entire life cycle (egg, larva, two nymphal stages and adult) is completed in about 35 days on a single host.

Geography

Worldwide.

Incidence and risk factors

Incidence is poorly described, but cheyletiellosis is uncommon in household dogs and cats. Subclinically infested dogs and cats can act as a source of infection. *Cheyletiella* spp. are most common in puppies, and in dogs and cats living in high-density housing (shelters, breeding facilities, catteries).[1] Adult dogs with a long duration of infestation (5–11 months) have been described.[2]

Common clinical signs

Both dogs and cats may be subclinical carriers with no overt signs. Clinical signs differ in dogs and cats. In dogs, diffuse scaling is most common (**Fig. 5.1**). Pruritus is typically mild, but may be severe in some individuals.[2, 3] In cats, crusted papules with an erythematous base (miliary dermatitis) are most common.[3, 4] These are often located on the dorsum and are typically pruritic. Initial signs are often dry scaling on the dorsum.

Diagnosis

A combination of direct exam (including handheld magnifying glasses) and cytologic examination of samples obtained by skin scraping, tape prep, hair plucks or vacuum cleaning is used to confirm infection.[2]

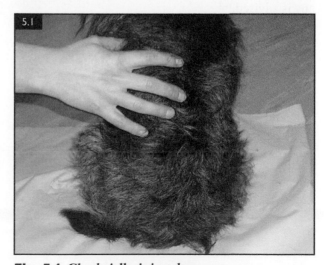

Fig. 5.1 Cheyletiellosis in a dog.

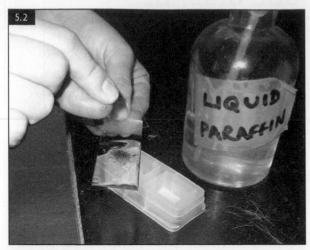

Fig. 5.2 Glass slide preparation for investigation of cheyletiellosis.

Table 5.1 **Treatment options for *cheyletiellosis***

AGENT	FORMULATION
Milbemycin	2 mg/kg PO weekly for 5–7 weeks
Ivermectin	Injections (0.2–0.3 mg/kg SC) repeated at 2-week intervals for 4–6 weeks
Fipronil	Spray (0.29%) applied to the whole dog every 2 weeks for 4–6 weeks, or 9.8% spot-on solution every 30 days, for 2 months total (i.e. two treatments)
Selamectin	Pour-on applied every 30 days for a total of three treatments

Collection of coat brushings (i.e. scales and hair accumulated on the examination table by rubbing the animal or by using a "toothbrush" or flea comb) is an effective means to obtain samples. Samples can be collected into a Petri dish (or on glass slides, **Fig. 5.2**) and covered with mineral oil. Diagnostic yield is improved with multiple sampling methods.[2] Mites (with characteristic hooks of accessory mouthparts), eggs and debris may be visible attached to hair.[2] Microscopic detection of mites can be an effective client therapy compliance tool.

Sometimes mites cannot be found, and trial therapy is advised.[5-7]

Therapy

Topical therapy for dogs and cats may consist of one of the following: fipronil, selamectin, milbemycin or ivermectin injection (*Table 5.1*).[8] Topical pyrethrin shampoo, spray or spot-on products may be used on dogs,[1] but not on cats because of toxicity concerns. Ivermectin should not be used in herding breeds, those with suspected or known multidrug-resistance gene (*MDR-1*) mutation, or in pets less than 6 months of age.

Environmental decontamination with a flea-type product or as for scabies, together with cleaning (or discarding) of bedding and all grooming equipment should be performed. All in-contact (household) pets will require concurrent therapy, along with monitoring for possible infection if they are negative.

Prognosis/complications

Typically, clinical improvement (reduced pruritus, resolution of mite infestation) is noted within a few days of therapy. Treatment failure is usually due to poor environmental cleaning, high animal density, poor treatment compliance or incorrect dosing. Treatment failure (or incomplete response) may also indicate the presence of an underlying dermatologic (e.g. atopy) or endocrine disease (e.g. hypothyroidism).

Prevention

Environmental cleaning and decontamination are integral for therapy and prevention of re-infestation.

Public health

Risks to humans are limited; however, an intensely pruritic self-limiting rash can develop in up to 20% of cases.

DEMODEX CANIS
Anette Loeffler

Definition
Demodicosis (demodectic mange) is a common inflammatory skin disease, associated with high numbers of *Demodex* mites in the skin. In dogs, disease severity ranges from localized, mild and self-resolving to very severe, but disease is rare in cats.

Etiology and pathogenesis
Demodex mites are normal skin commensals of dogs and cats. They are typically found in low numbers in the hair follicles or, with some species, living in the surface epidermis. In dogs, *D. canis*, *D. injai* and *D. cornei* (short form) are most common. In cats, *D. cati*, *D. gatoi* (short form) and an unnamed species have been described. Mites are acquired from the bitch or queen at birth or shortly thereafter. Development of skin disease is associated with an uncontrolled proliferation of mites due to underlying immune imbalances.

Geography
Worldwide.

Incidence and risk factors
Predisposed breeds include Staffordshire Terriers, Shar Peis, West Highland White Terriers and many others. In young dogs (<2 years), the immune imbalance tends to be mite specific and may spontaneously resolve (localized forms). In adult dogs, hyperadrenocorticism (iatrogenic and spontaneous) and neoplasia are important risk factors.

Physical examination and clinical signs
See **Figs. 5.3, 5.4** and *Table 5.2*.

Diagnosis
Cigar-shaped mites (adults, six-legged larvae and eight-legged nymphs) and lemon-shaped (fusiform) eggs (**Fig. 5.5**) can be found on hair plucks (**Fig. 5.6**). Skin scrapes (squeezing skin to extrude mites before scraping) or acetate tape impression smears may identify surface living mites. Histopathology from biopsy specimens may be required to diagnose demodicosis from chronically thickened skin, such

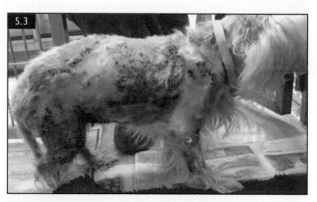

Fig. 5.3 Generalized juvenile demodicosis complicated by deep pyoderma in a 9-month-old West Highland White Terrier.

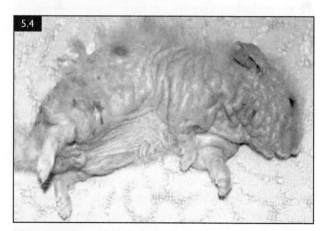

Fig. 5.4 Extensive alopecia in a 2-year-old hamster with demodicosis.

Table 5.2 **Clinical presentations of demodicosis**	
Localized	Mainly in puppies and young adults
	Individual patches of alopecia (<5), sometimes with scaling
	Often on the face or around the eyes
Generalized	Lymphadenopathy is common
	Numerous alopecic patches
	Erythema, comedones, hyperpigmentation ("blue tinge"), crusts, hemorrhagic crusts (indicating secondary deep pyoderma)
Pododemodicosis	Alopecia, swelling, erythema, lichenification, thickened skin, hyperpigmentation
Feline demodicosis	Alopecia and often intense pruritus

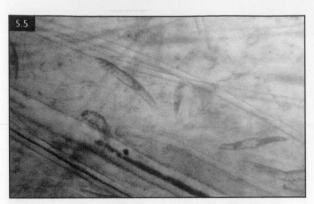

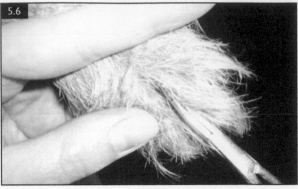

Fig. 5.5 Multiple *Demodex canis* adults and nymphs from a hair pluck. Note: diameter of hair shaft is similar to diameter of mites (×10 lens [×100 magnification] in liquid paraffin).

Fig. 5.6 Hair plucks will yield *Demodex* mites reliably in most cases of generalized demodicosis and are less invasive than skin scrapings, especially from challenging body sites such as paws and periocular skin.

as in pododemodicosis or from some individuals (e.g. Shar Peis).

If only one mite is seen in a sample more sampling is recommended, as this could represent a normal commensal burden. Identification of higher numbers of mites in an animal with skin lesions is compatible with demodicosis.

In all cases of adult-onset demodicosis, the main diagnostic challenge will be the identification of underlying causes. Therefore, the diagnostic work-up should include a comprehensive physical examination, blood sampling for hematology, biochemistry and endocrine assays, as well as imaging for neoplasia.

Cytology of skin lesions should be performed to investigate secondary pyoderma.

Therapy

Localized forms may be left untreated but need monthly monitoring for progression. All generalized cases require acaricidal and typically antibacterial treatment, together with correction of any underlying triggers.

Isoxazolines (e.g. afoxolaner, sarolaner, fluralaner) are showing promising results in the treatment of canine demodicosis,[9–11] and have the advantages of ease of administration and fewer safety concerns than avermectins.

Weekly 0.05% w/v amitraz dips have been the first-line treatment, and have excellent efficacy reported after correct application. Resistance to the drug has not been reported, but treatment failure is common with inappropriate use. Product instructions must be followed closely, and animals should be clipped to facilitate good penetration. Correct amitraz dilution and handling are required (the product is light sensitive). It needs to be used within a couple of hours after dilution and must not be rinsed off.

Good data exist on the efficacy and safety of oral milbemycin for canine demodicosis.[12] Ivermectin is also effective and easy to give. However, owing to potentially serious adverse effects, even in non-Collie breeds, this product should only be used with great care and when safer alternatives are not available. It should not be used in herding breeds, dogs with known or suspected ATP-binding cassette subfamily B member 1 (*ABCB1*)/multidrug-resistance gene (*MDR-1*) mutation, or in pets less than 6 months of age.

Topical (spot-on) treatment with imidacloprid/moxidectin is authorized in many countries for the treatment of generalized demodicosis at weekly intervals (instead of every 4 weeks, as is used for fleas) and amitraz collars directed against ticks have been used. However, efficacy has been disappointing and close monitoring of progress is required.

Treatment should continue until two sets of negative skin scrapes (or hair plucks) have been obtained 4 weeks apart. After this time the disease can be declared in remission. Animals can be considered cured if clinical signs do not reoccur within 1 year after stopping therapy.

Prognosis/complications

The prognosis for localized forms is excellent. The prognosis for generalized juvenile demodicosis can be good, but depends on response to therapy, compliance and general immune status of the patient. For adult-onset demodicosis, the prognosis depends primarily on management of the underlying cause and varies from good to grave.

Prevention

Animals diagnosed with demodicosis should be neutered once the skin disease has resolved. This helps reduce risk of demodicosis in their offspring (given the suspected genetic component) and of recurrence of disease during estrus in entire bitches. *D. canis* is not considered contagious, so no special measures are required.

DERMATOPHYTOSIS (RINGWORM)
Michelle Evason and Anette Loeffler

Definition

Dermatophytosis is a fungal infection of the hair, skin and claws of dogs and cats. Cutaneous signs consist of alopecia (focal to multifocal), scaling and crusting, most often on the head and legs. It can easily be misdiagnosed and is highly contagious and zoonotic.

Etiology and pathogenesis

Dogs and cats are most commonly infected with *Microsporum canis*, *Trichophyton mentagrophytes* or *M. gypseum*. Molds are spread between animals (or people) by direct contact, contact with infected hair, scale or crusts in the environment, or through contaminated fomites (e.g. grooming equipment). Typically, exposure is through direct contact with tiny fungal arthrospores. These spores can also be carried via dust or air and survive in the environment for many months.

In healthy individuals with intact skin, the fungus is eliminated without causing infection. In situations where there is a break in intact skin, arthrospores may attach tightly to keratin and invade skin, hair or claws. The life cycle is completed in about 7 days with growth of fungal hyphae. Clinical lesions develop 1–3 weeks later.[13]

Geography

Worldwide, especially warm and humid climates.

Incidence and risk factors

The prevalence of *M. canis*, *M. gypseum* and *Trichophyton* spp. varies according to geography, presence of clinical signs (vs. none) and patient demographics.[13–18] Overall prevalence is considered low, even in cats with skin disease.

Risk factors have been identified as warmth and humidity, very young or very old age, feral, high housing density (e.g. cattery, shelter), long haircoat and lack of normal skin defenses (e.g. wounds).

Dogs

Single-species infections are most common; however, more than one dermatophyte species may be involved. This is most commonly *M. gypseum* and *Trichophyton* spp.[19] A predisposition for *M. canis* in Yorkies has been found, and working and hunting dogs may be at higher risk owing to increased exposure to spores.[13, 20]

Cats

In cats, over 90% of infections are caused by *M. canis*.[19] Lesions may be compatible with those of miliary dermatitis. Persian cats appear predisposed to infection.[4, 13] Feline immunodeficiency virus (FIV)- or feline leukemia virus (FeLV)-positive status does not appear to increase risk.

Common clinical signs
Cats and dogs

Alopecia (focal or multifocal), scales, crusts and pruritus (variable) are most common on the face, ears and paws (**Fig. 5.7**). The classic ring lesion with central healing may occur. However, this is variable and dependent on hair follicle destruction, inflammation or secondary infection (e.g. *Demodex* or staphylococcal folliculitis).

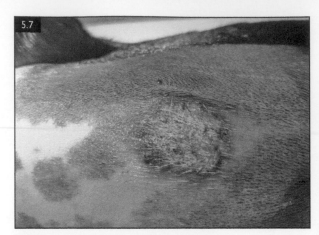

Fig. 5.7 Dermatophytosis in a dog.

Dogs

Dogs are more likely to develop a ring lesion. Lesions can be identical to those from other causes of focal hair loss in puppies and adult dogs. Deep pyoderma lesions, along with those resembling autoimmune disease (e.g. severe facial folliculitis and furunculosis), can develop.

Cats

Subclinical infections (carriage) are common, particularly in strays, multi-cat facilities and kittens. Pruritus can be severe (e.g. self-mutilation). Owners may complain of excess shedding, and some cats may have a history of vomiting hairballs. In kittens, hair loss and scaling commonly begin on the face and forelegs.

Diagnosis

Dermatophytosis is diagnosed on history (e.g. cattery origin), owner-reported lesions on people (especially children) (**Figs. 5.8, 5.9**) in the house, clinical signs and exclusion of differential diagnoses. A combination of culture, cytologic findings and sometimes Wood's lamp are used to confirm infection. Often described as the "great mimic", it is frequently over- or underdiagnosed.

A Wood's lamp can be used for quick screening for infection. This is more likely to be positive with *M. canis* infection, where an apple green fluorescence of individual hairs will be noted. Bathing care, scales and creams may give a more yellow fluorescence. If fluorescent hairs are seen, these should be plucked

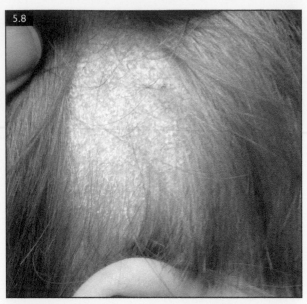

Fig. 5.8 Zoonotic dermatophytosis associated with scaling and alopecia.

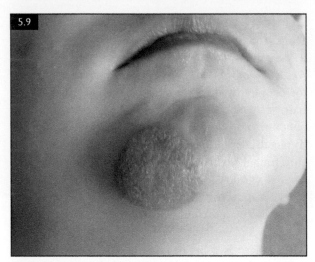

Fig. 5.9 Zoonotic dermatophytosis on the face of a child.

and submitted for culture. Warming the Wood's lamp before use, and ensuring it is of standard make, may improve sensitivity; however, false positives and negatives are common, due to poor equipment and training.

Cytology

Hair plucks, scale or skin scrapes from alopecic areas used for microscopic exam may reveal fungal hyphae or spores (**Fig. 5.10**). Use of 10–20% potassium

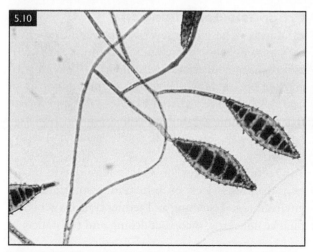

Fig. 5.10 *Microsporum canis*, showing large, spindle-shaped macroconidia (475× magnification). (Courtesy of Dr Lucille K. Georg, CDC)

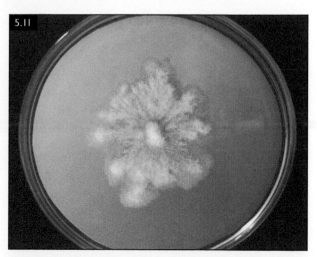

Fig. 5.11 Typical colony appearance of *Microsporum canis*. (Courtesy of Dr Lucille K. Georg, CDC)

hydroxide (KOH) aids visualization owing to removal of scale and debris; however, mineral oil is quick, readily available and works well.

Culture of hair and scale

Submission of hair pluckings and scales to a standardized lab is advised to allow speciation and reduce false-positive or -negative results (**Fig. 5.11**). Appropriate numbers of hair pluckings, or scale removal from lesions or by the "toothbrush" method will improve diagnoses. Positive culture and hyphae or spores on cytology from culture plates, along with clinical signs, are highly suggestive of the diagnosis.[13, 21] Fungal culture alone is not considered sufficient for diagnosis, because of the likelihood of false positives, false negatives and contamination.

PCR

PCR to detect fungal DNA may be used; however, this cannot distinguish between cases of active infection and those that have undergone successful treatment.

Histopathology

This is more often used with nodular disease. Biopsy is not considered as sensitive as culture; however, the presence of fungal elements on biopsy (using special stains such as periodic acid–Schiff) may be helpful for diagnoses.

Therapy

Therapy of clinically and subclinically affected dogs and cats is always advised. This will lower zoonotic risk and the risk of transmission to other animals, and decrease contamination of the environment.

Therapy should consist of specific treatment of the individual patient (topical and systemic) and environmental decontamination. All in-contact household pets require culture and possible therapy, along with monitoring for potential infection if they are negative.

Topical therapy

Clipping of the entire haircoat may facilitate topical antifungal therapy and environmental cleaning. Goals of clipping are removal of infected hair, facilitation of topical therapy and environmental cleaning, and reducing the load of overall infection. Sedation or anxiolytics may be required for clipping, particularly for cats. Proper disposal of hair and cleaning of clippers is critical to prevent spread and zoonotic risk.

Bathing, shampoos and dipping of the entire haircoat with topical antifungals can be used. Cats may be difficult to bathe; however, gentle handling, patience and medication can yield positive results. Topical therapy helps reduce environmental contamination.

Lime sulfur solutions, enilconazole and miconazole/chlorhexidine shampoos are effective for both dogs and cats. Twice-weekly application is advised.[13] Accelerated hydrogen peroxide was shown to be effective *in vitro*.[22] Enilconazole dips may cause severe side effects in cats, but work well in dogs. Chlorhexidine alone is less successful.[13]

Licking or grooming after topical therapy can be prevented through use of an E-collar or similar device.

Systemic antifungals

Systemic therapy alone is less successful than topical protocols. These drugs are used to speed disease resolution and should be used only when the diagnosis is certain. Itraconazole and terbinafine are well tolerated and considered most effective (*Table 5.3*).[13]

Monitoring

Monitoring with rechecks at 2- to 4-week intervals is critical for success. Clinical improvement and fungal culture should both be used to determine progress. Fungal cultures should be performed routinely to achieve a "mycologically cured" pet, with two consecutive negative cultures typically used to declare an animal dermatophyte free.[19] Repeating culture once the prior culture result is back may reduce expense without compromising therapy.

In a treated patient, a negative PCR or negative culture with no overt lesions is consistent with cure.[13] Clinical cure will occur before mycologic cure and this is an important client education point, as typically several months of therapy are needed despite clinical appearance. Photographs of the patient before and during the therapy course to "map" the disease process (and progress) are advised.

Prognosis/complications

Prognosis is based on severity of presenting clinical signs, and ability of clients to commit to the cost and management (time investment) associated with appropriate therapy. Typically, dermatophytosis in cats resolves in less than 100 days with appropriate therapy.[19] Clinical improvement (reduced pruritus, hair regrowth, less scale) is noted within 2–4 weeks of therapy.

Treatment failures (or relapses) are due to incorrect diagnosis, lack of infection resolution, poor environmental cleaning and reinfection, owner compliance concerns, incorrect dosing and resistance.

Infection control

Environmental cleaning and decontamination are integral to therapy and prevention. Removal of hair with physical cleaning (e.g. vacuum), disinfectants and disposal are strongly advised. Vacuums should be equipped with a high-efficiency particulate air filter to prevent airborne dissemination of spores. Disinfection procedures and removal of gross debris are indicated. Spores can survive in the environment for many months, and are resistant to most disinfectants.

Public health and infection control

Dermatophytosis is zoonotic, and children, older adults and those with immune-compromising conditions are considered at high risk. Clinical signs of disease in dogs or cats are not required for transmission to humans. Personal protective equipment (e.g. gloves, gown) should be worn when handling known or suspected cases. Scheduling appointments at the end of the clinic day may facilitate cleanup and reduce risk of spread.

Table 5.3 **Systemic antifungal options for the treatment of dermatophytosis**

ANTIFUNGAL	CANINE DOSE	FELINE DOSE
Itraconazole	5–10 mg/kg q24h given with food × 28 days, then every other week until cure achieved (or on a 1 week on, 1 week off basis)	5–10 mg/kg q24h given with food × 7 days for 3 alternating weeks. Persist for 3 weeks until cure achieved (or on a 1 week on, 1 week off basis)
Terbinafine	20–40 mg/kg q24h × 14 days	20–40 mg/kg q24h

LAGENIDIOSIS
Kenneth Cockwill

Definition

Lagenidiosis refers to disease caused by fungus-like *Lagenidium* and *Paralagenidium* spp. Dogs can be infected by *L. gigateum* forma *caninum* and *P. karlingii*, whereas *L. decidium* causes disease in cats.[23]

Etiology and pathogenesis

Little is known about the life cycles of these species, although it is speculated that disease is caused by flagellated zoospores that adhere to and encyst in damaged tissue.

Geography

Lagenidiosis is most common in the southeastern United States (particularly Florida and Louisiana). However, it has been reported in Texas, Tennessee, Alabama, Georgia, South Carolina, Maryland, Virginia, Indiana and Illinois.

Incidence and risk factors

The incidence is not well defined, but the disease is considered uncommon. Affected dogs are usually young to middle aged (1–6 years of age).[3] Prior exposure to local lakes and ponds may be a risk factor; however, association with immunosuppression has not been reported.[24] Anecdotally, infection has been reported in cats.

Clinical signs

Two clinical forms have been recognized in dogs. One involves aggressive clinical disease (caused by *L. gigateum* forma *caninum*). Primary signs include progressive, extensive cutaneous or subcutaneous (often multifocal) skin lesions involving the extremities and body. Multiple firm nodular (cutaneous to subcutaneous) lesions or ulcerated, thickened and edematous areas with necrosis and draining tracts may be present, along with regional lymphadenopathy and edema.[23, 24]

The other form is indolent clinical disease, caused by *P. karlingii*. This results in locally aggressive cutaneous lesions that are chronic and slowly progressive, or somewhat stable for more than 2 years.[23, 24]

Diagnosis

Cytology is inflammatory (neutrophilic, pyogranulomatous or eosinophilic) with or without fungal elements.[24, 25]

Immunoblot testing is available for serology, but it is not specific and cross-reacts with *P. insidiosum*. It should be interpreted in conjunction with *P. insidiosum* serology.

Culture is the preferred (and definitive) means of diagnosis, and can aid differentiation between the two pathological species and assist in determining prognosis.[24] Specific growth medium is needed (peptone–yeast–glucose agar amended with ampicillin and streptomycin). Characterization based on morphology is difficult and definitive diagnosis should be based on molecular techniques.

Histopathologically, pyogranulomatous and eosinophilic inflammation with broad, irregularly branching, sparse, septate hyphae are typically evident (**Fig. 5.12**). Hyphae are more visible on hematoxylin and eosin (H&E) sections. *L. gigateum* forma *caninum* hyphae average 12 µm, whereas *P. karlingii* hyphae are usually 7.5 µm.[25]

Molecular diagnostics (e.g. ribosomal [r]RNA gene sequencing or specific PCR) are now the methods of choice.

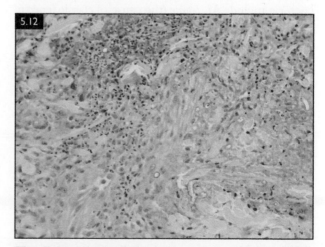

Fig. 5.12 Histopathology of a cutaneous *Lagenidium* lesion in a cat (H&E; 40× magnification). (Courtesy of Dr Michelle Dennis)

Therapy

Aggressive surgical resection is indicated. Before aggressive surgery, further investigation (radiographs, CT or abdominal ultrasound) to investigate for the presence of occult lesions is recommended in cases with known or suspected *L. gigateum* forma *caninum* infection.

Medical therapy alone is usually ineffective, although aggressive surgical resection followed by itraconazole 10 mg/kg PO q24h (3–9 months) and terbinafine 5–10 mg/kg PO q24h (3–9 months) cured two dogs that had no systemic involvement.

LEPROMATOUS MYCOBACTERIAL INFECTIONS
Michelle Evason

Definition

Feline leprosy syndrome and canine leproid granuloma syndrome (CLG) are rare causes of disease in cats and dogs, respectively. They typically result in cutaneous, focal-to-multifocal, nodular granulomatous or pyogranulomatous lesions. Nodules may (or may not) ulcerate and are frequently located on the head, neck or feet. Definitive diagnosis and therapy can be challenging.

Etiology and pathogenesis

Mycobacterium spp. are gram-positive, acid-fast and typically slow growing bacteria. Lepromatous mycobacteria include *M. leprae* (the cause of classic leprosy in humans), *M. lepraemurium* and additional poorly characterized, non-tuberculous, mycobacteria. Little is known about these pathogens and their associated disease syndromes. This is due to the challenges associated with culture growth and subsequent species identification.

Cats

Rats are the main sources of *M. lepraemurium*. Cats are likely infected through traumatic inoculation of the skin by rodent (rat) bites, or scratches and bites from affected cats. It is unclear whether concurrent immunosuppression due to feline immunodeficiency virus (FIV) and feline leukemia virus (FeLV) is a risk factor for disease. Feline leprosy syndrome has been classified as either lepromatous or tuberculoid.[27] However, both types can be present in a single patient.[27]

Mefenoxam (an agricultural fungicide) has a superior inhibition of growth of *Lagenidium* spp. *in vitro* and has been used successfully to treat pythiosis in one dog. This drug may prove effective in the future;[26] however, it is not approved.

Prognosis/complications

The prognosis is grave because of systemic spread. This can result in massive acute hemorrhage due to great vessel involvement and/or other systemic signs including edema.

An immune deficiency has been speculated on as a cause for the different clinical and histopathologic syndromes.[27–29]

Dogs

Species causing CLG syndrome have not yet been cultured, and much is unknown about the pathogen(s).[30] One report supports the *M. simiae* clade as the cause.[31] An insect vector has been theorized given the location of the lesions (e.g. head and neck) and possible seasonal association of disease.

Geography

Worldwide. In cats, disease is most commonly reported in the United Kingdom, Canada, Australia and New Zealand, Italy and Greece. Dogs with CLG and case clusters of disease have been reported in the western USA, Brazil, Europe, Australia and New Zealand.[27, 30, 32]

Incidence and risk factors

The incidence is unknown, and likely higher than estimated owing to lack of reporting and the challenge of diagnosis. Risk factors for cats are associated with increased exposure to (and trauma from) rats and other cats. These include outdoor access, rural environment, fighting behavior and history of bites or trauma. A possible breed predisposition for Boxer (and Boxer cross) dogs or Foxhounds housed together with those of similar genetic lines has been noted.[32] Short-coated and large breed dogs appear more commonly affected.[27, 30]

Common clinical signs

Cats and dogs may have single (or multiple) dermal or subcutaneous papular or nodular lesions on the head, neck and limbs (**Figs. 5.13, 5.14**). Ulceration (**Fig. 5.15**), alopecia and local lymphadenopathy may occur. Pruritus is rare.

In cats, tuberculoid leprosy presents clinically as firmly palpable focal or multifocal lesions. These may be widely distributed over the head, neck and limbs. Lepromatous leprosy is recognized as dermatitis with pyogranuloma lesions and panniculitis.[28]

Dogs develop skin lesions similar to those of feline tuberculoid leprosy. Lesions are typically found on the ears (pinnae) and may be noted on the head, limbs and thorax. Systemic illness has not been reported.

Diagnosis

Leprosy syndromes are difficult to diagnose via culture, and multiple criteria of diagnosis are required. These may include suggestive skin lesions and histopathology, and lack of systemic illness or response to prior therapy (e.g. antimicrobials). Finding acid-fast bacilli together with granulomatous disease is suggestive. However, species identification is needed to confirm the diagnosis and to provide guidance about potential zoonotic concerns associated with different *Mycobacterium* spp.

Cytology

Direct exam of impression smears or aspirates typically reveals pyogranulomatous inflammation with intracellular bacteria. These will stain pink with acid-fast techniques.

Culture

Culture is typically unrewarding because of the fastidious nature of these organisms.

Histopathology

Histopathology (skin biopsy) of either tuberculoid feline leprosy or CLG cases reveals pyogranulomas or tubercle lesions full of macrophages and concurrent inflammation, with possible calcification and a necrotic center. Acid-fast staining may reveal acid-fast organisms.

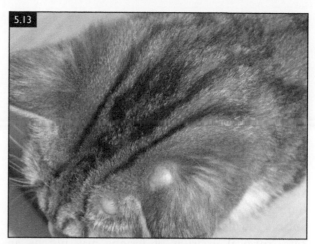

Fig. 5.13 Feline leprosy lesions on the head and ear. (Courtesy of Dr Margie Scherk)

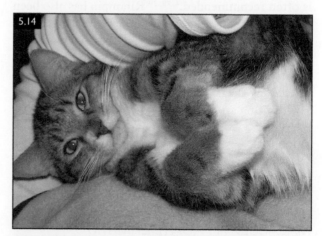

Fig. 5.14 Feline leprosy lesion on a forelimb. (Courtesy of Dr Margie Scherk)

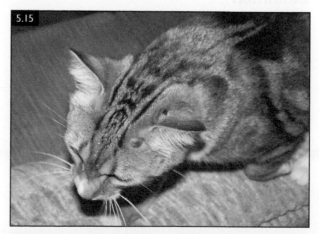

Fig. 5.15 Excoriated lesions of feline leprosy. (Courtesy of Dr Margie Scherk)

In lepromatous feline leprosy, a pyogranulomatous dermatitis and panniculitis with macrophages, neutrophils and multinucleate giant cells, along with organisms, has been noted.

PCR of histopathology samples may be useful when available and to aid identification of *Mycobacterium* spp.[28, 30] Species-specific PCR is required for confirmation.

Therapy
Cats
Surgical removal of lesions (if feasible) followed by antimicrobial therapy may be curative.[28] In some cats, surgical excision of lesions may not be an option. In these cases, combination therapy with clarithromycin, a fluoroquinolone and clofazimine is often recommended.[4, 28, 29] Rifampin has also been used as part of combination therapy.[4] Antimicrobial therapy should be continued until lesion resolution, and ideally 2–3 months after, in order to reduce recurrence. Cost and client capability may play a role in therapy decisions. In some cats, disease may be self-limiting and resolve spontaneously.[33]

Dogs
Disease may resolve spontaneously (without specific therapy) in dogs within 1–3 months. Antimicrobials used in dogs include clarithromycin and rifampin combination therapy, together with silver sulfasalazine. Surgical resection of isolated lesions may be successful.

Dogs and cats
Antimicrobial or topical therapy may be required for secondary bacterial pyoderma. Follow-up rechecks at 2- to 4-week intervals are critical for success and ensuring compliance.

Prognosis/complications
Complete cure with therapy has been achieved in both dogs and cats.[30, 33] Prognosis is based on initial presentation, disease extent, owner commitment and response to therapy. The prognosis can be good, and in dogs lesions do not typically reoccur.[30–32] In cats, recovery may take 3–6 months.[33]

Prevention
There is no vaccine; however, indoor housing (if feasible) may reduce disease associated with trauma, puncture and bites.

Infection control and public health
Feline and canine leprosy are not zoonotic.

MALASSEZIA PACHYDERMATIS
Charlie Pye

Definition
Malassezia pachydermatis is a lipophilic, non-lipid-dependent yeast normally found on the skin, vagina, anal sacs, external ear canals and mucosal surfaces of healthy cats and dogs. Disease occurs most commonly in dogs.

Etiology and pathogenesis
Malassezia pachydermatis is part of the normal skin microbiota of dogs and cats and is usually found in low numbers on healthy skin.[34] However, it is able to increase in number because of its ability to produce beneficial growth factors. These alter the cutaneous microenvironment and compromise the barrier function, thereby changing normal skin defenses.

Mucosal carriage may also play a role in infection due to licking of the skin. It is not uncommon for dogs to have concurrent bacterial pyoderma.

Geography
Worldwide.

Incidence and risk factors
There are specific breed predispositions noted in dogs including: West Highland White Terriers, Basset Hounds, Cocker, Springer and Cavalier King Charles Spaniels, Shih Tzus, English Setters, Toy/Miniature Poodles, Boxers, Australian and Silky Terriers, German Shepherd Dogs, Dachshunds and Shar Peis.

Over 70% of dogs with yeast dermatitis have concurrent dermatoses. The incidence of *Malassezia* spp. may increase over the summer months but it can occur year round. This increase during warmer weather is due to increased numbers of allergens and humidity.[35]

Many conditions predispose an individual to yeast overgrowth, such as allergic skin disease, endocrine disease and seborrheic skin disease. Specific predisposing skin factors for *Malassezia* dermatitis include excess moisture, warmth, increased humidity, skin folds and inflamed skin/ears.[35] Development of *Malassezia* dermatitis may be associated with prior antibiotic therapy; however, this has not been proven.[35]

There is a lower incidence of *Malassezia* dermatitis in cats than in dogs, although Persians are thought to be predisposed and may have higher incidence. Certain cats, such as Sphynx and Rex breeds, have a higher carriage of yeast on their skin normally. Devon Rex are predisposed to paronychia due to *Malassezia* spp.

Clinical signs

Pruritus is a major clinical sign. Erythema and alopecia are commonly noted along with scaling, yellow/brown crusting and odor. Porphyrin staining occurs as individuals lick their skin and hair. With chronicity of the disease, clinical signs such as hyperpigmentation and lichenification of the skin may be observed. In cats, pruritus remains a common clinical feature along with erythema, follicular casts and a scaly-to-waxy dermatitis.

Areas affected by *Malassezia* dermatitis tend to be locations where moisture and heat are trapped. Regions of the body commonly affected in dogs are the interdigital regions, ventral neck, axillae, ventral abdomen and ventral tail (**Figs. 5.16, 5.17**). In cats, clinical signs generally appear on the face and chin (chin acne). Both species can develop otitis externa and paronychia, where the nail beds are affected.[34, 36] Clinically this will be apparent with a brown line around the nail bed. The lower lip folds may also be affected in dogs.

Diagnosis

Diagnosis is via cytology performed on samples collected using cotton tipped applicators, acetate tape,

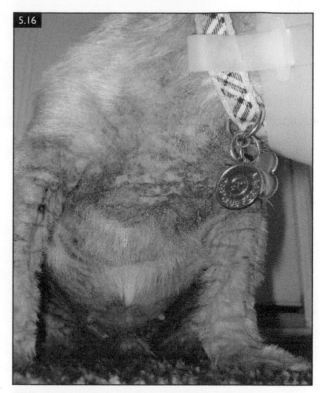

Fig. 5.16 *Malassezia* dermatitis in a dog, predominantly affecting the ventral neck, ventral abdomen and axillae.

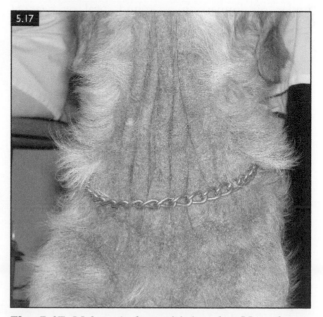

Fig. 5.17 *Malassezia* dermatitis in a dog. Note the lichenification and hyperpigmentation. (Courtesy of Dr Tony Yu)

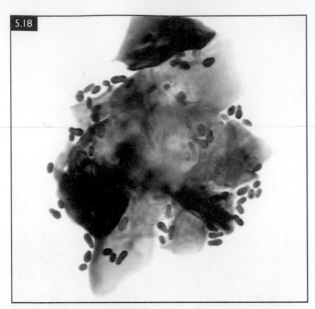

Fig. 5.18 Ear cytology from a dog with *Malassezia* otitis externa. Large numbers of yeast organisms are evident (Gram stain). (Courtesy of Dr Tony Yu)

Table 5.4 **Doses of systemic antifungals used in dogs**

ANTIFUNGAL	DOSE
Ketoconazole	5–10 mg/kg PO q24h
Itraconazole	5–10 mg/kg PO q24h or 5–10 mg/kg PO on the first 2 days of every week
Fluconazole	2.5–5 mg/kg PO q24h
Terbinafine	30 mg/kg PO q24h or 30 mg/kg PO on 2 consecutive days a week

toothpicks, scalpel blades or spatulas.[34, 37] Acetate tape preparations are more useful for dry lesions and difficult to sample areas, whereas cotton-tipped applicators are beneficial for moist and waxy lesions.[9]

Malassezia spp. can be viewed easily at 40× or under oil immersion as round, oval or peanut/footprint-shaped yeasts (**Fig. 5.18**). Small numbers of the organisms may be considered normal. However, if a yeast is found in larger numbers or in combination with clinical signs such as erythema and pruritus, then treatment should be considered. Diagnosis of hypersensitivity is via intradermal or serologic testing for IgE.[38] Identification of the concurrent dermatoses must also be undertaken.

Therapy
Treatment can involve topical antifungal therapy using shampoo, sprays, wipes, ointments and creams. Topical agents commonly used include miconazole 2%, enilconazole, chlorhexidine (2–4%), nystatin, clotrimazole, lime sulfur, ketoconazole and selenium sulfide 1%, every 1–3 days until resolution. Topical therapy is more beneficial for localized regions of the body or for yeast otitis externa. Some of the most common antifungal agents in otic preparations are clotrimazole, nystatin, miconazole and thiabendazole.[39]

Systemic antifungals (*Table 5.4*) should be selected if the yeast dermatitis is generalized; they are not used for localized disease. For cats, the recommended systemic antifungal is itraconazole. Pulse therapy with oral azoles/terbinafine is sometimes recommended for patients known to be hypersensitive to *Malassezia* spp. Treatment of concurrent dermatoses and simultaneous bacterial pyoderma is also important.

At the end of therapy, cytology should be repeated to verify the cytologic and clinical cure of the infection.

Prognosis/complications
Prognosis is good, and infection is usually responsive to antifungal therapy. It is important to address concurrent dermatoses as well as treating the yeast. Some animals may not be cured but their condition is able to be controlled with topical or intermittent systemic therapy.

Prevention
If the underlying disease allowing the yeast to proliferate is controlled, recurrent yeast infections should be preventable. In cases where the disease cannot be identified, or a yeast hypersensitivity is suspected or known, routine topical therapy may be useful to keep numbers of *Malassezia* spp. to a minimum. For recurrent yeast otitis externa, routine cleaning with a solution containing dilute acetic acid, salicylic acid, chlorhexidine or boric acid may be helpful to acidify the ear canal.[39]

NECROTIZING FASCIITIS
J Scott Weese

Definition

Necrotizing fasciitis is a severe, acute, rapidly progressive infection of the lower layers of the skin and subcutaneous tissue. Severe systemic illness may be present and infections can quickly progress from minor to life threatening.

Etiology and pathogenesis

Streptococcus canis is most often implicated. Staphylococci, anaerobes and gram-negative bacteria such as *Pasteurella* and *Escherichia coli* are less common causes.[40–42]

Incidence and risk factors

This is a rare and sporadic condition. Risk factors include events associated with entry of bacteria into tissue, such as bites and penetrating wounds. However, inciting causes are often minor and may not be noticed. Anaerobic infections can occur from significant tissue trauma without skin breaks if tissue damage creates a local anaerobic environment that allows dormant clostridial spores to germinate and grow.

Reasons for progression of minor wounds to necrotizing fasciitis are poorly understood. Enrofloxacin use is strongly associated with *S. canis* necrotizing fasciitis, through drug-mediated upregulation of toxin production.[43, 44] This does not appear to be a concern with other fluoroquinolones.

Clinical signs

Necrotizing fasciitis usually starts as a small skin or soft tissue infection, with minor erythema, swelling and pain, followed by rapid local and systemic progression. Margins are usually well defined and expansion of the affected area can be observed over minutes to hours (**Fig. 5.19**). Fever is often absent initially but develops once more overt signs of systemic involvement are apparent. Discoloration, pronounced pain on palpation and edema are often present. Although the appearance of the skin surface is variable, extensive deeper damage is often present, with widespread necrosis, thrombosis and purulent exudate (**Fig. 5.20**). Pain and systemic illness are frequently disproportionate to the severity of the evident skin lesion.

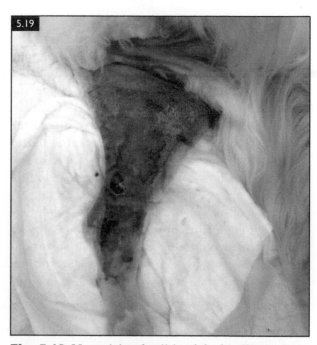

Fig. 5.19 Necrotizing fasciitis of the hindlimb of a dog caused by *Pasteurella* spp. following a cat bite. Note the line of demarcation proximally. (Courtesy of Dr Ameet Singh)

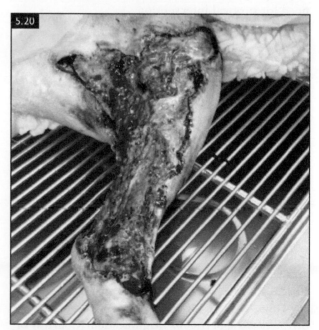

Fig. 5.20 Hindlimb of the dog in Fig. 5.19 after resection of necrotic skin. Note the marked inflammation and purulent debris. (Courtesy of Dr Ameet Singh)

Concurrent toxic shock syndrome or multi-organ failure may occur.

Diagnosis

Necrotizing fasciitis is diagnosed clinically based on the extent of evident tissue infection, severity of systemic disease and rapidity of spread. Imaging (e.g. ultrasound) may be required to gauge the extent of tissue involvement and identify areas in need of surgical attention. Hematology is required to assess systemic and organ compromise and to guide supportive care. Culture is required and samples are best collected from deep aspirates. Surgical samples can also be submitted for culture but preoperative and pre-antimicrobial samples are ideal. Cytological examination of aspirates should be performed, and can help differentiate gram-positive cocci (streptococci, staphylococci) from less common gram-positive rods (e.g. clostridia) and gram-negative rods (e.g. *E. coli*) (**Fig. 5.21**). At surgery, the condition is characterized by fascia that is necrotic, does not bleed and yields easily to blunt dissection.

The extent of the affected area should be marked on the patient and the degree of spread monitored. Rapid progression provides further indication of a need for surgical intervention.

Therapy

Aggressive supportive care may be required to stabilize the patient. Immediate and thorough surgical intervention is needed to resect compromised tissue and establish drainage. At surgery, necrotic tissue is removed and drainage is established. Large open wounds and soft tissue defects may remain and require significant wound care (**Figs. 5.22, 5.23**). Infections localized to a limb may be best treated by prompt amputation, before there is spread to the abdomen or thorax.

Antimicrobials should be started immediately. Ampicillin, clindamycin or a combination of the two is ideal for empirical therapy of suspected *S. canis* and staphylococcal infections. Gram-negative involvement is uncommon but addition of a fluoroquinolone (not enrofloxacin) or third-generation cephalosporin can be considered while cultures are pending.

Prognosis/complications

The prognosis is guarded because of the typical severity of disease and rapid progression. With prompt intervention, survival is possible. Long-term sequelae may occur from the amount of tissue damage (from infection or surgical resection) and consequences of severe systemic illness (e.g. renal compromise).

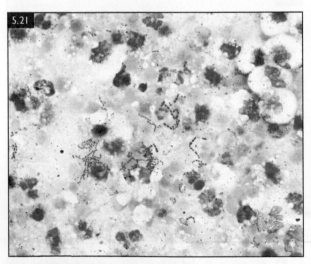

Fig. 5.21 Necrotizing fasciitis cytology. Note the Gram-positive cocci in chains, consistent with *Streptococcus* spp. (1,000× magnification) (Courtesy of Dr Noel Clancy)

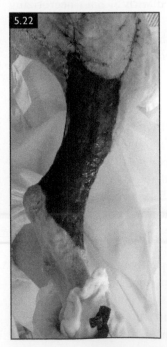

Fig. 5.22 Healthy granulation tissue following treatment of necrotizing fasciitis in the dog in Fig. 5.19. The large defect is present because of the need for extensive resection of necrotic skin. (Courtesy of Dr Ameet Singh)

Fig. 5.23 Hindlimb of the dog in Fig. 5.19 after skin grafting, once the infection had been controlled and a healthy bed of granulation tissue was present. (Courtesy of Dr Ameet Singh)

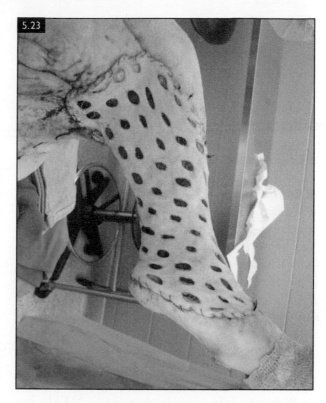

Prevention

There are few preventive measures because infection likely occurs following relatively benign breaks in the skin. Enrofloxacin should never be used for treatment of a soft tissue infection if *S. canis* might be the cause.

NON-TUBERCULOUS MYCOBACTERIA
Beth Hanselman

Definition

Mycobacteria can be differentiated into tuberculous (e.g. *Mycobacterium bovis*, *M. tuberculosis*) and non-tuberculous groups. Non-tuberculous mycobacteria (NTM) include slow growing species (*M. avium-intracellulare* complex [MAC], *M. kansasii*, *M. genavese*, *M. terrae* complex, *M. simiae*, *M. malmoense*, *M. mageritense*) and rapid growing species (*M. thermoresistible*, *M. xenopi*, *M. chelonae-abscessus* group, *M. fortuitum* group, *M. phlei*, *M. smegmatis* group). Infections can occur in dogs and cats.

Etiology and pathogenesis

Mycobacterium is a genus of aerobic, non-spore-forming, non-motile, gram-positive bacilli that are morphologically similar but are subdivided into several groups and individual species. NTM are saprophytes commonly found in the environment that may cause opportunistic infections.

NTM infections vary according to the species involved, host immune responses and route of infection. Disease is uncommon in cats and rare in dogs. Localized or disseminated subcutaneous infections are most typical; these rarely progress to systemic disease.[45] NTM infections may form granulomas that are indistinguishable clinically from tuberculous mycobacterial infections.

Mycobacteria become phagocytosed by macrophages, causing granulomatous and pyogranulomatous inflammatory responses in the organ affected.[45] In some circumstances, infection may become quiescent and then re-emerge following immunosuppression. If there is severe immunosuppression, bacteremia and dissemination to multiple organs may occur.[46]

Geography

NTM are ubiquitous in the environment and have a worldwide distribution in soil, water and decaying vegetation.[46, 47]

Incidence and risk factors

The incidence of NTM infection is low. However, molecular techniques are allowing recognition of more cases, which may suggest that infection has been underdiagnosed. Recent information from human medicine suggests an increase in the incidence of NTM infections, including those in people without apparent risk factors. Whether a parallel increase is occurring in companion animals is unclear.

NTM infection has been reported more frequently in adult, non-pedigree, neutered male cats with outdoor access. Siamese and Abyssinian breeds appear to be over-represented.[47, 48] In dogs, Basset Hounds and Miniature Schnauzers have a higher incidence of infection, giving rise to the suspicion of unrecognized defects in cell-mediated immunity.[46]

The main risk factor for infection is wound contamination from mycobacteria present in the soil or introduction from bites or scratches when playing with infected prey.[48] Infectious aerosols are a likely source of pulmonary NTM infections.

Clinical signs

Infection with NTM most often results in skin lesions characterized as dermal nodules, subcutaneous swelling, ulceration and non-healing wounds with fistulous tracts (**Figs. 5.24, 5.25**).[45, 49] Local or generalized lymph node enlargement and soft tissue calcification may be identified.[45, 46] A British study of 339 NTM cases reported that 75% of cats had single or multiple cutaneous lesions and 47% had lymph node involvement (typically submandibular lymph nodes).[48] Infection may spread locally or disseminate hematogenously.

Systemic infection is rare with NTM, but may occur more frequently with MAC infections or immunosuppression.[45, 46] Weight loss, abdominal organomegaly or mass, ascites and generalized lymphadenopathy may be present in disseminated disease. Ocular, CNS, gastrointestinal or bone involvement occurs rarely, and may present clinically as paraspinal hyperesthesia, paresis, lameness, anterior uveitis, chorioretinitis and corneal granuloma.[45, 46] Systemic infections may be insidious and not noted until disease is advanced.

Diagnosis

Identification may be challenging depending on clinical presentation, especially if skin lesions are absent. Clinical laboratory findings are non-specific and suggestive of chronic inflammation. Moderate leukocytosis, lymphopenia, anemia (often non-regenerative), hypoalbuminemia, hyperglobulinemia, hypercalcemia due to granulomatous disease and increased liver enzyme activity may be identified.[46, 48]

Thoracic radiographs are non-specific and variable (**Fig. 5.26**). Osteolysis or sclerosis, diskospondylitis, osteoarthritis, periostitis, soft tissue calcification and hypertrophic osteopathy (associated with pulmonary disease) are rarely reported.[46, 47] Abdominal imaging may reveal hepatomegaly, splenomegaly, lymphadenopathy, gastrointestinal wall thickening or effusion.[45, 46]

Cytology (fine-needle aspirate or impression smears) of skin lesions, lymph nodes, fluid or hepatosplenomegaly may allow presumptive diagnosis. The high lipid content of the mycolic acid in the cell wall that stains red with acid–alcohol fastness (**Fig. 5.27**) enables identification of mycobacteria

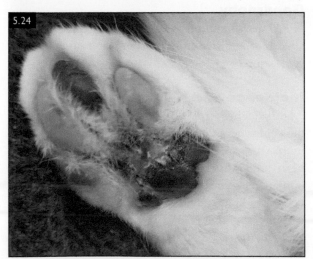

Fig. 5.24 *Mycobacterium microti* foot lesion in a cat. (Courtesy of Drs Louise Powell and Danielle Gunn-Moore)

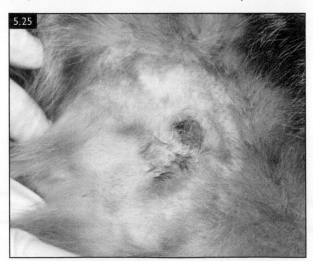

Fig. 5.25 Cutaneous *Mycobacterim avium* complex skin lesion in a Bengal cat. (Courtesy of Drs Viktoria Tsari and Danielle Gunn-Moore)

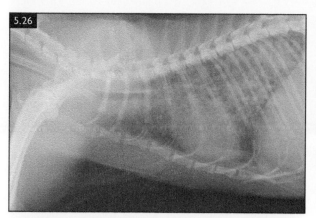

Fig. 5.26 Lateral thoracic radiograph of a cat with pulmonary *Mycobacterium microti* infection. (Courtesy of Drs Sally Aylward and Danielle Gunn-Moore)

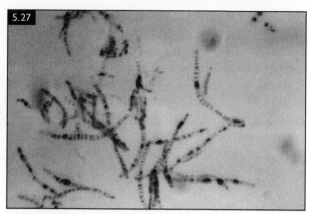

Fig. 5.27 Numerous acid-fast organisms, stained with modified Ziehl–Neelsen stain, consistent with mycobacteria.

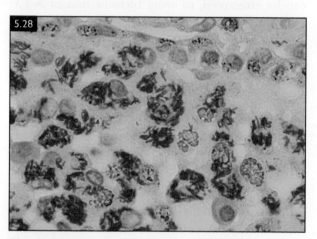

Fig. 5.28 Acid-fast stain from a cat with non-tuberculous mycobacterial infection (1,000× magnification). (Courtesy of Drs Kathryn Ling, Nekesa Morey and Danielle Gunn-Moore)

within macrophages.[45, 46] However, cytology has variable sensitivity depending on species and host immune response. Therefore, negative cytology does not exclude infection.[50]

If NTM infection is suspected, fresh tissue samples should be collected for histopathology, culture and PCR. Histopathology shows a pyogranulomatous or granulomatous inflammatory pattern with acid-fast bacteria (**Fig. 5.28**), although some NTM may not be detected by staining.[45, 50]

Culture and/or PCR allows identification of the *Mycobacterium* species involved, which impacts treatment, prognosis and counseling on zoonotic risk. Results may be delayed for up to 4–6 weeks with slow growing mycobacteria, and some species may fail to grow. Susceptibility testing is not widely available, and if it is needed the assistance of a reference laboratory may be required. Susceptibility testing is most important if a poor response to treatment or relapse occurs. Some NTM strains, such as the *M. chelonae-abscessus* group, are more likely to be multidrug resistant.[45] Tuberculin skin testing is unreliable in dogs and cats.

Therapy

Treatment of NTM is challenging, and prolonged therapy with multiple antimicrobials is usually required for resolution of infection. The ability of the owners to treat long term must be considered when determining whether to treat.

Cutaneous lesions should be treated with complete resection if feasible, or surgical debulking followed by multiple drug therapy over several months.[49]

Antimicrobial monotherapy or short courses of treatment are not advocated owing to the potential development of resistance and relapse of disease with possible systemic spread. Double or triple antimicrobial therapy is recommended, with typical combinations of rifampin (10–15 mg/kg PO q24h) with a fluoroquinolone (e.g. marbofloxacin 2 mg/kg PO q24h) and a macrolide (clarithromycin 7–15 mg/kg PO q12h or azithromycin 5–15 mg/kg PO q24h). Treatment should be given for at least 6–9 months, with suggested administration of triple therapy for

2 months, followed by continuation of two drugs for an additional 4–7 months.[45]

MAC infections may be more resistant to treatment and fluoroquinolones are not as effective.[50] A few cases with good outcomes have been reported in response to first-line therapy using clarithromycin with clofazimine (4–8 mg/kg PO q24h), rifampin or doxycycline (5 mg/kg PO q12h or 10 mg/kg PO q24h).[45, 46] Rifampin use is advised for CNS infections because it has good penetration. Abyssinian cats with disseminated infection have been treated similarly with clofazimine and clarithromycin, with or without doxycycline.

Prognosis/complications

Prognosis is variable to guarded depending on the *Mycobacterium* species and severity of disease.

Localized skin disease with NTM has a favourable prognosis if appropriate treatment is given.

In a case series of 10 cats with cutaneous infection, 5 achieved clinical resolution with antimicrobial therapy (± surgical debulking) for a median duration of 7 months (range of 3–21 months).[49] In a case series of 339 cats, 56% responded favourably to treatment and 42% had complete remission, whereas 32–52% progressed to develop pulmonary or systemic involvement.[50]

Disseminated infection has been generally associated with a poor prognosis.[45, 46, 48]

Prevention

Given that it is a relatively ubiquitous environmental opportunist, avoidance of NTM is difficult or impossible. Preventing contact with wild rodents can be attempted, to avoid introduction of NTM through bites or scratches.[45] NTM infections in dogs and cats are not considered to be of zoonotic relevance.

OTITIS EXTERNA
Anette Loeffler

Definition

Otitis externa is inflammation of the external ear canal arising from numerous causes and factors. It is frequently associated with bacterial or fungal (yeast) infection or parasitic infestation. Specific parasitic causes are addressed elsewhere in this chapter.

Etiology and pathogenesis

Typically, bacterial and fungal pathogens involved in microbial otitis are commensals or opportunists. They will only cause otitis secondary to disturbances of the ear canal skin barrier. The majority of otitis externa cases in dogs involve gram-positive cocci (predominantly staphylococci, >50%) or *Malassezia* spp. (40%). Gram-negative bacteria are more frequently found in chronic otitis. The presence of marked inflammation, exudate accumulation and biofilm complicates management.

There are primary and secondary causes leading to microbial otitis. In addition, predisposing and perpetuating factors that contribute to or promote otitis by altering canal structure or physiology need to be identified (*Table 5.5*).

Geography
Worldwide.

Incidence and risk factors

Otitis externa is common in small animal practice, with around 15% of dogs and 5% of cats affected. Predisposing factors increase the risk of otitis externa; however, disease is the result of the underlying primary and secondary causes. Recurrent otitis is recognized as a risk factor for *Pseudomonas* otitis because this organism tends to be associated with damaged tissue and moisture. Involvement of *Pseudomonas* spp. is frequently associated with ulceration, rupture of the tympanic membrane and middle-ear infection (otitis media).

Clinical signs

Clinical signs vary, depending on the primary cause, pathogen and chronicity. Yellow exudate may be associated with bacterial infection due to staphylococci or streptococci. Brown or black, sometimes dry crumbly exudate can indicate *Malassezia* overgrowth. Marked inflammation, erosions, ulcerations

Table 5.5 **Causes and risk factors for otitis**

CAUSES		FACTORS	
PRIMARY	**SECONDARY**	**PREDISPOSING**	**PERPETUATING**
Create disease in a normal ear	Create disease in an abnormal ear	Occur before development of otitis	Occur in response to otitis
May be subtle but alter environment and frequently lead to secondary causes	Easily identified and eliminated	Increase the risk of otitis	Mostly seen in chronic cases
Identification and elimination are critical for successful management and prevention of recurrence	Difficult to prevent unless primary causes corrected	Will not cause disease on their own	Prevent resolution if left untreated. May lead to changing clinical presentation over time
• Allergic skin diseases • Immune-mediated diseases • Endocrinopathies • Keratinization disorders • Foreign bodies • Ectoparasites	• Bacteria • Fungi and yeast • Medication (adverse reaction) • Over-cleaning	• Excessive hair • Pendulous pinnae • Stenosis • High humidity • Polyps • Primary secretory otitis media • Trauma	• Stenosis • Excessive debris • Tympanic membrane disease • Sebaceous gland abnormality • Calcification of fibrous tissue • Otitis media • Osteomyelitis

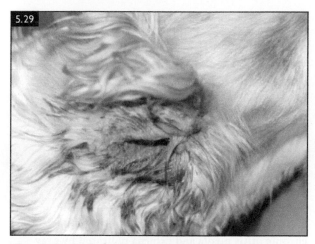

Fig. 5.29 Elderly Cocker Spaniel with a 2-year history of recurrent bilateral otitis recently complicated by *Pseudomonas aeruginosa*, indicated by large amounts of yellow–green pus (combined with malodor, ulceration and pain).

and large amounts of malodorous yellow–green or bloody discharge are hallmarks of *Pseudomonas* infection (**Fig. 5.29**).

Erythema, hyperpigmentation and lichenification of the concave aspects of the pinnae are common and their extent gives an indication of severity and chronicity.

Diagnosis

Cytology

In-house cytology of ear canal exudate or debris is the first diagnostic step (**Fig. 5.30**). Most animals will allow sampling of the ear canals more readily than otoscopy (**Fig. 5.31**). Smears can be stained with rapid stains and examined as for pyoderma (×100 lens, oil immersion). Microscopy will show squames and amorphous waxy material, and confirm adequate sampling. The presence of inflammatory cells (degenerate neutrophils, macrophages) together with microbes confirms infection. The most common findings are cocci (typically staphylococci or streptococci), rods (most often *Pseudomonas* spp., *Proteus* spp.) and peanut-shaped yeasts (*Malassezia* spp.). Melanin granules (brownish, occur only within squames, lack the clustering of dividing cocci) in pigmented animals need to be differentiated from cocci.

Culture

Bacterial culture and antimicrobial susceptibility testing does not replace cytology. Swabs from the external ear canal should be submitted when rods are seen on cytology and systemic treatment is chosen. Laboratory testing allows identification of *Pseudomonas* spp., which may be associated with a less

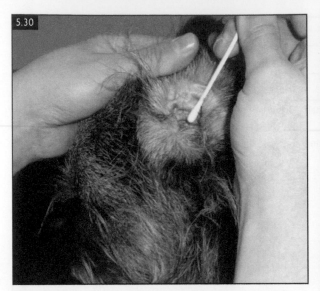

Fig. 5.30 Sampling of the ear canal for cytologic examination of exudate or debris. The pinna is pulled up and toward the examiner to straighten the canal. The wrist is kept in contact with the patient's head to compensate for sudden movement.

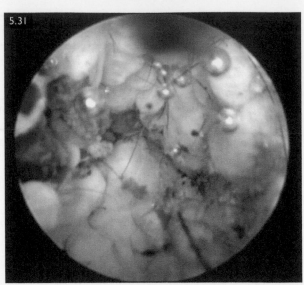

Fig. 5.31 Horizontal canal of dog with *Pseudomonas* otitis. Note the stenosis, ulceration, and large amounts of debris and exudate.

favorable prognosis. For topical therapy, *in vitro* susceptibility testing is not usually required. Currently, there are no breakpoints for topically used agents. As such, drugs to which a bacterium is reported as being resistant may still be effective given the high local levels that are achieved.

Otoscopy

Otoscopy can help to identify foreign bodies, stenosis and type of exudate. Hair, stenosis and exudates, along with pain, discomfort and lack of patient compliance may hamper visibility. Assessment of the ear drums can be very difficult or impossible in the conscious patient. General anesthesia and imaging (radiography, CT) are indicated to assess deeper structures and provide a prognosis (**Fig. 5.32**).

Therapy

Treatment aims to remove exudate and debris, resolve microbial infection, kill pathogens, decrease inflammation and restore a healthy microclimate in the canal to prevent recurrence

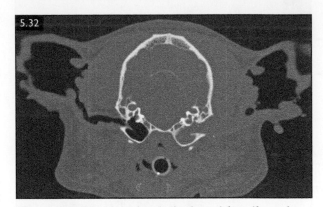

Fig. 5.32 CT of the head of a dog with unilateral chronic otitis media and externa indicated by gray material filling the bulla and canal. Note the air-filled (black) bulla and canal on the contralateral side.

Topical treatment is preferred in most cases; however, this requires compliant patients. Owners need to be shown how to restrain their pet and apply products.

Ear cleaning is essential in the management of purulent or ceruminous otitis. This is done at home to remove debris, improve access of

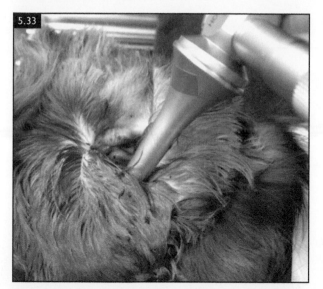

Fig. 5.33 Thorough flushing with hand-warm saline under general anesthesia will remove debris and allow visualization of deeper structures. (Courtesy of Dr Anette Loeffler)

medication, support antimicrobial treatments and prevent recurrences. Most ear-cleaning products include a combination of ceruminolytic, surfactant, astringent (drying) and antimicrobial components. Ear flushing (lavage) under anesthesia may be required for chronic or severe cases to facilitate assessment of deeper structures (e.g. the middle ear, including myringotomy) and guide prognosis (**Fig. 5.33**).

Antimicrobial treatment is best achieved using topical preparations. Veterinary polypharmacy eardrop products are generally safe and effective in resolving infection, provided there are intact eardrums, good compliance and absence of perpetuating factors. Such products tend to be antibacterial, antifungal and anti-inflammatory combinations. Selection should be based on identification of the target pathogen using ear cytology. For example, fusidic acid or mupirocin (depending on country-specific authorization) are good choices against cocci, whereas azoles will be effective against

Malassezia spp. Aminoglycosides or fluoroquinolones are indicated if rods predominate. Eardrops should be used until clinical signs have resolved and microbiological cure is confirmed through cytology. Five to seven days of application are often recommended, but chronic cases may require 2–4 weeks of treatment, particularly while underlying causes are addressed.

Systemic antimicrobial treatment is rarely necessary for otitis externa. Systemic treatment will be indicated in some cases of severe stenosis, ulcerative otitis or otitis media, and in bacterial otitis. Selection should always be based on susceptibility testing.

Paradoxically, systemic glucocorticoids are frequently indicated to reverse the inflammatory changes (e.g. swelling, hyperplasia, stenosis) that often promote microbial infection and hinder proper ventilation and drainage.

Treatment of primary causes needs to be initiated as soon as these are identified. Treatment of microbial infection alone, without addressing primary triggers, will rarely be successful. If a cause cannot be accurately diagnosed, owners need to be warned about the risk of recurrence.

Prognosis/complications

For microbial otitis externa, the prognosis depends on underlying primary causes and predisposing and perpetuating factors. If complicated by otitis media, medical management can still be successful but will be more involved and potentially costly and lengthy. Surgery must be considered for chronic cases involving the middle ear (e.g. total ear canal ablation and bulla osteotomy). Surgery is indicated for "end-stage otitis" (e.g. chronic proliferative changes in the horizontal canal, neoplasia in the canal or bulla, irreversible stenosis, calcification, osteomyelitis, pain).

Prevention

Primary causes must be identified and corrected, even if clinical signs are subtle.

OTODECTES CYNOTIS (EAR MITES)
Michelle Evason and Anette Loeffler

Definition
Otodectes cynotis is a common, highly contagious pathogen of cats and dogs that affects the external ear canals. Clinical signs range from subclinical pruritus (typically very young animals) to severe pruritus. Many cats have intense pruritus around the ears, leading to self-trauma and otitis. Unlike most mites, *Otodectes* spp. are not host specific and can infest other animals and rarely humans.

Etiology and pathogenesis
Otodectes cynotis is spread by direct contact with infested animals, subclinical carriers or through contact with contaminated materials (e.g. grooming equipment, bedding). Adult mites cause local inflammation through bites and feeding deep within the ear canal (**Fig. 5.34**).

Geography
Worldwide.

Incidence and risk factors
Incidence is variable. Reportedly, mites accounted for 25% of diagnosed otitis externa in cats[51, 52] and 7% in dogs.[51] Mixed infestations of *Otodectes cynotis*

with *Sarcoptes* spp., *Demodex* spp., ticks, fleas and dermatophytes have been detected in an additional 6.5% of cats and 4.5% of dogs.[51]

Infestations are most common in young cats and dogs, or those in high-density housing (shelters, breeding facilities, catteries). Cats appear more susceptible than dogs.

Common clinical signs
Kittens or puppies frequently have mild clinical signs, and many mites. Adult cats and dogs typically have few mites, and a suspected associated hypersensitivity.

Pruritus ranges from mild to severe. Secondary otitis may be due to concurrent bacterial infection (e.g. staphylococcal infection). Intense head shaking and scratching can result in aural hematomas.

Dark "coffee-ground" discharge (dried blood, dead mites, squamous cells and wax) and local inflammation in the affected ear canal(s) are common (**Fig. 5.35**). This has been noted in 84% of infested cats.[52]

The pruritus threshold varies among individual cats, and may be unrelated to mite numbers.[52] This is considered a hypersensitivity reaction to the mites.[4] Feline acne may be present in 10% of affected cats.[52]

Skin lesions and associated pruritus may be found on the neck, hindquarters or tail with severe infestations (ectopic ear mite infestation). Rarely, neurologic signs (incoordination), deafness, fever and death have been reported.[51]

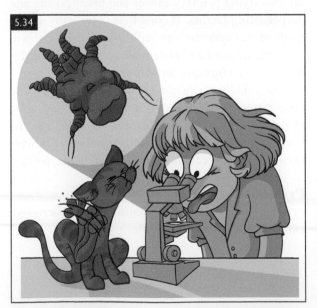

Fig. 5.34 Diagnosis of ear mites (*Otodectes cynotis*).

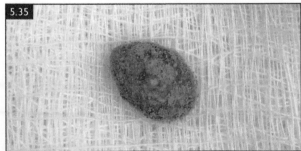

Fig. 5.35 Ear plug composed of mites and inflammatory debris secondary to *Otodectes* infestation. (Courtesy of Atlantic Veterinary College)

Diagnosis

Typically, clinical signs, direct otoscopic exam and cytological findings are confirmatory.

Cytology

A direct ear swab frequently reveals mites and debris at low power (×40). Mites are light sensitive and can be seen as white–gray specks moving away from the otoscope light source. Client microscopic exam of mites can be an effective therapy compliance tool.

Therapy

See *Table 5.6*. Kittens and puppies are usually easy to treat with a spot-on acaricide and contact advice. For this group, polypharmacy eardrops and ear canal cleaning are not advised unless severe debris is present.

In adult animals, mites are easy to kill; however, associated inflammatory otitis may require specific therapy and topical eardrops (with glucocorticoid) may be insufficient. In these cases, a short course of an anti-inflammatory dose of glucocorticoids may be needed.

In cases where gentle ear canal cleaning is indicated, administration of sedatives, anxiolytics and pain medications may improve ease and thoroughness for both the patient and the vet teams. Care and selection of appropriate ear-cleaning medication are essential, particularly with concern for ruptured tympanums.

Environmental decontamination should be performed concurrently. Bedding and all grooming equipment should be cleaned or discarded. Ear mites can be a challenging parasite to eradicate in a high pet-density environment. Direct conversations with owners about outcome, expectations and cost are needed. Additionally, all in-contact animals will require therapy and monitoring.

Table 5.6 *Otodectes* treatment options and reported response rates			
DRUG	**FORMULATION**	**ADMINISTRATION**	**CURE**
Ivermectin	Eardrops	0.5 mL of 0.01% drops once	Kittens cured at 72 h, based on 10- to 12-h checks. Drug will take effect as early as 10–12 h
	Eardrops	1% drops given once every 3 days	At 2 weeks post-treatment: 83% of cats and 66% of dogs cured
Fipronil	Topical spot-on	Two drops of 10% solution. May need to be repeated 2–4 weeks apart in dogs	Dogs and cats
Selamectin	Pour-on	Applied to skin at manufacturer dose and label recommendation	Kittens cured at 72 h based on 10- to 12-h rechecks. Drug will take effect as early as 10–12 h
		Apply to skin, 6–12 mg/kg in cats and dogs once	Clinical cure at 2 weeks post-treatment: cats 96%, dogs 77%
Doramectin	Subcutaneous (SC)	1 mL/50 kg body weight injected SC once	Clinical cure at 2 weeks post-treatment: cats 90%, dogs 75%
10% imidacloprid + 2.5% moxidectin	Topical	Two topical treatments at label dose, i.e. given 28 days apart for a total of two treatments	Dogs: 78% mite clearance at 28 days, 82% at 56 days
Sarolaner	Oral	One or two oral treatments	Dogs: 2 mg/kg as a single oral dose resulted in 98.2% reduction at day 30 and two doses of sarolaner, administered 1 month apart, resulted in 99.5% reduction in ear mites
Fluralaner	Topical or oral	One treatment	Cats (topical): 100% mite clearance 28 days after treatment. Dogs (topical or oral): 99.8% reduction 28 days after treatment

Topical therapy

Topical ivermectin is commonly used.[51, 53] Fipronil, selamectin and imidacloprid/moxidectin have also been used. Ivermectin should not be used for herding breeds, dogs with known or suspect multidrug resistance-1 gene (*MDR-1*) mutation, or in pets less than 6 months of age. Follow-up exams and cytologic rechecks are helpful to ensure successful eradication of infection.

Prognosis/complications

Prognosis is excellent with uncomplicated infestation. Typically, clinical improvement (reduced pruritus, resolution of discharge and inflammation) is noted within a few days of therapy.

PAPILLOMAVIRUS
Jason W Stull

Definition

Papillomaviruses (PVs) are non-enveloped DNA viruses (family Papillomaviridae) that cause skin and mucosal growths. Numerous distinct canine and several feline PV diseases have been reported. Dogs and cats may display a variety of PV-associated skin disorders including benign warts and plaques, which are generally self-limiting. Rarely these lesions can progress to malignant tumors.[55] Patients with oral papillomatosis are likely infectious while lesions are present, and therefore should be kept separated from other susceptible animals. Many animal species are affected (including dogs and cats), but PVs are species specific.

Etiology and pathogenesis

Infection can be transmitted by direct contact with the papilloma of an infected animal or contact with the virus in the environment. Transmission occurs through cutaneous or mucosal inoculation of the virus through trauma (micro-abrasions). Virus is shed when infected cells exfoliate from the skin or mucous membranes. An incubation period of approximately 4 weeks before the onset of clinical signs is suspected;[55, 56] however, dogs may be infectious without visible lesions.[55]

Treatment failures most commonly involve poor environmental cleaning, high-pet density scenarios, treatment compliance concerns or incorrect dosing. Lack of clinical resolution (despite apparent eradication of mites) usually reflects ongoing hypersensitivity reactions to mite antigen or otitis due to other primary (e.g. atopy) or perpetuating (bacterial, yeast infections) factors.

Prevention/infection control

Environmental cleaning and decontamination are integral to therapy and prevention of reinfection.

Public health and infection control

Ear mites are zoonotic, although this is very rare aside from deliberate self-infection.[54]

Geography

Likely worldwide.

Incidence and risk factors

Exposure to papillomaviruses is likely widespread and underreported in the dog and possibly cat populations.[57] Canine oral papillomas (**Fig. 5.36**) are commonly observed, whereas other types are less common (**Fig. 5.37**).

A number of risk factors for papillomas have been suggested. Oral papillomas most commonly occur in young dogs. Cocker Spaniels and Kerry Blue Terriers may be predisposed to cutaneous papillomas, and Pug and Miniature Schnauzer breeds are predisposed to pigmented plaques. Additionally, immunosuppression or chronic infections can increase risk for clinical PV infection, especially for severe disease.[58]

PV infections, including sarcoids and plaques, are uncommonly reported in cats. Cats affected by feline sarcoids are often less than 5 years of age and have a history of living outdoors in rural environments. Cattle are theorized to be a reservoir for feline sarcoids.[59] Feline plaques are most common in older and immunosuppressed cats (e.g. feline immunodeficiency virus infected).

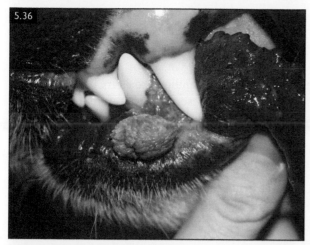

Fig. 5.36 Oral papilloma in a dog. (Courtesy of the Ohio State University, College of Veterinary Medicine Dermatology Service)

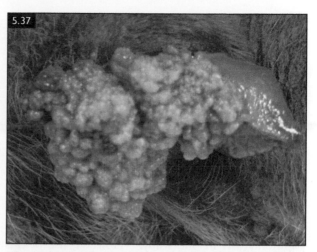

Fig. 5.37 Papilloma in a 5-year-old mixed breed dog who presented for bloody discharge from the penis. (Courtesy of the Ohio State University, College of Veterinary Medicine Dermatology Service)

DISEASE	CLINICAL SIGNS
Table 5.7 Overview of clinical signs associated with canine papillomavirus infection in dogs and cats	
Dogs	
Oral papillomatosis	Early lesions white and smooth. Enlarge over several weeks to become pedunculated (cauliflower like; **Fig. 5.36**). May be pigmented. Generally seen on the mucosal tissue of the lips, oral cavity, and occasionally eyelids and skin
Cutaneous exophytic papillomas (warts)	Generally occurring as solitary masses (**Fig. 5.37**). May appear anywhere on the body, but most frequently observed on the lower limbs and footpads
Cutaneous endophytic papillomas (inverted warts)	Cup-shaped, unpigmented solitary lesions with a central depression. Single or multiple lesions can occur anywhere on the body, but most often on the ventral abdomen
Pigmented cutaneous plaques	Cutaneous, flat, pigmented lesions. Typically present on the ventrum or medial aspects of the limbs. Usually non-regressing
Cats	
Viral plaques	Cutaneous, flat, often pigmented, sometimes ulcerated. Generally occur on the head, neck, dorsal thorax or abdomen
Sarcoids	Solitary, firm, sometimes ulcerated nodules. Often noted on the nose, lips, digits or tail tip

Clinical signs

Clinical signs vary with each PV disease, anatomic site affected and immune status of the animal (*Table 5.7*).

Physical exam

Single or multiple lesions are most commonly identified in the mouth or on the skin. Findings vary depending on disease. Severe disease is often associated with immunosuppression.[58] Canine oral papillomatosis lesions may be accompanied by halitosis, pytalism, oral bleeding and discomfort, and in rare cases respiratory difficulty.

Diagnosis

History and gross appearance of oral papillomas in dogs are generally sufficient for diagnosis. For other papillomas and plaques, the diagnosis can be confirmed with biopsy and histopathology.

A full-thickness biopsy that includes adjacent normal skin should be collected.

Therapy

For oral papillomatosis (especially in young dogs) and cutaneous exophytic papillomas, specific therapy is not indicated as these lesions will spontaneously regress. Underlying immunosuppression should be investigated with lesions in cats and severe disease in dogs and, when possible, treated (e.g. remove/reduce immunosuppressive medications). Lesions can be removed surgically but may reoccur. Treatment with azithromycin appeared to be effective for oral papillomatosis in one study.[60] However, use of this approach is controversial because of limited need in most situations and concerns about use of antimicrobials for non-antimicrobial effects.

Prognosis/complications

Oral and cutaneous papillomas in young dogs generally regress spontaneously over 3 months; however, it may take longer.[61] Patients that have recovered from oral papillomatosis are considered immune.[61] Lesions in older dogs, or when there is underlying immune compromise, may persist and occasionally progress to malignancy. Pigmented plaques in both dogs and cats tend to persist and, although rare, can progress to carcinomas.[10] Feline sarcoids often recur locally after surgical removal, but metastasis does not appear to occur.

Prevention

Patients with oral papillomatosis are likely infectious while lesions are present and therefore should be kept separated from other susceptible animals. Vaccines are not available for dogs or cats. Prevention of immunosuppressive conditions, such as retrovirus infections in cats, and cautious use of immunosuppressive drugs may reduce the chance of papillomas. For feline sarcoids, separation between cats and cattle may reduce occurrence.

Public health and infection control

Outbreaks have been reported in dog colonies and similar environments in which many dogs co-mingle (e.g. dog daycare).[62] As non-enveloped viruses, PVs are not killed by many chemical disinfectants; bleach and other oxidizing agents (e.g. accelerated hydrogen peroxide, potassium peroxymonosulfate) are effective. Environments in which PVs are expected (e.g. dog daycare, especially those with young dogs) or when transmission is suspected should consider using practices that may assist in reducing transmission, such as actively checking animals for disease, exclusion of animals with active or recent infection and establishing semi-permanent groups of dogs (cohorts).[63]

PYODERMA
Anette Loeffler

Pathogens

Staphylococcus pseudintermedius and, less commonly, other staphylococcal species such as *S. aureus*, *S. schleiferi* or coagulase-negative staphylococci are usually implicated.

Definition

Pyoderma is a bacterial infection of the skin most often involving staphylococci. Infection can involve all layers of the skin and the hair follicles. Bacterial infection can complicate virtually any skin disease, otitis and wounds. Pyoderma is always associated with an underlying problem that disrupts the normal skin barrier.

Etiology and pathogenesis

Staphylococci are commensals of all mammals and birds. They cause infection when concurrent or underlying primary problems disrupt the skin barrier, either physically or immunologically (opportunistic pathogens). Methicillin (meticillin)-resistant *S. pseudintermedius* (MRSP) and *S. aureus* (MRSA) have emerged as highly drug-resistant pathogens. Although they are no more virulent than their susceptible counterparts, they may present treatment challenges if involved in deep infections. They are associated with zoonotic risks, MRSA more so than MRSP.

Geography

Worldwide.

Incidence and risk factors

Bacterial skin infections are among the top three dermatologic conditions diagnosed in dogs and cats in first opinion practice.[64] Common primary causes that can lead to pyoderma include allergic skin diseases (flea allergy dermatitis, food allergy, atopic dermatitis), ectoparasite infestations, endocrinopathies such as hypothyroidism or hyperadrenocorticism, immune-mediated, metabolic and neoplastic conditions.

Clinical signs

The clinical presentations of pyoderma vary widely depending on depth of infection, chronicity and coat type. Pyodermas are most commonly classified by depth of infection in the skin surface (*Table 5.8*). This classification helps diagnostics, treatment decisions and prognosis.

Signs of surface pyoderma (**Fig. 5.38**) include most skin lesions, such as erythema, hyperpigmentation, swelling, exudate, erosion, scaling, crusting and lichenification.

The hallmark clinical signs of canine superficial pyoderma (folliculitis) are papules, pustules and epidermal collarettes (target lesions), most commonly found on the ventral abdomen and medial thigh (**Fig. 5.39**). Hemorrhagic crusts, draining sinuses, furuncles and nodules indicate dermal involvement (blood vessels are located in the dermis) and deep pyoderma (**Fig. 5.40**). Pruritus is common with canine superficial pyoderma. Deep pyoderma may be pruritic and may also be painful.

A less common presentation is superficial pyoderma in short-coated dog breeds. This presents as a "moth-eaten" appearance resulting from small focal areas of alopecia on the trunk (subsequent to epidermal collarettes). This form may resemble dermatophytosis, and fungal culture is needed to confirm/rule out this diagnosis.

Table 5.8 Comparison of surface, superficial and deep pyoderma

DEPTH	EXAMPLES	TREATMENT APPLICATION	COMMENT
Surface pyoderma: infection involves only the outermost layers of the skin	• Acute moist dermatitis (pyotraumatic dermatitis, "hot spots") • Skin-fold pyoderma (intertrigo) • Mucocutaneous pyoderma • Bacterial overgrowth syndrome	• Topical (cleansing, astringents) • Minimal antibacterial therapy usually required but underlying problems need to be resolved (anti-inflammatory therapy, flea control, surgical correction of folds, etc. as indicated)	Underlying causes to consider: ectoparasites, hypersensitivities, otitis, anal sac disease. Anatomic breed predispositions, obesity for intertrigo
Superficial pyoderma	• Bacterial folliculitis (pustule formation around and into hair follicles)	Topical therapy provided dog and owner are compliant, ± systemic antimicrobials	Very common in dogs
	• Impetigo (pustules affecting epidermis between hair follicles)	Topical therapy and supportive management	Uncommon. Puppies, ventral abdomen, resolves quickly after puberty
Deep pyoderma: infection extends into the dermis (furunculosis) and subcutis (cellulitis)	• Localized folliculitis and furunculosis: muzzle, callus, paws (pododermatitis, interdigital nodules), nasal, chin acne (dogs and cats), acral lick dermatitis • Generalized deep pyoderma • Cellulitis (extending into subcutis)	Systemic antimicrobials (± antibacterial soaks and washes provided not too painful)	Rarer than surface and superficial forms but serious, lengthy, expensive. Underlying causes include demodicosis (commonly) and hypersensitivities, but also consider more serious diseases such as endocrinopathies and neoplasia. Joint disease, behavior for acral lick dermatitis
	• Abscess (e.g. cat bite)	Lancing and topical therapy alone in uncomplicated cases such as localized disease without systemic signs of infection (Federation of Companion Animal Veterinary Associations [FECAVA] guidelines)*	Frequently involves non-staphylococcal pathogens

*Available at: https://www.fecava.org/en/policies-actions/guidelines

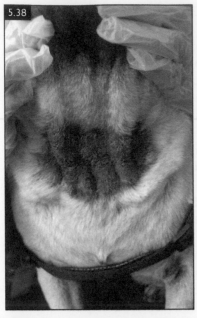

Fig. 5.38 Surface pyoderma in an atopic Pug. Alopecia, hyperpigmentation and lichenification on the ventral neck associated with pruritus and malodor. (Courtesy of Dr Anette Loeffler)

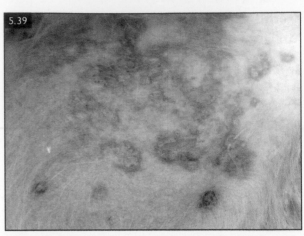

Fig. 5.39 Superficial pyoderma (bacterial folliculitis) in a Cocker Spaniel with underlying hypothyroidism. Erythematous papules, small pustules and epidermal collarettes on the ventral abdomen. (Courtesy of Dr Anette Loeffler)

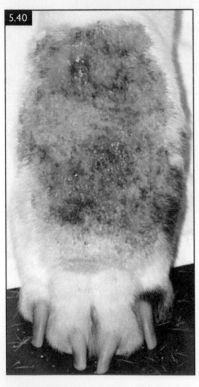

Fig. 5.40 Deep pyoderma due to acral lick dermatitis on the front leg of a Dalmatian with chronic osteoarthritis pain. (Courtesy of Dr Anette Loeffler)

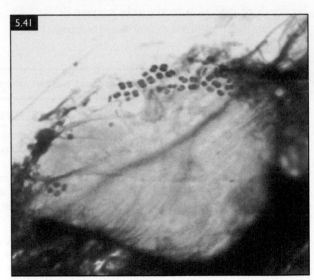

Fig. 5.41 High-power microscopy (×100 oil immersion lens) of a tape-strip preparation from the neck of the Pug in Fig. 5.38 (Diff-Quik stain). Multiple pairs of actively dividing cocci in proximity to a keratinocyte (pale blue) surrounded by degenerate neutrophil material (purple). (Courtesy of Dr Anette Loeffler)

Diagnosis

Confirmation of bacterial infection requires cytologic examination of tape strip or smear preparations (**Fig. 5.41**). Samples are stained with rapid Romanovsky-type stains (e.g. Diff-Quik) and examined at high power (×100 lens oil immersion). Lesions will show cocci with variable numbers of neutrophils. Submission of a swab to a laboratory for bacterial culture (**Fig. 5.42**) and antimicrobial susceptibility testing will enable identification of bacterial species and their resistance pattern, along with focus therapy. However, bacterial

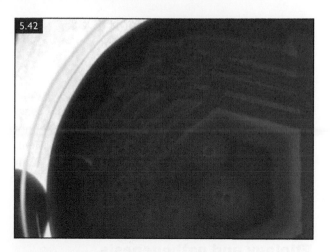

Fig. 5.42 *Staphylococcus pseudintermedius* colonies on sheep blood agar showing characteristic double-hemolysis zone. This isolate was subsequently identified as MRSP through species confirmation by matrix-assisted laser desorption/ionization–time of flight (MALDI-TOF) mass spectrometry and antimicrobial susceptibility testing. Accurate species identification by the laboratory is important because the epidemiology varies between MRSP (dog adapted) and MRSA (primarily a human pathogen).

isolates reported from a culture may represent the commensal staphylococcal skin flora, so bacterial infection needs to be confirmed as described above. The best lesions to sample are those most likely to represent active infection, such as pustules (pricked) and exudate. Collarettes and papules will also yield pathogens. For deep pyoderma, sampling the surface needs to be avoided. Pus from draining sinuses or tissue obtained by aspiration or biopsy will be needed in these cases. Pathogens in deep infection differ substantially from those on the surface.[65]

Therapy

Antibacterial therapy is needed to resolve pyoderma lesions. A wide range of topical and systemic antibacterial drugs are authorized for use in canine and feline pyoderma. These should be used according to recommendations specific for each country and following guidelines for responsible use of antimicrobials in skin disease.[66, 67] Underlying causes need to be treated in parallel to prevent recurrent infection.

Topical therapy

For localized areas, creams, gels and ointments containing fusidic acid, mupirocin and silver sulfadiazine may be effective. If large areas are affected, shampoos containing chlorhexidine (2–3%) or benzoyl peroxide (up to 2.5%) can be used 2–3 times per week with a 10-minute contact time. Mousse, foam or spray products may enhance owner compliance as they do not need to be rinsed off, particularly on difficult-to-treat areas such as the paws.

Systemic therapy

In view of the global threat from increasing antimicrobial resistance, the choice of antimicrobial needs to be based on culture and susceptibility testing and a tier-based approach whenever possible. Guidelines for responsible use of antimicrobials in pyoderma are widely available.[66, 67] If MRSP or MRSA is isolated, treatment choices will be substantially limited, and infections should be treated topically whenever possible. If systemic therapy is indicated for a multidrug-resistant bacterium, involvement of a dermatologist or infectious disease specialist is recommended.

Follow-up examinations including cytology are needed to determine progress. Good information on duration of therapy for pyoderma is lacking, but 3 weeks are traditionally recommended for superficial pyoderma and 6–8 weeks for deep pyoderma.

Prognosis/complications

The prognosis depends primarily on owner compliance and underlying causes. If multidrug-resistant staphylococci are involved, the prognosis can be good provided topical therapy can be used. Prognosis may be less favorable for deep infection, because drugs associated with higher toxicity may have to be used.

Prevention

Pyoderma prevention is based on identification and correction of primary causes, such as rigorous flea control and anti-inflammatory or dietary therapy of underlying allergic disease. Infections due to multidrug-resistant bacteria are prevented through reduced need for repeated antibiotic therapy, antimicrobial stewardship and strict hygiene measures.

PYTHIUM INSIDIOSUM (PYTHIOSIS)
Kenneth Cockwill

Definition
Pythiosis refers to disease caused by the fungal organism *Pythium insidiosum*. *P. insidiosum* causes one of two severe disease entities, which do not occur together in the same canine or feline patient: (1) chronic, progressive gastrointestinal disease, or (2) cutaneous disease characterized by an ulcerative, nodular lesion with draining tracts.[25, 68] Dogs are more often affected than cats.

Etiology and pathogenesis
The motile infective zoospore form of *P. insidiosum* is found in wet environs and is thought to cause infection by encysting on cut or damaged edges of the skin and presumably also via the gastrointestinal (GI) tract. Germ hyphae develop, then invade the body.[68, 69] Most infected dogs (and cats) have frequent exposure to standing freshwater (lakes, ponds, irrigation fields), although disease has been reported in pets living in suburban environments with no exposure.[68, 70–73] Exposure and transmission are through direct contact and skin penetration (after swimming or wading in water) for the cutaneous form, or drinking contaminated water for the gastrointestinal form.

Geography
Pythiosis occurs in tropical, subtropical and some temperate regions of the world, with most cases occurring in the Gulf coast states of the USA. Pythiosis has also been identified in New Jersey, Virginia, North and South Carolina, Illinois, Indiana, Kentucky, Tennessee, Missouri, Oklahoma, Kansas, Arizona and California.[25, 26, 68, 70, 71, 73]

Incidence and risk factors
This is a sporadic disease. Young animals (9 months to 8 years) are most commonly affected, with 1–2 years being the main age range. Large breed dogs (especially Labrador Retrievers) are most often involved.[25, 68, 70, 71, 73, 74] Most but not all dogs have an exposure to warm standing water.[25, 68, 70, 71, 73] There are insufficient case numbers to determine risk factors.

Clinical signs
Cutaneous form
Skin disease is characterized by the presence of non-healing wounds with ulcerated nodules and draining tracts and a mass-like appearance found at the base of the tail or on the extremities, ventral neck and perineum.[25, 68]

Gastrointestinal form
Chronic progressive weight loss with hyporexia or anorexia, vomiting and diarrhea can be present (**Fig. 5.43**). Regurgitation, dysphagia and hematochezia can also occur, depending on the location of the lesions.[25, 26, 68, 71, 73–75] A palpable abdominal mass and thin body condition may be noted.[68] Signs of systemic illness are uncommon, unless complications occur (GI perforation or obstruction).[25, 26, 68, 70, 71, 73]

Diagnosis
Diagnosis is typically made through a combination of clinical suspicion based on geography and disease presentation, abdominal imaging, serology and in some cases histopathology. Histopathology does not reliably differentiate pythiosis from lagenidiosis and zygomycosis. Imaging is also used to determine the extent of surgery required, guide prognosis, and obtain samples for cytology or histology.[68]

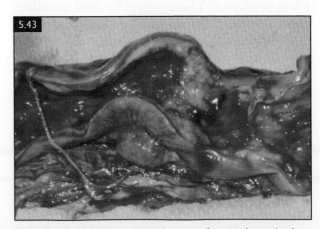

Fig. 5.43 Gross necropsy image of gastrointestinal pythiosis. Note the marked change in the mucosa in the middle of the picture. (Courtesy of Dr Nikki Sereda)

Laboratory abnormalities

Eosinophilia, anemia, hypoalbuminemia and hyper-globulinemia may be noted.[25, 26, 68, 70, 71, 73, 74]

Imaging

Marked segmental GI thickening may be observed in multiple locations. Intestinal obstruction may be noted, along with mesenteric lymphadenopathy.[25, 68, 70] Disease is most common in the stomach, small intestine, colon and rectum but can also involve the esophagus and pharynx.

CT and/or thoracic radiographs are preferred when clinical signs are more consistent with esophageal or pharyngeal disease. CT may also be used to assess the extent of dermatologic lesions.[68]

Cytology

Cytology from aspirates or impression smears of lesions may show fungal hyphae and eosinophilic or pyogranulomatous inflammation. This does not differentiate pythiosis from closely related fungal pathogens.[68]

Culture

Culture can be performed, but specific handling is needed for samples. The best results are through submission of an unrefrigerated biopsy specimen (wrapped in sterile moistened gauze) and shipped at ambient temperature. Samples must arrive promptly (within 24 hours) at a laboratory that has experience with culture of specific fungal pathogens.[68] Consultation with the laboratory is recommended before sample collection.

Histopathology

Histopathology on biopsy samples is characterized by pyogranulomatous inflammation with multifocal areas of necrosis and significant infiltration of tissues with neutrophils, eosinophils, macrophages and fungus (**Fig. 5.44**).[25, 26, 68, 70, 71] In the GI tract, pathology is located within the submucosal and muscularis layers, and may be missed if only superficial biopsies are obtained.[68] Hyphae are not seen with hematoxylin and eosin (H&E) staining but are usually visualized with Gomori's methenamine silver.[25, 68]

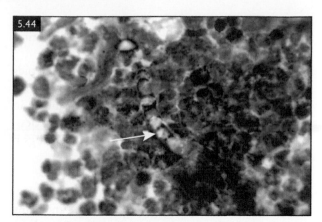

Fig. 5.44 Microscopic image of gastrointestinal pythiosis. Note the hyphae in the center of the image in the middle of the inflammation (arrow) (100× magnification).

Serology

Serology is highly recommended when possible, because it allows non-invasive diagnosis through the use of a highly sensitive and specific enzyme-linked immunosorbent assay (ELISA) that detects anti-*P. insidiosum* antibodies in dogs.[72]

Therapy

Therapy consists of aggressive surgical resection of all infected tissue with wide surgical margins.[25, 68, 70] Evaluation of regional lymph nodes is strongly recommended, as lymphadenopathy may represent spread of disease as opposed to reactive lymph nodes.

In addition to aggressive surgical intervention (or in cases where surgery is not pursued), treatment with itraconazole (10 mg/kg PO q24h) and terbinafine (5–10 mg/kg PO q24h) for 2–3 months is recommended. This has been curative in some cases, although the response rate is very low and it is rarely successful.[25, 26, 68, 70, 71, 73, 74, 76] A recent report of successful therapy of GI pythiosis with mefenoxam, an agricultural fungicide, in addition to itraconazole and terbinafine, holds promise, but use of this drug is currently extra-label and it is difficult to acquire.[26]

Serology can also be used to monitor treatment efficacy, particularly in dogs that have undergone complete surgical removal of affected tissue. There should be a dramatic decrease in antibody level due to removal of active infection within 2–3 months postoperatively. Dogs with a persistently high titer may be more likely to relapse.[68]

Palliation with anti-inflammatory glucocorticoids (prednisone 1 mg/kg) can be used to improve clinical signs for a short time. This may be considered in cases without surgical or financial options, particularly with GI disease, as in a small number of dogs it has been curative.[68]

Prognosis/complications

The prognosis is extremely guarded in dogs, and many die soon after diagnosis and/or surgery. Cures have been reported in cases that were amenable to either surgery or medical management.[25, 68, 70, 71, 73] Cats appear to have a more favorable response than dogs to surgical removal.[77] Local recurrence appears common, particularly when wide surgical margins cannot be obtained.[68]

Prevention

A vaccine has been developed for pythiosis, but its use is currently not recommended in dogs or cats owing to limited efficacy.[68, 78] Avoiding exposure to warm standing water in endemic areas, if possible or practical, is perhaps the most effective preventive measure.

SARCOPTES SCABIEI AND *NOTOEDRES CATI*
Anette Loeffler

Definition

Scabies (sarcoptic or fox mange) is caused by the burrowing mite *Sarcoptes scabiei* var. *canis*. Foxes are the most frequently reported source. The disease typically affects dogs, and is contagious and zoonotic. Skin disease due to burrowing mites is rare in cats.[79] The burrowing mite *Notoedres cati* (family Sarcoptidae) may affect pet cats in some areas, but it more commonly spreads among wildlife. The pathogenesis, clinical signs and treatment of notoedric mange in cats are as for sarcoptic mange.

Etiology and pathogenesis

Scabies mites dig tunnels in the epidermis where they deposit eggs (and feces). The severe pruritus associated with typically small numbers of mites supports a hypersensitivity to mites or their fecal antigens.

Geography

Worldwide.

Incidence and risk factors

There is no known age or breed predisposition. Contact with infested animals or vectors (e.g. in parks, grooming parlors, woods) may predispose to infection. Scabies mainly infests dogs; cats are rarely affected. Notoedric mange affects cats.

Common clinical signs

Elbows, hocks, pinnal margins, and the ventral abdomen and face are commonly affected areas (**Figs. 5.45, 5.46**). There is a mostly widespread lesion distribution. Crusted, erythematous papules and intense pruritus are the hallmarks of scabies. Thick yellow crusting can be seen in chronic cases (**Figs. 5.47, 5.48**). Scabies can be considered the most itchy canine skin disease. Excoriations, secondary bacterial infections and peripheral lymphadenopathy are common.

Atypical presentations with either localized lesions or relatively lesion-free pruritus may occur.

Diagnosis
Skin scrapings

Mites, eggs or fecal pellets may be identified on skin scrapings (**Fig. 5.49**). A single mite, egg or cluster of feces is diagnostic because *Sarcoptes* spp. are obligate parasites and not found on normal skin. However, skin scrapings have a sensitivity of only around 60%. Multiple scrapings should be taken if scabies is suspected. To enhance recovery of mites, areas need to be chosen carefully (non-excoriated, ideally crusty areas at predilection sites). If affected, sampling above the elbows is preferred because there is a higher likelihood of finding mites.

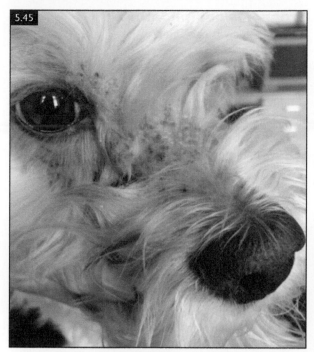

Fig. 5.45 Facial dermatitis in a dog with scabies. Note the alopecia, erythematous papules and crusting. (Courtesy of Dr Anette Loeffler)

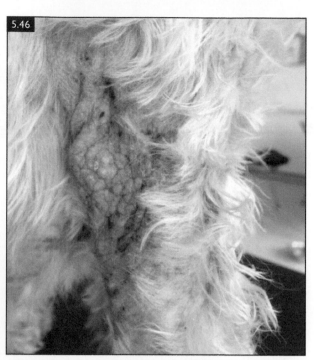

Fig. 5.46 Marked alopecia, erythematous papules and crusting over the elbow of a dog with scabies. (Courtesy of Dr Anette Loeffler)

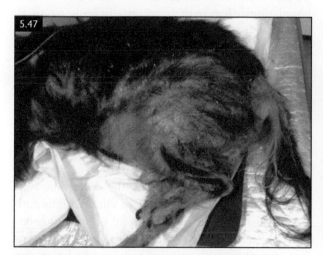

Fig. 5.47 Extensive yellow crusting, erythema and alopecia in a Cocker Spaniel with scabies. The scratch reflex is prompted by rubbing of the pinna (pinnal–pedal reflex). (Courtesy of Dr Anette Loeffler)

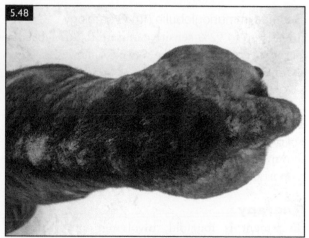

Fig. 5.48 Weight loss and widespread alopecia, severe erythema and crusting in a Staffordshire Bull Terrier with a several months' history of intense pruritus due to sarcoptic mange. (Courtesy of Dr Anette Loeffler)

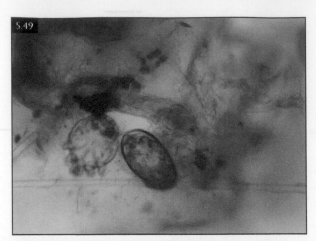

Fig. 5.49 Skin scraping from a dog with scabies showing an adult *Sarcoptes* mite next to an egg and several fecal pellets (×10 magnification). (Courtesy of Dr Anette Loeffler)

Pinnal–pedal reflex
Dogs will start to scratch with a hind leg when the pinna/tip of the pinna (not the base of the pinna) is rubbed between the fingers. This test has been positive in 75–90% of dogs with scabies, with an overall specificity of 93%, and can easily be done (e.g. during history taking).

Scabies immunoglobulin (Ig) G serology
This is up to 92% sensitive and up to 96% specific. Seroconversion may take 5 weeks, however, so its diagnostic utility is limited.

Trial therapy
Resolution of typical clinical signs using appropriate acaricidal therapy may support a diagnosis of scabies and may present a cost-effective way to rule out this important differential in a pruritic patient.

Therapy
Treatment is fourfold, involving mite treatment with systemic or topical acaricide (e.g. fluralaner),[80] treatment of secondary bacterial skin infections (as described for pyoderma), anti-inflammatory treatment with glucocorticoids for 7–14 days to relieve pruritus, and environmental treatment with an acaricidal product, including treatment of the house, car and other indoor contact areas. Care must be taken because products may be toxic to non-mammals (e.g. fish, cage birds, reptiles).

Prognosis/complications
The prognosis is excellent.

Prevention
In areas where foxes and/or scabies are prevalent, products used for ectoparasite prophylaxis against fleas should include anti-mite agents. These may be combination or dual action with insecticidal and acaricidal activity and should be used all year round.

Infection control
Environmental cleaning and decontamination are an integral part of therapy and prevention of reinfection. All in-contact pets in the house will require therapy and monitoring.

Public health and infection control
Sarcoptic mites can be transferred between dogs (and cats) and humans. Clients need to be advised to consult their physician if they notice skin lesions on themselves or family members. Typically, this consists of itchiness and a papular rash on the forearms or trunk.

Notoedric mange should be identified in domestic cats early to avoid spread to vulnerable wildlife populations that may be more difficult to treat. Speciation of mites may require expert advice.

SPOROTRICHOSIS
Michelle Evason

Definition
Sporotrichosis is an uncommon and geographically variable fungal (yeast) infection affecting cats, and less frequently dogs, caused by the dimorphic fungus *Sporothrix schenckii*. Typically, clinical signs consist of subacute or chronic dermal or subcutaneous focal to multifocal nodules on the head, trunk or feet, together with generalized lymphadenopathy. Lesions are frequently ulcerated and draining. It is often misdiagnosed and is both contagious and a zoonotic pathogen.

Etiology and pathogenesis
Sporothrix schenckii causes infection after being inoculated into the skin through traumatic contact with the fungus (mold phase) found in soil or

decaying vegetation. Direct infection of the yeast form from an infected animal can also occur through bites, scratches and contact with infectious fluids.[81, 82] After host tissue invasion, *S. schenckii* reproduces, causes local skin disease, and then may disseminate into the lymphatic system and further into other body organs, particularly the liver or lungs. Three clinical forms are recognized and may present concurrently: the localized cutaneous, cutaneo-lymphatic, and disseminated or systemic forms.[81–83]

Dogs

Dogs appear to have relatively low susceptibility to infection,[83, 84] and most commonly have the cutaneous or cutaneo-lymphatic form.

Cats

Cats are considered more susceptible, and more likely to have cutaneo-lymphatic or disseminated disease or both.[83] Contamination of the oronasal cavity and nail beds appears common, and is likely associated with risk of disease and spread.[82,84] Concurrent immunosuppression with feline immunodeficiency virus (FIV) and feline leukemia virus (FeLV) can occur, but it is not clear whether this is a risk factor for disseminated disease.

Geography

Worldwide, especially warm and humid climates.

Incidence and risk factors

The incidence of reported cases is highest in North and South America, and occasional outbreaks of infection (in humans and cats) have been reported.[81, 82] The true incidence is unknown and likely higher than reported. Reported risk factors involve activities that increase the risk of puncture wounds, such as having outdoor access and, for dogs, being used for hunting.

Clinical signs

Dogs and cats develop similar skin lesions (**Fig. 5.50**), although dogs may more often have respiratory involvement. Lesions can be firm on palpation, focal or multifocal, and widely distributed over the head and trunk (localized cutaneous form).[4] Draining fluid and ulceration are common, and ulceration,

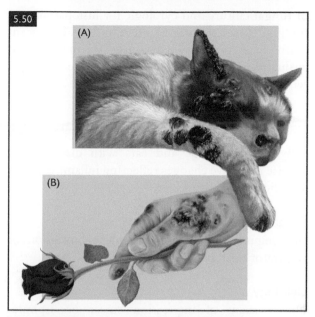

Fig. 5.50 (A) Feline sporotrichosis: nodular and ulcerated skin lesions in a cat. (B) Human sporotrichosis: transmission (mold phase) is commonly associated with inoculation during gardening.

alopecia and drainage of serosanguineous fluid may occur and be confused with an abscess. Lesions may arise over the lymphatics and travel over an affected limb (cutaneo-lymphatic form). Lymphadenopathy is common. In cats, lesions are often first noted on the distal aspects of the body and frequently confused with cat-bite abscesses.

Nasal lesions (bridge of nose, between eyes), with concurrent respiratory signs (disseminated form), can occur. These systemic signs may include cough, nasal discharge, sneezing or respiratory compromise, lethargy, depression, fever and anorexia.[83, 84]

Less commonly, cats or dogs may develop disseminated or systemic disease with multiple organ involvement, such as the liver, spleen, lungs, kidneys and lymph nodes. This is more common in cats than dogs.[83] In these animals, fever, poor appetite, vomiting, weight loss and lymphadenopathy may be noted.

Diagnosis

Sporotrichosis is typically diagnosed on the history, index of suspicion, clinical signs and lack of response to prior therapy (e.g. antimicrobials). A combination of fungal culture and cytologic (or histopathologic) findings is used to confirm infection.[83, 85] Fluorescent antibody testing may aid diagnosis. It is important to evaluate patients, especially cats, for evidence of systemic disease.

Laboratory abnormalities

CBC, serum biochemistry and urinalyses are typically normal. Dogs and cats with disseminated disease may have changes reflecting inflammation or specific organ dysfunction.

Diagnostic imaging

Imaging is frequently normal, unless bony lesions or respiratory compromise is present.[86]

Cytology

Direct exam of impression smear or aspirates may reveal free yeast (**Fig. 5.51**) or yeast located within neutrophils or macrophages.[85] This finding appears less reliable in dogs, and in both dogs and cats negative cytology does not rule out infection. A skilled pathologist with a high index of suspicion is needed, as confusion with other fungal organisms (e.g. *Cryptococcus* spp., *Candida* spp.) may occur. Preferred samples include exudate or fluid taken from draining tracts, or submission of suspect tissue (e.g. skin biopsy). Precautions should be taken to avoid sharps injury or inoculation of infected tissues or fluids into broken skin when obtaining samples, owing to zoonotic concerns.

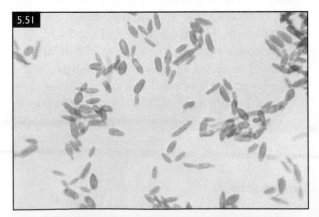

Fig. 5.51 Yeast phase of *Sporothrix schenckii* (970× magnification). (Courtesy of Dr Lucille K. Georg)

Culture

Fungal culture can confirm diagnosis. Communication with the diagnostic laboratory is important to ensure that they are aware of the potential for sporotrichosis and are able to use the required biosafety practices.

Histopathology

Skin biopsies typically reveal pyogranulomatous inflammation. The presence of fungal (yeast) elements in a biopsy is helpful for diagnosis, particularly when culture results are difficult to interpret. Finding *Sporothrix* spp. appears to be more frequent in cats than dogs.[83, 85]

It is important to communicate with the pathologist or dermatopathologist regarding suspicion of disease, so that fungal stains (periodic acid–Schiff or Grocott's methanamine silver) can be used if needed to improve diagnosis.

Serology

Enzyme-linked immunosorbent assay for human and feline disease is available and may be helpful.[81–83]

Therapy

The current recommended treatment of choice for both dogs and cats is systemic antifungal therapy with itraconazole.[83, 84, 86] Both fluconazole and ketoconazole have also been used successfully.[83] Additional options include sodium or supersaturated potassium iodide, terbinafine and amphotericin B.[4, 84]

Duration of treatment is not well established but is typically extended for 1 month beyond clinical cure. It is essential that owners are aware that therapy is typically needed for 4–6 months.[83, 84] Cost may play a role in therapy choice and should be discussed with clients. Amphotericin is typically reserved for cases that are refractory to itraconazole, owing to toxicity concerns. [84]

Local thermo- or cryotherapy may also be an option for focal disease, along with surgical excision. Antimicrobials may be required because of concurrent or secondary bacterial infections. Most common bacterial pathogens are those that cause other types of skin infection, particularly staphylococci.

Follow-up exams and rechecks at 2- to 4-week intervals are critical for success, and to ensure compliance with therapy.

Prognosis/complications

Prognosis and treatment duration are based on severity of presenting clinical signs, and ability of owners to commit to the cost and management (time investment) associated with appropriate therapy. Cats had a good prognosis for complete cure (65–70%) in one study, regardless of extent of lesions.[83] Dogs have an excellent prognosis for cure with itraconazole or ketoconazole, after a median 2–4 months of therapy.[83, 84, 86]

Prevention

There is no vaccine; however, indoor housing, when feasible, may reduce disease occurrence due to trauma or puncture.

Infection control and public health

Sporotrichosis is zoonotic, and avoidance of bites and scratches, proper sharps handling and good wound care are critical. Particular care should be taken when handling infected cats because of the potential for bite-associated infection.[82, 87]

ZYGOMYCOSIS
Kenneth Cockwill

Definition

Zygomycosis refers to disease caused by fungi in the class Zygomycetes. Dogs and cats can be affected.

Etiology and pathogenesis

Zygomycetes includes fungi from the genera *Basidiobolus* and *Conidiobolus* from the order Entomophthorales, and the genera *Rhizopus*, *Mucor* and *Rhizomucor* in the order Mucorales.[25, 88–90] *Basidiobolus* and *Conidiobolus* spp. are saprophytes found in the soil and decaying plant matter. *Basidiobolus* spp. can be isolated from insects and feces of amphibians and reptiles. Cutaneous infection likely occurs via direct inoculation from the environment or possibly insect bites. Hard palate lesions may be the result of direct inoculation.

Geography

Basidiobolus spp. and *Conidiobolus* spp. have a widespread distribution but most reports appear to be from the southeastern United States.

Incidence and risk factors

Zygomycosis is rare. Incidence is poorly defined and highly variable geographically.

Clinical signs and physical exam
Basidiobolomycosis

Ulcerative draining skin lesions which resemble pythiosis and lagenidiosis are most common, with rare reports of tracheobronchitis and disseminated disease.

Conidiobolomycosis

Respiratory signs, including nasopharyngeal disease (which can be invasive), with ulcerative lesions of the nasal planum and hard palate occur most commonly. Pneumonia, primary nasal cavity disease or multifocal nodular draining subcutaneous lesions can occur.

Diagnosis
Culture

Culture and identification of the pathogen is the optimal means of diagnosis. These fungi grow well on routine fungal media.

Histopathology

Pyogranulomatous and eosinophilic inflammation, with broad, thin-walled hyphae, is present. The hallmark of zygomycosis is the presence of a wide eosinophilic sleeve around the hyphae, which is not present in lagenidiosis or pythiosis. Hyphae are larger than for pythiosis: *Basidiobolus* spp. (mean 9 μm diameter) and *Conidiobolus* spp. (mean 8 μm diameter).

Therapy

Optimal treatments are not clearly defined. Most often, aggressive surgical resection of cutaneous lesions (if possible) followed by itraconazole

(5–15 mg/kg for 2–3 months) is recommended. Amphotericin B or itraconazole can be considered if resection is not possible. One cat was successfully treated for a cutaneous *Mucor* infection with posaconazole.[89]

Prognosis/complications

Zygomycosis is less aggressive than cutaneous pythiosis or lagenidiosis. Cure is possible but progressive lesions and systemic dissemination can occur.

REFERENCES

1 Scott, DW *et al.* (1987) Zoonotic dermatoses of dogs and cats. *Vet Clin North Am Small Anim Pract* **17**:117–44.

2 Saevik, BK *et al.* (2004) *Cheyletiella* infestation in the dog: observations on diagnostic methods and clinical signs. *J Small Anim Pract* **45**:495–500.

3 Moriello, KA (2003) Zoonotic skin diseases of dogs and cats. *Animal Health Research Reviews/Conference of Research Workers in Animal Diseases* **4**:157–68.

4 Nuttall, TJ *et al.* (2009) *A Colour Handbook of Skin Diseases of the Dog and Cat.* Manson Publishing Ltd, London.

5 Paradis, M (1998) Mite dermatitis caused by *Cheyletiella blakei. J Am Acad Dermatol* **38**:1014–15.

6 Paradis, M *et al.* (1990) Efficacy of ivermectin against *Cheyletiella blakei* infestation in cats. *J Am Anim Hosp Assoc* **26**:125–8.

7 Paradis, M *et al.* (1988) Efficacy of ivermectin against *Cheyletiella yasguri* infestation in dogs. *Can Vet J* **29**:633–5.

8 Curtis, CF (2004) Current trends in the treatment of *Sarcoptes, Cheyletiella* and *Otodectes* mite infestations in dogs and cats. *Vet Dermatol* **15**:108–14.

9 Beugnet, F *et al.* (2016) Efficacy of oral afoxolaner for the treatment of canine generalised demodicosis. *Parasite* **23**:14.

10 Fourie, JJ *et al.* (2015) Efficacy of orally administered fluralaner (Bravecto™) or topically applied imidacloprid/moxidectin (Advocate®) against generalized demodicosis in dogs. *Parasit Vectors* **8**:187.

11 Six, RH *et al.* (2016) Efficacy of sarolaner, a novel oral isoxazoline, against two common mite infestations in dogs: *Demodex* spp. and *Otodectes cynotis. Vet Parasitol* **222**:62–6.

12 Mueller, RS *et al.* (2012) Treatment of demodicosis in dogs: 2011 clinical practice guidelines. *Vet Dermatol* **23**:86–96, e20–1.

13 Moriello, KA *et al.* (2016) Review of dermatophyte diagnosis and treatment studies in small animals (1900–2016) summary and conclusions. World Association of Veterinary Dermatology Consensus Statement. http://www.wavd.org/media/k2/attachments/Review_of_Dermatophyte_Diagnosis_and_Treatment_Studies_1900-2016_Summary_and_Recommendations.pdf. Accessed June 15, 2017.

14 Cafarchia, C *et al.* (2004) The epidemiology of canine and feline dermatophytoses in southern Italy. *Mycoses* **47**:508–13.

15 Iorio, R *et al.* (2007) Dermatophytoses in cats and humans in central Italy: epidemiological aspects. *Mycoses* **50**:491–5.

16 Moriello, KA *et al.* (1994) Isolation of dermatophytes from the haircoats of stray cats from selected animal shelters in two different geographic regions in the United States. *Vet Dermatol* **5**:57–62.

17 Proverbio, D *et al.* (2014) Survey of dermatophytes in stray cats with and without skin lesions in Northern Italy. *Vet Med Intern* **2014**:565470.

18 Sparkes, AH *et al.* (1993) Epidemiological and diagnostic features of canine and feline dermatophytosis in the United Kingdom from 1956 to 1991. *Vet Rec* **133**:57–61.

19 Greene, C (2012) Cutaneous fungal infections. In *Infectious Diseases of the Dog and Cat*, 4th ed. CE Greene, ed. Elsevier, St. Louis, MO, pp.588–602.

20 Cafarchia, C *et al.* (2006) Isolation of *Microsporum canis* from the hair coat of pet dogs and cats belonging to owners diagnosed with *M. canis* tinea corporis. *Vet Dermatol* **17**:327–31.

21 Moriello, KA *et al.* (2006) Recommendations for the management and treatment of dermatophytosis in animal shelters. *Vet Clin North Am Small Anim Pract* **36**:89–114, vi.

22 Moriello, KA (2017) In vitro efficacy of shampoos containing miconazole, ketoconazole, climbazole or accelerated hydrogen peroxide against *Microsporum canis* and *Trichophyton* species. *J Feline Med Surg* **19**:370–4.

23 Spies, CFJ *et al.* (2016) Molecular phylogeny and taxonomy of *Lagenidium*-like oomycetes pathogenic to mammals. *Fungal Biol* **120**:931–47.

24 Grooters, AM *et al.* (2003) Clinicopathologic findings associated with *Lagenidium* sp. infection in 6 dogs: initial description of an emerging oomycosis. *J Vet Intern Med* **17**:637–46.

25 Grooters, AM (2003) Pythiosis, lagenidiosis, and zygomycosis in small animals. *Vet Clin North Am Small Anim Pract* **33**:695–720, v.

26 Hummel, J *et al.* (2011) Successful management of gastrointestinal pythiosis in a dog using itraconazole, terbinafine, and mefenoxam. *Med Mycol* **49**:539–42.

27 Malik, R *et al.* (2013) Ulcerated and nonulcerated nontuberculous cutaneous mycobacterial granulomas in cats and dogs. *Vet Dermatol* **24**:146–53, e132–43.

28 Malik, R *et al.* (2002) Feline leprosy: two different clinical syndromes. *J Feline Med Surg* **4**:43–59.

29 Sykes, J (2014) Mycobacterial infections. In *Canine and Feline Infectious Diseases*. J Sykes, ed. Elsevier, St. Louis, MO, pp.418–36.

30 Conceição, LG *et al.* (2011) Epidemiology, clinical signs, histopathology and molecular characterization of canine leproid granuloma: a retrospective study of cases from Brazil. *Vet Dermatol* **22**:249–56.

31 Dedola, C *et al.* (2014) First report of canine leprosy in Europe: molecular and clinical traits. *Vet Rec* **174**:120.

32 Smits, B *et al.* (2012) Case clusters of leproid granulomas in foxhounds in New Zealand and Australia. *Vet Dermatol* **23**:465–88.

33 Laprie, C *et al.* (2013) Feline cutaneous mycobacteriosis: a review of clinical, pathological and molecular characterization of one case of *Mycobacterium microti* skin infection and nine cases of feline leprosy syndrome from France and New Caledonia. *Vet Dermatol* **24**:561–9, e133–4.

34 Kennis, RA *et al.* (1996) Quantity and distribution of *Malassezia* organisms on the skin of clinically normal dogs. *J Am Vet Med Assoc* **208**:1048–51.

35 Plant, JD et al. (1992) Factors associated with and prevalence of high *Malassezia pachydermatis* numbers on dog skin *J Am Vet Med Assoc* **201**:879–82.

36 Colombo, S *et al.* (2007) Prevalence of *Malassezia* spp. yeasts in feline nail folds: a cytological and mycological study. *Vet Dermatol* **18**:278–83.

37 Lo, KL *et al.* (2016) Evaluation of cytology collection techniques and prevalence of *Malassezia* yeast and bacteria in claw folds of normal and allergic dogs. *Vet Dermatol* **27**:279–e267.

38 Bond, R *et al.* (2002) Intradermal test reactivity to *Malassezia pachydermatis* in atopic dogs. *Vet Rec* **150**:448–9.

39 Negre, A *et al.* (2009) Evidence-based veterinary dermatology: a systematic review of interventions for *Malassezia* dermatitis in dogs. *Vet Dermatol* **20**:1–12.

40 Banovic, F *et al.* (2013) Cat scratch-induced *Pasteurella multocida* necrotizing cellulitis in a dog. *Vet Dermatol* **24**:463–e108.

41 Weese, JS *et al.* (2009) *Staphylococcus pseudintermedius* necrotizing fasciitis in a dog. *Can Vet J* **50**:655–6.

42 Worth, AJ *et al.* (2005) Necrotising fasciitis associated with *Escherichia coli* in a dog. *NZ Vet J* **53**:257–60.

43 Ingrey, KT *et al.* (2003) A fluoroquinolone induces a novel mitogen-encoding bacteriophage in *Streptococcus canis*. *Infect Immun* **71**:3028–33.

44 Miller, CW *et al.* (1996) Streptococcal toxic shock syndrome in dogs. *J Am Vet Med Assoc* **209**:1421–6.

45 Lloret, A *et al.* (2013) Mycobacterioses in cats: ABCD guidelines on prevention and management. *J Feline Med Surg* **15**:591–7.

46 Greene, CE (2012) Mycobacterial infections In *Infectious Diseases of the Dog and Cat*, 4th ed. CE Greene, ed. Elsevier, St. Louis, MO, pp.462–77.

47 Bennett, AD *et al.* (2011) Radiographic findings in cats with mycobacterial infections. *J Feline Med Surg* **13**:718–24.

48 Gunn-Moore, DA *et al.* (2011) Mycobacterial disease in cats in Great Britain: I. Culture results, geographical distribution and clinical presentation of 339 cases. *J Feline Med Surg* **13**:934–44.

49 Horne, KS *et al.* (2009) Clinical outcome of cutaneous rapidly growing mycobacterial infections in cats in the south-eastern United States: a review of 10 cases (1996–2006). *J Feline Med Surg* **11**:627–32.

50 Gunn-Moore, DA *et al.* (2011) Mycobacterial disease in a population of 339 cats in Great Britain: II. Histopathology of 225 cases, and treatment and outcome of 184 cases. *J Feline Med Surg* **13**:945–52.

51 Salib, FA *et al.* (2011) Epidemiology, genetic divergence and acaricides of *Otodectes cynotis* in cats and dogs. *Vet World* **4**:109–12.

52 Sotiraki, ST *et al.* (2001) Factors affecting the frequency of ear canal and face infestation by *Otodectes cynotis*. *Vet Parasitol* **96**:309–15.

53 Nunn-Brooks, L *et al.* (2011) Efficacy of a single dose of an otic ivermectin preparation or selamectin for the treatment of *Otodectes cynotis* infestation in naturally infected cats. *J Feline Med Surg* **13**:622–4.

54 Weese, JS *et al.* (2011) Parasitic zoonoses. In *Companion Animal Zoonoses*. JS Weese, MB Fulford, eds. Wiley, Ames, IA, pp.47–8.

55 Lange, C *et al.* (2011) Canine papillomaviruses. *Vet Clin N Am Small Anim Pract* **41**:1183.

56 Chambers, VC *et al.* (1959) Canine oral papillomatosis. I. Virus assay and observations on the various stages of the experimental infection. *Cancer Res* **19**:1188–95.

57　Lange, CE *et al.* (2009) Detection of antibodies against epidermodysplasia verruciformis-associated canine papillomavirus 3 in sera of dogs from Europe and Africa by enzyme-linked immunosorbent assay. *Clin Vaccine Immunol* **16**:66–72.

58　Goldschmidt, MH *et al.* (2006) Severe papillomavirus infection progressing to metastatic squamous cell carcinoma in bone marrow-transplanted X-linked SCID dogs. *J Virol* **80**:6621–8.

59　Munday, JS *et al.* (2010) Amplification of feline sarcoid-associated papillomavirus DNA sequences from bovine skin. *Vet Dermatol* **21**:341–4.

60　Yağci, BB *et al.* (2008) Azithromycin therapy of papillomatosis in dogs: a prospective, randomized, double-blinded, placebo-controlled clinical trial. *Vet Dermatol* **19**:194–8.

61　Sancak, A *et al.* (2015) Antibody titres against canine papillomavirus 1 peak around clinical regression in naturally occurring oral papillomatosis. *Vet Dermatol* **26**:57–9, e19–20.

62　Yhee, J-Y *et al.* (2010) Characterization of canine oral papillomavirus by histopathological and genetic analysis in Korea. *J Vet Sci* **11**:21–5.

63　Stull, JW *et al.* (2016) Risk reduction and management strategies to prevent transmission of infectious disease among dogs at dog shows, sporting events, and other canine group settings. *J Am Vet Med Assoc* **249**:612–27.

64　Hill, PB *et al.* (2006) Survey of the prevalence, diagnosis and treatment of dermatological conditions in small animals in general practice. *Vet Rec* **158**:533–9.

65　Shumaker, AK *et al.* (2008) Microbiological and histopathological features of canine acral lick dermatitis. *Vet Dermatol* **19**:288–98.

66　Hillier, A *et al.* (2014) Guidelines for the diagnosis and antimicrobial therapy of canine superficial bacterial folliculitis (Antimicrobial Guidelines Working Group of the International Society for Companion Animal Infectious Diseases). *Vet Dermatol* **25**:163–e143.

67　Beco, L *et al.* (2013) Suggested guidelines for using systemic antimicrobials in bacterial skin infections: part 2 – antimicrobial choice, treatment regimens and compliance. *Vet Rec* **172**:156–60.

68　Grooters, AM (2014) Pythiosis, lagendiosis and zygomycosis. In *Canine and Feline Infectious Diseases*. J Sykes, ed. Elsevier, St. Louis, MO, pp.668–78.

69　Gaastra, W *et al.* (2010) *Pythium insidiosum*: an overview. *Vet Microbiol* **146**:1–16.

70　Berryessa, NA *et al.* (2008) Gastrointestinal pythiosis in 10 dogs from California. *J Vet Intern Med* **22**:1065–9.

71　Fischer, JR *et al.* (1994) Gastrointestinal pythiosis in Missouri dogs: eleven cases. *J Vet Diagn Invest* **6**:380–2.

72　Grooters, AM *et al.* (2002) Development and evaluation of an enzyme-linked immunosorbent assay for the serodiagnosis of pythiosis in dogs. *J Vet Intern Med* **16**:142–6.

73　Helman, RG *et al.* (1999) Pythiosis of the digestive tract in dogs from Oklahoma. *J Am Anim Hosp Assoc* **35**:111–14.

74　Dycus, DL *et al.* (2015) Surgical and medical treatment of pyloric and duodenal pythiosis in a dog. *J Am Anim Hosp Assoc* **51**:385–91.

75　Bonenberger, TE *et al.* (2001) Rapid identification of tissue micro-organisms in skin biopsy specimens from domestic animals using polyclonal BCG antibody. *Vet Dermatol* **12**:41–7.

76　Thieman, KM *et al.* (2011) Diagnosis and treatment of truncal cutaneous pythiosis in a dog. *J Am Anim Hosp Assoc* **239**:1232–5.

77　Rakich, PM *et al.* (2005) Gastrointestinal pythiosis in two cats. *J Vet Diagn Invest* **17**:262–9.

78　Mendoza, L *et al.* (2003) An improved *Pythium insidiosum*-vaccine formulation with enhanced immunotherapeutic properties in horses and dogs with pythiosis. *Vaccine* **21**:2797–804.

79　Hardy, JI *et al.* (2012) Feline sarcoptic mange in the UK: a case report. *Vet Rec* **171**:351.

80　Romero, C *et al.* (2016) Efficacy of fluralaner in 17 dogs with sarcoptic mange. *Vet Dermatol* **27**: 353–e388.

81　Barros, MB *et al.* (2004) Cat-transmitted sporotrichosis epidemic in Rio de Janeiro, Brazil: description of a series of cases. *Clin Infect Dis* **38**: 529–35.

82　Barros, MB *et al.* (2008) An epidemic of sporotrichosis in Rio de Janeiro, Brazil: epidemiological aspects of a series of cases. *Epidemiol Infect* **136**:1192–6.

83　Crothers, SL *et al.* (2009) Sporotrichosis: a retrospective evaluation of 23 cases seen in northern California (1987–2007). *Vet Dermatol* **20**:249–59.

84　Sykes J (2014) Sporotrichosis. In *Canine and Feline Infectious Diseases*. J Sykes, ed. Elsevier, St. Louis, MO, pp.624–32.

85　Pereira, SA *et al.* (2011) Sensitivity of cytopathological examination in the diagnosis of feline sporotrichosis. *J Feline Med Surg* **13**:220–3.

86　Whittemore, JC *et al.* (2007) Successful treatment of nasal sporotrichosis in a dog. *Can Vet J* **48**:411–14.

87 Weese, JS *et al.* (2011) Fungal diseases. In *Companion Animal Zoonoses*. JS Weese, MB Fulford, eds. Wiley, Ames, IA, pp.291–3.

88 Hawkins, EC *et al.* (2006) Treatment of *Conidiobolus* sp. pneumonia with itraconazole in a dog receiving immunosuppressive therapy. *J Vet Intern Med* **20**: 1479–82.

89 Wray, JD *et al.* (2008) Infection of the subcutis of the nose in a cat caused by *Mucor* species: successful treatment using posaconazole. *J Feline Med Surg* **10**:523–7.

90 Greene, CE *et al.* (2002) Infection with *Basidiobolus ranarum* in two dogs. *J Am Vet Med Assoc* **221**: 528–32.

ACTINOMYCES AND *NOCARDIA* SPP.
J Scott Weese

Definition
These are unrelated bacteria that are often considered together because of similarities in the types of disease they produce. They are opportunists which cause a range of infections that can be hard to treat. Dogs are affected more often than cats.

Etiology and pathogenesis
The two bacterial genera are compared in *Table 6.1*. Both are filamentous bacteria that typically cause suppurative and/or granulomatous inflammation.

Actinomycosis is usually associated with trauma, bites or migrating foreign bodies (e.g. grass awns). Co-infections with other opportunists are common.

Nocardiosis is less common and typically a mono-infection acquired from environmental exposure.

Geography
Actinomyces sp. is a relatively ubiquitous commensal. *Nocardia* sp. is an environmental organism that is most common in arid regions such as parts of Australia and the southwestern United States.

Clinical signs
Both organisms can cause similar infections, characterized by the presence of exudates, draining tracts, abscesses and/or dense fibrous masses (**Fig. 6.1**). These can be slowly progressive and often not fully investigated until empirical treatments have failed. Sometimes the lesions can appear similar to neoplasia, with their dense composition and slow growth. Chronic draining tracts are particularly common. Sulfur granules may be visible, especially with actinomycosis.

Table 6.1 **Comparison of *Actinomyces* and *Nocardia* spp.**

	***ACTINOMYCES* SPP.**	***NOCARDIA* SPP.**
Bacterium	Anaerobic Gram positive Non-acid fast Filamentous	Aerobic Gram positive Partially acid fast Filamentous
Main source	Commensal microbiota	Environment
Most common infection type	Mixed infection	Mono-infection
Frequency	Uncommon	Rare
Infection spread	Direct spread	Hematogenous spread
Mortality	Low	Moderate to high
Patient population most commonly affected	Outdoor dogs Bite victims Foreign body cases	Young animals Immunocompromised patients
Exudates	May contain sulfur granules	May contain sulfur granules

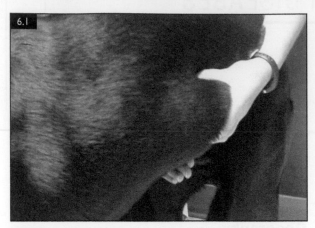

Fig. 6.1 Large, firm mass on the flank of a dog with actinomycosis. (Courtesy of Johanna Heseltine)

Table 6.2 **General categorizations of actinomycosis, and likely causes**

DISEASE TYPE/ LOCATION	LIKELY INCITING CAUSE
Cervicofacial	Bite wound Penetrating foreign body
Thoracic	Aspiration or inhalation of foreign materials Migrating foreign body Penetrating (esophageal) foreign body
Abdominal	Penetrating ingested foreign body Migrating foreign body
Subcutaneous	Bite Trauma Penetrating or migrating foreign body

Table 6.3 **Classification of human nocardiosis**

SITE	TYPE	COMMENTS
Skin	Superficial	Presence of ulcers, pustules, abscesses, cellulitis and/or granulomas
	Lymphocutaneous	Ulcerated papules that progress to lymphangitis and subcutaneous nodules
	Mycetomas	Indurated masses with fibrosis, necrosis and draining tracts
	Secondary	Disseminated infection also affecting skin, usually from pulmonary nocardiosis
Lungs	Pulmonary	Chronic to peracute Mild to severe Pneumonia, abscessation and/or pyothorax
Various	Disseminated	Disease involving two or more body sites Usually associated with pulmonary nocardiosis

Clinical presentation varies with the location of infection. Presenting signs may relate to direct effects of the infection (e.g. visible mass or draining tract), systemic sequelae (e.g. weight loss) or the effects of a space-occupying lesion.

Actinomycosis is sometimes classified according to location, which can indicate likely sources of exposure (*Table 6.2*). In humans, nocardiosis is classified by site into categories that are probably reasonable to consider in animals (*Table 6.3*).

Diagnosis

Misdiagnosis as neoplasia can occur if testing is not performed. *Actinomyces* sp. is sometimes overlooked if co-infection with another pathogen is present, because the other bacterium may grow more readily. This highlights the importance of cytology.

Cytology of aspirates or exudates can provide a suspicion of these organisms based on their filamentous appearance (**Figs. 6.2–6.4**). Acid-fast staining can help differentiate *Actinomyces* sp. (negative) from *Nocardia* sp. (often positive) because differentiation cannot be made solely by appearance.[1] Histological analysis of biopsies may also be useful, particularly with firm masses where neoplasia is a concern.

Culture is required for definitive diagnosis, but it can be challenging. Exudates, aspirates or tissue samples can be tested. However, deep samples are preferred to avoid confusion with contaminants and the skin microbiota. Anaerobic culture is required for *Actinomyces* sp. and it may be readily overgrown because of its slow growth. Negative culture results cannot rule out actinomycosis and the diagnosis should still be considered when clinical signs and

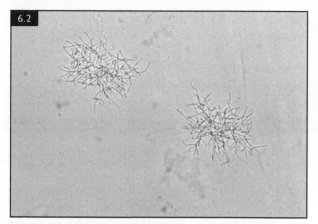

Fig. 6.2 Morphology of *Actinomyces* sp. Note the long thin filamentous appearance (500× magnification). (Courtesy of Lucille K Georg)

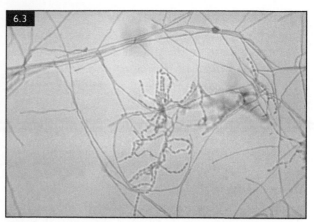

Fig. 6.3 Morphology of *Nocardia* sp. (Courtesy of Lucille K Georg)

cytology are supportive. *Nocardia* sp. is aerobic but isolation may still be a challenge because it is slow growing and plates must be kept longer than for typical cultures. Overgrowth of contaminants can result in false-negative results.

Antimicrobial susceptibility testing is rarely provided.

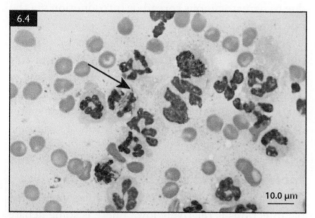

Fig. 6.4 Actinomycosis cytology. Note the filamentous bacteria within neutrophils (arrow). (Courtesy of Johanna Heseltine)

Therapy

Differentiating *Actinomyces* and *Nocardia* spp. and other atypical organisms like *Mycobacterium* spp. is important for determination of optimal drugs and durations (*Table 6.4*). Duration of treatment is poorly characterized but is prolonged. A year or more may be required for systemic or complicated nocardiosis. Surgery may be indicated to remove or debulk infected sites, to establish drainage or to correct an underlying problem (e.g. foreign body).

Table 6.4 **Antimicrobial treatment of actinomycosis and nocardiosis**		
	***ACTINOMYCES* SPP.**	***NOCARDIA* SPP.**
Recommended antimicrobial	Amoxicillin: 20 mg/kg PO q8–8h	Trimethoprim sulfonamide: 15–30 mg/kg PO q12h
Other antimicrobial options	Erythromycin Clindamycin Doxycycline Chloramphenicol Third-generation cephalosporins	Third-generation cephalosporins Amoxicillin Doxycycline Amikacin
Duration	Weeks to months	Months to years
Other	Drainage of abscesses and effusions Resection of affected tissue	Drainage of abscesses and effusions Resection of affected tissue

Prognosis/complications

Prognosis is guarded because of the commonness of advanced disease by the time of diagnosis, as well as the cost and difficulties of prolonged treatment. There is little guidance to provide good survival estimates; however, severity of disease and initial response to treatment are the main prognostic factors.

Prevention

There are no specific preventive measures.

ANAEROBIC BACTERIAL INFECTIONS
Jinelle A Webb and Lee Jane Huffman

Definition

Anaerobic bacteria cannot grow well (or at all) in the presence of oxygen. Clinical signs are related to site of infection and anaerobic infection should be suspected after trauma (e.g. bite wounds) and with periodontal disease.

Etiology and pathogenesis

Anaerobic bacteria comprise a large percentage of the normal bacterial microbiota of the oral, gastrointestinal and genital tracts of animals. The main anaerobic bacterial pathogens in dogs and cats include *Clostridium* spp., *Bacteroides* spp., *Fusobacterium* spp., *Prevotella* spp., *Porphyromonas* spp., *Propionibacterium* spp. and *Peptostreptococcus* spp. Some anaerobic bacteria (e.g. *Clostridium* spp.) are sporeformers, and the hardy spores can exist in a dormant state in the body (including in healthy tissues) and the environment. Entrance into the dog or cat is usually via a penetrating injury, most commonly from a bite wound or penetrating foreign object. Anaerobes can also gain entrance if mucosal barriers are compromised, and rarely by hematogenous spread. Brain abscessation can be seen after direct extension of tooth root infection or otitis. Bacterial cholangiohepatitis can occur due to hematogenous spread or introduction via the bile duct.[2]

Anaerobic bacteria have been implicated as a significant cause of periodontal disease, skin and soft tissue infections/abscessation, retrobulbar abscesses, pyothorax, peritonitis, pyometra and some forms of bacterial pneumonia (**Figs. 6.5, 6.6**).[3, 4] Many sites of infection contain a mixed population of anaerobic and facultative bacteria.[3, 4]

Incidence and risk factors

The apparent incidence of clinically relevant anaerobic infections is relatively low. There is some debate about whether the apparent low incidence truly

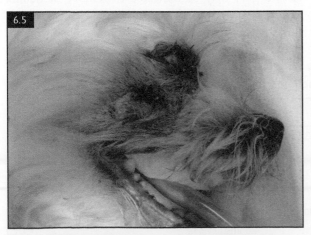

Fig. 6.5 Ruptured tooth root (tooth 108) abscess in a small dog. Tooth 108 had a complicated (pulp-exposed) slab fracture allowing bacterial entry.

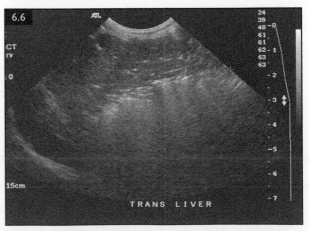

Fig. 6.6 Ultrasound image of gas within a septic focus in a liver lobe in a 9-year-old Dachshund.

means that anaerobic infections are uncommon or whether they are often undiagnosed.

Risk factors for penetrating anaerobic infections include bite wounds and active outdoor pets that are exposed to penetrating foreign objects. Advancing age is correlated with increased incidence of periodontal disease.

Clinical signs

Clinical signs are closely correlated with site of infection and can range from mild to imminently life threatening (*Table 6.5*).

Diagnosis

Diagnosis of an anaerobic bacterial infection is through a combination of typical history, clinical signs, physical examination, presence of purulent material or abscessation (often with a foul odor), gas production within an organ or deep abscess, and bacterial culture.

Bacterial culture

It can be difficult to obtain a positive culture for anaerobic bacteria if samples are not properly collected and transported, or if the laboratory is not adept at anaerobic culture. The presence of bacteria on cytology with a negative culture suggests an anaerobic bacterial infection.

False negatives are common and, to increase the chance of obtaining a positive culture, fluids or tissues should be submitted in an anaerobic transport device.[5] Additionally, some anaerobic infections result in gas formation, whereas foul odor and gas production do not always occur with anaerobic infections.

Therapy

Antimicrobials are the mainstay of therapy for anaerobic bacterial infections (*Table 6.6*). Rendering the local environment inhospitable by drainage of purulent material and/or debridement of affected

---

Table 6.5 Common clinical presentations of anaerobic infections

DISEASE	COMMON SIGNS	PHYSICAL EXAMINATION
Periodontal disease	Halitosis, plaque/calculus, tooth or jaw mobility, tooth loss, pain response on or avoidance of handling mouth/face or chewing, face pawing/rubbing, soft tissue hyperemia, swelling ± fistulation ± discharge, nasal/oral purulent or bloody discharge, lethargy	Plaque/calculus, apparently missing teeth, pain, facial swelling, discharge
Retrobulbar abscess	Unilateral exophthalmos, protruding nictitans, ocular discharge, pain or difficulty opening the mouth, inappetence or anorexia, facial swelling	Unilateral exophthalmos, ocular discharge, pain, facial swelling
Soft tissue infections	Firm or fluctuant subcutaneous swelling, lethargy, inappetence, pain. Serosanguineous-to-purulent material may be produced from swelling	Firm or fluctuant subcutaneous swelling with associated pain, variable discharge
Pyothorax/ pneumonia	Dyspnea, tachypnea, coughing, nasal discharge, lethargy, inappetence	Decreased lung sounds focally or ventrally, crackles, wheezes, increased lung sounds, harsh lung sounds
Peritonitis	Abdominal pain, severe lethargy, vomiting, diarrhea, recumbency	Abdominal pain and fluid wave, dehydration, tachycardia, poor peripheral pulses
Cellulitis/fasciitis	Localized signs of inflammation and pain, with or without discharge or crepitus. Pyrexia, dullness. Signs of systemic involvement (e.g. fever, anorexia, toxemia) may also be present	Localized signs of inflammation may be present, with or without discharge or crepitus. The presence of crepitus is neither pathognomonic for an anaerobic infection nor always present, but is strongly suggestive. Signs of systemic involvement (e.g. fever, anorexia, toxemia) may also be present
Cholangiohepatitis	Pyrexia, lethargy, anorexia, vomiting, weight loss	Pyrexia, lethargy, icterus, vomiting, weight loss

Table 6.6 **Suggested drugs with doses for anaerobic bacterial infections**

ANTIMICROBIAL	DOGS	CATS
Metronidazole	10–15 mg/kg IV or PO q12h	10–20 mg/kg IV or PO q24h
Amoxicillin/clavulanic acid	13.75 mg/kg PO q12h	12.5 mg/kg PO q12h
Clindamycin	5.5–33 (generally 5.5–11) mg/kg IV, SC, IM or PO q12h; IM less bioavailable and locally tolerable than SC such that painful IM injection not recommended	11–33 (generally 11–22) mg/kg IV, SC, IM or PO q24h; can be divided and given q12h; IM less bioavailable and locally tolerable than SC such that painful IM injection not recommended
Chloramphenicol	40–50 mg/kg IV, IM, SC or PO q8h	10–20 mg/kg IV, IM, SC or PO q24h (maximum 50 mg/cat dose)

tissues will improve resolution. Although resistance to antimicrobial drugs is possible with anaerobic bacteria, it is uncommon,[2, 3, 6] and poor response to treatment is usually the result of disease factors, not antimicrobial resistance.

Prognosis/complications

Prognosis is based on location of the infection and the ability to drain or debride affected tissue and remove an inciting nidus. Septicemia is rare, although likely underdiagnosed.[2–4, 7, 8]

ANGIOSTRONGYLUS VASORUM (FRENCH HEARTWORM)
Michelle Evason and Gary Conboy

Definition

Angiostrongylus vasorum is a slender nematode found in the pulmonary arteries and heart of infected wild and domestic dogs. Clinical signs range from mild-to-severe cardiorespiratory disease or coagulopathy. Domestic and wild dogs (e.g. foxes, wolves and coyotes) can be affected.

Etiology and pathogenesis

Canids are the main definitive hosts. Infection occurs after ingestion of the intermediate host (snail, slug or frog) containing third-stage larvae. Once consumed, larvae leave the intestine and enter the pulmonary artery (**Fig. 6.7**) and right ventricle where maturation to the adult stage occurs. After reproduction, eggs enter and become lodged in the lung capillaries (**Fig. 6.8**), where they develop into L1 larvae, are coughed up and swallowed by the dog. The life cycle is completed after larvae are excreted and subsequently ingested from the soil or feces by the intermediate host. Adult worms begin egg production 28–108 days after infection and can live as long as the dog.

Geography

This parasite can be found in parts of Africa, North and South America, and Europe. Endemic foci within countries or geographic locations are common and it is considered an emerging infection in some regions. Canine importation presents a risk for establishment in new locations.

Incidence and risk factors

Prevalence in dogs is variable, and likely impacted by geography and local wild canid populations. Higher incidence has been reported in specific regions.[9, 10]

Risk factors may include hunting and older age, both of which may increase exposure.[9, 10] Recent history of deworming (milbemycin oxime) has been associated with reduced risk.[10]

Common clinical signs

Clinical signs vary widely from subclinical infection to fatal disease (e.g. respiratory failure, severe blood loss anemia and coagulopathy). Duration of clinical signs may range from 14–66 days[9] to years (chronic disease).

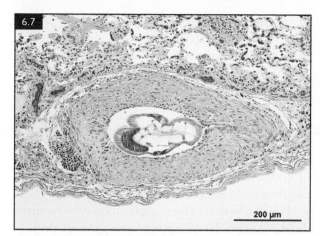

Fig. 6.7 Section of an adult *Angiostrongylus vasorum* in a pulmonary artery of an infected dog (H&E). (Courtesy of Gary Conboy)

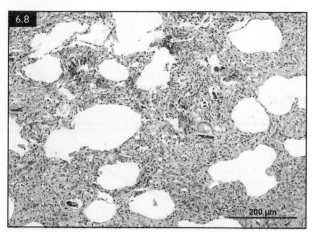

Fig. 6.8 Section of lungs from a dog infected with *Angiostrongylus vasorum* (H&E). Note the developing eggs, larvae and granulomatous inflammatory response. (Courtesy of Gary Conboy)

Classic disease is cardiorespiratory, with the lungs being most affected. Cough (acute or chronic), dyspnea, gagging and exercise intolerance due to interstitial pneumonia, coagulopathy, congestive right heart failure or pulmonary hypertension may occur.[9–11]

Bleeding tendencies are frequently reported and may include anemia, melena, epistaxis, prolonged bleeding from wounds, hemoabdomen, conjunctival hemorrhage, CNS bleeds, hemothorax or hemorrhage thought to be secondary to consumptive coagulopathy (disseminated intravascular coagulopathy, DIC).

Anorexia, lethargy, vague gastrointestinal signs (vomiting or diarrhea) and weight loss are common. In one study, half of cases with bleeding or non-pulmonary signs had concurrent respiratory disease.[10]

Neurologic signs may occur and appear to be associated with bleeding. These can range from ataxia, seizures and collapse to cranial nerve deficits.[10, 11]

Parasite aberrant migration may occur. Clinical signs may be related to inflammation within the eye, abdominal organs and skeletal muscle.[10, 11]

Diagnosis

Diagnosis is based on history, clinical signs and fecal Baermann identification of larvae (**Fig. 6.9**) or through evidence of adult worms (**Fig. 6.10**) in the dog.[9–11]

Laboratory findings

The CBC and serum biochemistry may be normal, or in more severe cases reveal thrombocytopenia, anemia (blood loss or regenerative), eosinophilia, hypoalbuminemia and hypoproteinemia, or increased globulins.[11, 12] Proteinuria may be detected.[11] Increased prothrombin time and activated partial thromboplastin time may be noted.[11]

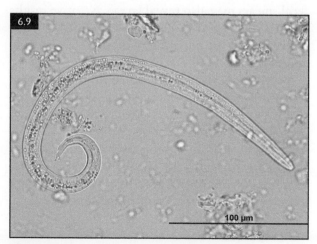

Fig. 6.9 First-stage larvae of *Angiostrongylus vasorum* recovered from the feces of a dog by Baermann fecal examination. Larvae are 340–399 × 13–17 µm in size and have a distinctive kinked tail with a small dorsal spine. (Courtesy of Gary Conboy)

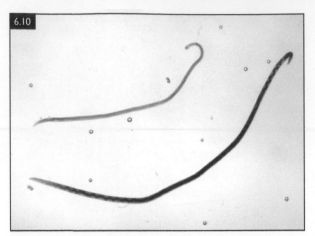

Fig. 6.10 Adult male (upper) and female (lower) *Angiostrongylus vasorum* recovered from the pulmonary artery of an infected red fox (*Vulpes vulpes*) from Newfoundland, Canada. Worms range in size from 14 mm to 21 mm in length (about a tenth of the size of *Dirofilaria immitis*). Note that the male has a small genital bursa at the caudal end and the blood-filled red intestine entwined with the white reproductive tract gives a "barber pole" appearance to the female. (Courtesy of Gary Conboy)

Fecal examination

Baermann technique is the method of choice.[10] Multiple fecals on consecutive days will improve sensitivity. Fecal flotation by centrifugation or direct fecal smears may also reveal larvae. Negative results do not rule out infection, as larvae may be shed intermittently or not at all with severe disease and lack of feces.

Fecal exam may also determine whether infection (or co-infection) with *Crenosoma vulpis* is present.

Respiratory sample cytology

Transtracheal wash or bronchoalveolar lavage may be helpful to identify L1 larvae. Alternatively, fine-needle aspiration of lung tissue or urine sediment exam may enable organism identification.[11]

Imaging

Thoracic radiographs may be normal or show an alveolar or interstitial pattern; this may progress to a denser bronchial or interstitial pattern with chronicity. Residual abnormalities may be noted on films despite therapy and apparent clinical resolution.[11]

Echocardiogram may reveal pulmonary hypertension, right ventricular dilation and changes in pulmonary flow patterns.[11] CT and MRI may show consolidation and patchy opacities in the lungs. MRI may be helpful for assessment of cerebral or spinal hemorrhage.[11]

Therapy

Therapy is advised in all cases (even with an absence of clinical signs), owing to the severity of disease progression in some cases (*Table 6.7*).

Transfusion with blood or plasma may be required during the first 24–48 hours of anti-parasitic therapy. Bleeding tendencies should subside after this time;[11] however, dyspnea may be noted after therapy. Treatment is directed at management of ascites or respiratory compromise, and may include bronchodilators, diuretics or corticosteroids for reduction of inflammation or lung fibrosis. Strict cage rest for the first 2–3 days is advised after anti-parasitic treatment, particularly for severely compromised dogs.[11]

Follow-up Baermann fecal examination (over 3 consecutive days) after clinical cure, or at the end of treatment, is helpful to ensure successful eradication of infection.[11] Additional Baermann testing after 3 months, and repeated twice annually, is advised to monitor for reinfection.[11] After this time frame, testing should be repeated if clinical signs reoccur.

Prognosis/complications

Prognosis can be excellent with appropriate management. Clinical improvement is typically noted within a few days of therapy. Severely ill dogs may require intensive hospitalization and transfusion; prognosis is guarded in these cases. Death is typically due to coagulopathy, and in the referral setting the mortality rate may be 10–15% despite therapy.[13] Some dogs may continue to cough and have reduced exercise tolerance even with therapy.[11]

Table 6.7 **Recommended therapy for *Angiostrongylus vasorum* (French heartworm)**		
DRUG	**DOSE**	**DURATION**
Milbemycin	0.5 mg/kg once weekly	4 weeks
Fenbendazole	25 mg/kg PO q24h	14–21 days

BABESIA SPP. (BABESIOSIS)
Michelle Evason

Definition

Babesiosis is an increasingly recognized hemo-protozoal infection of dogs and cats. Disease ranges from mild to severe, and typically manifests as lethargy, hemolytic anemia (**Fig. 6.11**) and splenomegaly. Subclinical, chronically infected or recovered animals may act as reservoirs of infection.

Etiology and pathogenesis:

In dogs, *Babesia* spp. of clinical importance include *B. canis* (subspecies *vogeli*, *canis*, *rossi*), *B. gibsoni* and *B. conradae* (**Fig. 6.11**). In cats, *B. felis* and *B. cati* have been recognized. Ticks (*Table 6.8*, **Fig. 6.11**) can transmit *Babesia* spp. to their vertebral host during release of sporozoites from the tick mouthparts.[14] A minimum of 2–3 days of feeding (tick attachment) is needed for transmission.[14] Sporozoites invade host red blood cells (piroplasm form) and undergo merogony. After this, merozoites infect additional red blood cells and the cycle repeats. Transmission of *B. gibsoni* is thought to occur primarily from infected dog to dog through bites or fighting behavior (**Fig. 6.11**), vertically or through blood transfusion (**Fig. 6.12**).[15, 16]

Table 6.8 **Geography, tick vectors and various *Babesia* spp. in dogs**

***BABESIA* SPP.**	**GEOGRAPHY**	**TICK VECTORS**
B. canis vogeli	Warm humid locations in Africa, Asia, Australia, Europe, North and South America	*Rhipicephalus sanguineus*
B. canis canis	Europe (particularly France) and Africa	*Dermacentor reticulatus, R. sanguineus*
B. canis rossi	Africa	*Haemaphysalis elliptica*
B. gibsoni	Asia, North and South America, Africa, Australia and Europe	*H. bisponosa, H. longicornus, R. sanguineus* (?)
B. conradae	California, USA	Unknown

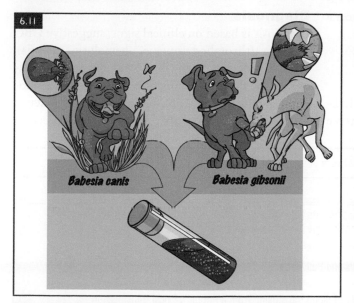

Fig. 6.11 Transmission of *Babesia* spp. and resultant clinical disease in dogs: transmission of sporozoites from the tick mouthparts to a dog or dog-to-dog transmission of *B. gibsoni* through bites. Hemolytic anemia is common.

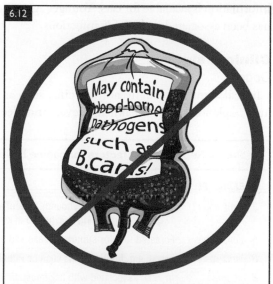

Fig. 6.12 Transmission of *Babesia* spp. occurring through blood transfusion. Testing blood or blood products is encouraged in endemic regions and in at-risk dogs.

Clinical disease is largely due to hemolysis. Platelets may also be targeted, through either immune-mediated thrombocytopenia or a consumptive coagulopathy.

Dog age, immune status and infecting *Babesia* spp. determine severity of clinical disease. However, clinical signs can vary among individual dogs regardless of strain. For example, *B. canis rossi* may cause severe disease in some dogs, while causing subclinical infection in others.[17, 18] Subclinical or chronic infections may become clinically apparent after immunosuppression or splenectomy.[14, 15] Disease can be severe in these cases.

Geography

Worldwide. In dogs, the species distribution varies geographically (*Table 6.8*). In cats, infection with *B. felis* has mainly been reported in southern coastal regions of Africa,[19] and sporadically in other regions (e.g. France, India).

Incidence and risk factors

Studies reporting clinical disease or prevalence (serology or PCR) are limited to specific geographic areas, kennels and dog breeds. Babesiosis is believed to be an emerging disease, likely due to expansion of tick vector range globally and increasing canine importation.[14, 15] Risk factors for dogs are presented in *Table 6.9*. Less information is available for cats. Younger age (<3 years) has been associated with *B. felis* infections.[19, 20]

Clinical signs
Dogs

Clinical signs are usually non-specific, such as lethargy, splenomegaly, weakness, fever and decrease in appetite. Pallor due to anemia is common.[14, 16, 18, 21] Jaundice, poor body condition, pigmenturia and lymphadenopathy may be noted.

Disease can range from hyperacute (e.g. disseminated intravascular coagulation [DIC], sudden death), acute or chronic to intermittent, with waxing and waning fever and anorexia. Subclinical or chronically infected animals (particularly Pitbulls or Greyhounds) may have no signs of disease.[14, 15, 21]

Less commonly, glomerulonephritis (immune) can lead to renal failure and associated proteinuria. Severe systemic inflammatory response (SIRS) or multiple organ dysfunction syndrome (MODS) may result with *B. canis canis* and *B. canis rossi*. Severe hypotension, renal failure, neurologic or respiratory signs, DIC and acute respiratory distress syndrome can occur.[14, 17, 18]

Cats

Lethargy, anorexia, weight loss, weakness and poor hair coat may result.[19] Pallor due to severe anemia can occur. Low-grade, chronic disease is most often reported, and may be precipitated by stress.[19] Fever, constipation, pica and icterus are uncommon manifestations.[19, 20]

Diagnosis

Diagnosis is based on clinical signs, suggestive CBC changes (thrombocytopenia, hemolytic anemia), cytologic identification (**Fig. 6.13**) and paired serology with PCR. Co-infections with other pathogens (e.g. *Bartonella* spp., feline immunodeficiency virus [FIV]) can occur.[18–20, 22] In dogs, infection

BABESIA SPP.	RISK FACTORS
B. canis vogeli	Older age, breed (Greyhound), lack of appropriate tick prevention, blood transfusion, and living in kennels or groups, e.g. racing Greyhound in kennels more likely infected than pet Greyhounds
B. canis canis	Forested rural or suburban areas and possibly breed
B. canis rossi	Breed, e.g. fighting dogs such as Pitbulls and Bull Terriers
B. gibsoni	In Asia: associated with tick infestation In North America: breed (Pitbull), history of blood transfusion from a Pitbull, vertical transmission (transplacental or perinatal) and fighting dogs or history of bite, kennel with history of infection
B. conradae	Coyote bites

Table 6.9 **Reported risk factors for canine babesiosis**

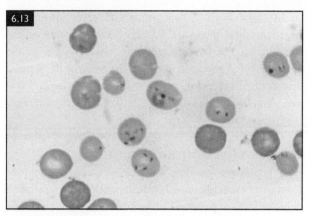

Fig. 6.13 *Babesia* sp. within red blood cells. (Courtesy of Dr George Healy)

may be misdiagnosed as immune-mediated hemolytic anemia, immune-mediated thrombocytopenia or infection by another vector-borne pathogen if babesiosis is not considered alongside other tests for those conditions.

CBC and biochemistry

Moderate-to-severe thrombocytopenia occurs in most clinically affected dogs, with or without anemia.[14–16, 18, 21] Anemia may or may not be regenerative, and range from mild to rapidly progressive and hemolytic.[15, 16] White cell count may be increased (e.g. neutrophilia) or decreased. Serum biochemistry may be non-specific for a sepsis-like response (e.g. hyper- or hypoglycemia) and inflammation, such as elevated or reduced globulin, hypoalbuminemia and concurrent hypocalcemia. Elevated bilirubin, alkaline phosphatase (ALP) and alanine aminotransferase (ALT) can occur, and are more consistent with *B. canis canis* or *B. canis rossi* infection.[14, 18]

Cats typically have regenerative anemia, normal platelet numbers, elevated bilirubin and ALT, with normal ALP and gamma-glutamyl transferase (GGT).[14, 19, 20] Anemia is not a consistent finding.[20]

Coagulation testing

Coagulation testing may be consistent with DIC and thrombocytopenia (i.e. increased activated partial thromboplastin time, prothrombin time and red cell adhesion). Autoagglutination or a positive Coombs test may be found.[14, 18, 20]

Urinalysis

Urinalyses may be normal, or reveal bilirubinuria or proteinuria.

Diagnostic imaging

Evidence of splenic enlargement or lymphadenopathy may be present.

Cytology

Cytology of whole blood or buffy coat smears, lymph node, spleen, liver or other organ aspirates may reveal piroforms.[14, 23] However, negative findings do not rule out infection, and repeated (multiple) samples may improve diagnoses. A skilled interpreter is needed to make the diagnosis, and *Babesia* spp. cannot be differentiated with cytology. Peripheral blood collection (e.g. nail-bed or ear-tip sampling) may improve diagnosis.[14, 17]

Culture

Culture is not widely available or practical for diagnoses.

Serological testing

Serology (immunofluorescent assay) is ideally performed on acute and convalescent samples to improve diagnoses, with a fourfold increase in titer supporting infection. False negatives can occur with acute or chronic infection, and false positives may result from prior exposure. *B. canis* or *B. gibsonii* titers of 1:64 or greater are suggestive of infection.[14] Cross-reactivity among strains usually necessitates the use of PCR for identification.

PCR

Currently, PCR testing of whole blood or splenic aspirates is considered the most sensitive and specific means to diagnose active infection.[14, 23] Results (and sensitivity) may, however, vary among *Babesia* species.[15] Multiple samples (serial tests 2–4 weeks apart) may improve sensitivity, especially with chronic infections.

Therapy

Imidocarb dipropionate is the treatment of choice for *B. canis* and is believed to eliminate infection. It may also reduce morbidity and parasitemia in dogs infected with *B. gibsonii*; however, it is not curative. Imidocarb may be given as a single dose (6.6 mg/kg IM) and repeated at 14 days, or this imidocarb dose given at the same time as diminazene (3.5 mg/kg).[14, 15] Side effects associated with imidocarb include injection site pain and cholinergic effects. Pre-treatment with atropine (0.5 mg/kg SC 30 minutes before administration) can reduce adverse effects.

For *B. gibsoni* and *B. conradae*, combination oral therapy for 10 days with azithromycin (10 mg/kg q 24h) and atovaquone suspension (13.5 mg/kg q8h with a fatty meal) is considered optimum.[14, 15] This treatment has been used to reduce parasitemia, but is not curative.[16]

In cats, treatment with the antimalarial primaquine phosphate (0.5 mg/kg PO q24h for 1–3 days or 1 mg/cat IM q36h for 6 days) is recommended, and the response can be good.[19, 20] However, severe side effects may occur at close to the required dose (1 mg/kg) and the response can be variable. Infection is infrequently cured with a single treatment course, and chronic (or repeated) therapy may be required.[19, 20]

For both dogs and cats, additional supportive therapy for critically ill animals may include IV fluid support and blood transfusions for severe anemia.

Monitoring
Clinical improvement typically occurs in 24–72 hours, but some dogs and cats may take 4–7 days (and some dogs <14 days) for disease resolution.

Ongoing monitoring of CBC (e.g. platelet counts) should occur until all changes have resolved. Antibody titers can decrease 3–5 months post-treatment; however, they may remain elevated for years.

In dogs with *B. gibsoni*, PCR tests should be performed at 60 and 90 days after combination atovaquone and azithromycin therapy to assess efficacy.[14, 16] Anecdotally, dogs that remain PCR positive are unlikely to respond to additional therapy and are suspected to have drug resistance. Consultation is strongly advised in these cases.

Prognosis/complications
The prognosis for dogs and cats can vary, and may (or may not) correlate with severity of presenting clinical signs or level of parasite burden.[18, 19] Most dogs infected with *B. canis* will recover completely with appropriate therapy, although mortality can be high in those with severe laboratory changes (leukopenia, thrombocytopenia), SIRS or MODS.[17, 18] Cats, and some dogs, with *B. gibsoni* infection may be resistant to treatment.[16, 19] Recovered animals appear more susceptible to reinfection and become chronic carriers (i.e. partially recovered, or have occasional relapses). Owners should be counseled that treatment might be ineffective.

Prevention and infection control
Recovery from infection does not appear to confer long-lasting immunity, and there is no cross-protection among strains.[14] Vaccination against *B. canis* is available in Europe, and may limit parasitemia and reduce severity of clinical signs.

Prevention is dependent on effective tick control. This is critical for recovered dogs and cats that serve as a source of infection for naïve ticks. Recovered animals should ideally be kept indoors and treated to reduce transmission to ticks. Reduction of fighting behavior may help decrease or prevent infection.

BARTONELLA SPP. (BARTONELLOSIS)
Michelle Evason

Definition
Infection with various *Bartonella* species can cause endocarditis in dogs. The bacteria may also be the cause of (or contributor to) other inflammatory disorders. Subclinical (and chronic) infections are common, particularly in cats. *Bartonella* spp. are zoonotic, and transmission to humans is most strongly associated with contact with cat fleas and flea dirt, although other means of blood-borne transmission, such as needlestick injuries and bites, are of increasing concern.

Etiology and pathogenesis
Bartonella spp. are gram-negative, intracellular bacteria transmitted predominantly through biting insect vectors. Fleas (mainly *Ctenocephalides felis*) are

Table 6.10 *Bartonella* spp., reservoir hosts and clinical disease

SPECIES	RESERVOIR HOSTS	CATS AND DOGS	HUMANS
Bartonella henselae	Cats, dogs, humans	Subclinical infections most common, endocarditis and myocarditis (primarily dogs), canine bacillary peliosis, vasculitis and thrombosis	Cat scratch disease (CSD), endocarditis, bacillary angiomatosis and peliosis, neuroretinitis, vasculitis and potentially a range of neurocognitive disorders, subclinical disease
B. vinsonii subsp. *berkhoffii*, *B. rochalimae*	Coyotes, dogs, cats, humans	Canine endocarditis and myocarditis, multiple inflammatory diseases, e.g. granulomatous disease, bacillary angiomatosis	Limited cases
B. clarridgeiae	Cats, dogs	Subclinical in cats, canine endocarditis	Possible role in CSD
B. koehlerae	Cats, dogs, humans	Subclinical in cats, canine endocarditis	Endothelioma
B. quintana	Humans, primates	Canine endocarditis	Trench fever, urban trench fever, bacillary angiomatosis, endocarditis
B. bacilliformis			Verruga peruana ("Peruvian warts")

the most common vectors.[24, 25] However, other biting insects (e.g. lice, keds and flies) may transmit the bacteria, and ticks may be the most common vector in dogs, particularly for *B. vinsonii* subsp. *berkhoffii*.[26] Transmission may also be directly blood borne, from blood transfusion or bites in cats and dogs.

Bartonellosis occurs in multiple species (*Table 6.10*). In cats, *B. henselae* is the most important species and the two main genotypes vary geographically, with type I more common in Asia, and type II in the USA, Europe, the UK and Australia. *B. clarridgeiae* and *B. koehlerae* can be found in both healthy and diseased cats. In dogs, *B. vinsonii* subsp. *berkhoffii* and *B. hensalae* are most common, and *B. vinsonii* subsp. *berkhoffii* may be an emerging pathogen.

Bacterial replication primarily takes place in the red blood cells, resulting in bacteremia. This is commonly subclinical and chronic in cats, lasting for months to years.[27, 28]

Geography

The bacterium can be found worldwide, although the prevalence is highest in subtropical and tropical regions.

Incidence and risk factors

Seroprevalence rates in cats and dogs vary depending on sampled population and region, and are highest in stray, shelter and feral animals, and those in warmer climates. Reported seroprevalence in cats can be high, ranging from 25% to 90%.[24, 25, 27, 29, 30] Risk factors for infection in cats include younger age, stray or feral lifestyle and multi-cat household. Seropositive status is more common with increased age, likely due to increased risk of exposure over time. Risk factors in dogs include tick, flea or cattle exposure, outdoor lifestyle (e.g. hunting dog) and strays.

Clinical signs

Subclinical infections in cats and dogs are considered common, particularly in cats with *B. henselae*, and most have no signs of disease.[31]

Bartonellosis is an important cause of infectious endocarditis or myocarditis in dogs,[32-34] but this occurs rarely in cats. Clinical signs of endocarditis include heart murmur, cough, dyspnea, multisystemic signs such as lethargy, inappetence, fever and weight loss, lameness or neurologic manifestations (e.g. seizures). Fever is less common than with other types of infective endocarditis.[34] Septic thromboemboli can result and clinical signs reflect the location of the thrombus (e.g. kidney, brain, muscles or the respiratory tract).[35]

In cats, bartonellosis can cause ocular disease (e.g. uveitis) and stomatitis.[31]

The range of other clinical signs due to various *Bartonella* spp. is currently unclear and it is possible that bartonellosis is a component of various diseases, particularly chronic inflammatory disorders such as pancreatitis, lymphadenopathy, neurologic disease, epistaxis, pyogranulomatous or granulomatous disease, splenomegaly, polyarthritis and vasculoproliferative disorders (e.g. peliosis hepatitis and bacillary angiomatosis).

Diagnosis

Bartonellosis should be considered in animals with non-specific signs or non-resolving illness, or those with a history of flea or tick exposure. The diagnosis can be difficult to confirm, because of limitations of current tests and the high prevalence of seropositivity in some healthy populations. Repeated testing (or a combination of diagnostics) to ensure presence of infection and avoid false positives is usually required.

Typically, diagnosis is confirmed by consistent clinical signs, together with positive PCR or culture from blood or tissues.[24, 25, 35, 36]

Laboratory abnormalities

Laboratory assessment reveals mild change or is normal. Abnormalities may include mild non-regenerative anemia, neutrophilia, eosinophilia and thrombocytopenia. Mild hypoalbuminemia, hyperglobulinemia and azotemia can occur. Urinalysis may show pyuria, hematuria and proteinuria.

Coagulation function testing may be abnormal in dogs with endocarditis.

Culture of blood or tissues may prove definitive; however, false negatives can occur due to intermittent bacteremia. False positives may be associated with subclinical infection in healthy animals or sample contamination.

Histopathology may show inflammation or bacteria. As with culture, bacterial presence may not equate with disease causation. Results must be interpreted in the light of the clinical signs.

Radiographs of animals with endocarditis may show pulmonary edema and cardiac enlargement consistent with congestive heart failure. Abdominal or cardiac ultrasonographic findings may vary widely or appear normal. The aortic (most common), the mitral or both valves may be affected with endocarditis. Splenic, liver or lymph node enlargement may be noted, in addition to echocardiographic abnormalities.

Serological testing (immunofluorescent assay, enzyme-linked immunosorbent assay and western blot assay) is an important aid to diagnoses, but care must be taken not to overinterpret results. False-positive (typically due to previous or current subclinical infection in healthy animals) and false-negative results are a common concern due to lab variability and intermittent bacteremia.[27] Cross-reactions among *Bartonella* spp. can occur. Chronic infection is common, and therefore acute and convalescent titers do not aid diagnosis unless an acute case is suspected and a rise in convalescent titer occurs. Serology is not advised for diagnosis in cats;[25] however, it may help define disease in culture- and PCR-negative dogs with endocarditis.

PCR after enrichment culture and real-time-PCR can be performed on blood, lymph node and splenic aspirates or tissue samples, and will detect either live or dead organisms. False-positive results can occur in healthy animals or with contamination and, as with serology, PCR must be interpreted together with clinical signs.

Awareness of assay limitations, the ability to detect and differentiate *Bartonella* spp. and an understanding of lab variations in testing are essential.

Therapy

Antimicrobial therapy is advised only for patients with overt clinical signs related to bartonellosis. In dogs and cats with endocarditis, therapy is directed at stabilization of cardiac disease or congestive heart failure (e.g. furosemide) along with antimicrobials. Doxycycline (10 mg/kg PO q12h) or a combination of antimicrobials, such as doxycycline together with rifampin (5 mg/kg PO q12h), azithromycin and a fluoroquinolone, or a fluoroquinolone with amoxicillin has been used.[35]. For other canine presentations of bartonellosis, doxycycline with a fluoroquinolone has been advised.

In cats with clinically significant disease due to bartonellosis, doxycycline, amoxicillin/clavulanic acid or a fluoroquinolone given for 4–6 weeks may be used to reduce bacterial load and alleviate clinical signs.[27, 31] However, incomplete responses are common and efficacy has not been established for any antimicrobial regimen. Enrofloxacin should not be used in cats owing to retinal toxicity concerns.

Prognosis/complications

Prognosis is guarded to poor in dogs and cats with endocarditis related to *Bartonella* spp. infection.[35] Many of these animals develop congestive heart failure. Survival times for infective endocarditis in dogs have ranged from 4 days to greater than 1,000 days, with a mean of 54.

Clinically normal bacteremic and chronically infected animals typically live normal lives. Prognoses associated with other presentations of bartonellosis are unknown.

Prevention

At this time, there is no effective vaccine for *Bartonella* spp. Protective immunity does not appear to develop after infection.

Prevention of bites, scratches and use of ectoparasite control are the most effective strategies.

Cats should be tested and if positive excluded as blood donors.[37]

Public health and infection control

Various *Bartonella* spp. are zoonotic and *B. henselae* is one of the most common causes of zoonotic bartonellosis. Although most commonly manifested as cat scratch disease, *B. henselae* infection in humans can cause a range of other diseases, including endocarditis, bacillary angiomatosis, neuroretinitis and potentially a range of neurocognitive disorders. Veterinarians and clinic staff may be at higher risk of infection because of increased exposure to fleas and flea dirt, particularly when handling young or fractious cats that may scratch or bite. Education of clients about flea and tick control, bite and scratch avoidance, and bite and scratch first aid are important to reduce zoonotic transmission.

COCCIDIOIDES IMMITIS AND *C. POSADASII* (COCCIDIOIDOMYCOSIS, VALLEY FEVER)
Jinelle A Webb and Michelle Evason

Definition

Coccidioidomycosis is a fungal disease that develops when *Coccidioides* spp. arthroconidia are inhaled from dry soil or, rarely, via inoculation (**Fig. 6.14**). There is a resultant local pyogranulomatous reaction, and the endospores may then disseminate. In dogs, subclinical disease is most common; however, lower respiratory tract signs and less commonly disseminated disease may occur.

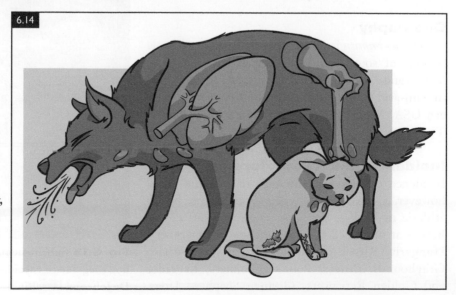

Fig. 6.14 Clinical signs of coccidioidomycosis in a dog associated with the respiratory, lymphatic and musculoskeletal (bone and spine pain) systems. In cats, skin lesions and lymphadenopathy are most common.

Etiology and pathogenesis

Coccidioides immitis and *C. posadasii* are dimorphic fungi. They are present as arthroconidia within vegetative mycelia (colonies of arthroconidia) in semi-arid to arid soil. Within the soil, arthroconidia are highly resistant; however, heavy rainfall followed by a dry period favors growth. Arthroconidia are released when the soil is disturbed and dispersed by wind.[38, 39]

Arthroconidia are the infective form. They enter the body via inhalation, and mature within a spherule to produce 200–300 endospores.[38] The endospores are released after rupture of the spherule, and endospores can then form new spherules. Infection may remain localized within the pulmonary tissue, spread to the hilar lymph nodes or less commonly disseminate.

Dissemination occurs in 20% of clinically affected dogs and 50% of clinically affected cats, and is considered most likely to occur in immunocompromised animals within 10 days of inhalation.[38, 40] Any organ or tissue can be affected, although the bones, CNS, skin, lymph nodes, heart and eyes are the most common organs to be involved in dissemination. Rarely, infection occurs via inoculation, which may lead to coccidioidomycosis localized only to the skin.[39–41]

Onset of clinical signs can occur months to years after exposure, and a large number of infected pets (70% of dogs in one study) will remain subclinical.[38–40]

Geography

Coccidioides immitis is primarily distributed in endemic regions of south-central California (hence "valley fever") and Arizona, whereas *C. posadasii* can be found in semi-arid to arid areas of the southwestern to western USA, Mexico, and Central and South America. The geographic range in the USA may be expanding.

Incidence and risk factors

Incidence can be high in dogs in endemic areas; however, disease is rare in cats. Young, large breed, athletic male dogs are most commonly affected.[39] Breeds at increased risk may include Weimaraners, Hungarian Viszlas, Norfolk Terriers, Dalmatians, Greyhounds, Boxers, Poodles, Pointers, Labrador and Golden Retrievers, German Shepherd Dogs, Australian Shepherds, Scottish Terriers, Dachshunds and Beagles.[39, 42] Risk factors include being housed outdoors, roaming, walking in the desert, digging behavior and history of travel to an endemic region.[38, 40, 43] The use of immunosuppressive therapy has been associated with relapse.[40]

Clinical signs

Fever, cachexia, increased or decreased lung sounds, decreased heart sounds, peripheral lymphadenopathy, draining skin lesions, subcutaneous masses (**Fig. 6.15**), painful bones, spine and/or joints, chorioretinitis, uveitis, keratitis, endophthalmitis, absent menace reflex, postural reaction deficits or organomegaly may be present.

Dogs

Subclinical disease is most common.[44] The most common presenting sign is a cough, which can be harsh and dry or moist. Systemic signs such as fever, inappetence, lethargy and weight loss can be present

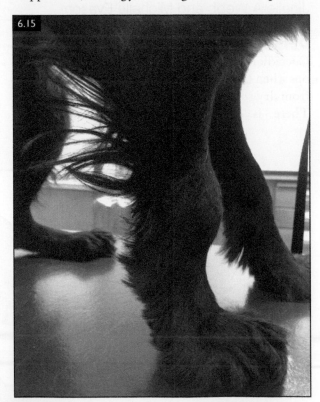

Fig. 6.15 Subcutaneous and bony swelling on a dog's leg due to coccidioidomycosis. (Courtesy of Dr Johanna Heseltine)

or occur intermittently.[44] In animals with disseminated coccidioidomycosis, clinical signs vary depending on the site(s) of dissemination and may include weakness, lameness, draining skin lesions, ocular lesions including blindness, seizures, ataxia, circling, behavioral changes, tetraparesis, pain associated with bones and/or spine, and/or signs of left- or right-sided heart failure. Gastrointestinal signs are rare.

Cats

The most common signs are skin lesions, respiratory effort and lameness, respectively. Cats often do not present with pulmonary signs even though the pathogenesis does not differ from that in the dog. The lack of pulmonary signs may be related to lower activity levels in affected cats.

Diagnosis

Typically, diagnosis is made through a combination of consistent clinical signs, radiographs, patient history (e.g. living in or travel to an endemic region), and cytology, culture or serologic testing. Confirmation of coccidioidomycosis is typically made via direct visualization of the organism on aspirated or biopsied material. However, organisms are often not visible in tissue, leading to the use of serology and fungal culture in many cases.

In endemic regions, the presentation of a chronic cough, with variable thoracic radiographic findings including nodular pulmonary disease and cardiomegaly, warrants further investigation for coccidioidomycosis. The presentation can mimic neoplasia, especially in an older dog.

Laboratory abnormalities

Non-regenerative anemia, neutrophilia ± left shift and monocytosis may be identified, along with hyperglobulinemia and hypoalbuminemia. Proteinuria, which can be severe, may also be noted.[45]

Diagnostic imaging

Thoracic radiographs may be normal or display a wide range of non-specific lung patterns, such as nodular, diffuse interstitial or alveolar. Solitary nodules are most common in the periphery of the lung field. Hilar lymphadenopathy is common, and cardiomegaly is variably present.

Echocardiography may reveal pericardial effusion and a thickened pericardium. Mass lesions and lymphadenopathy in the thorax or abdomen can result in a suspicion of neoplasia.[40, 46, 47] Bony lesions may be noted, and similarly mistaken for neoplasia (**Fig. 6.16**).

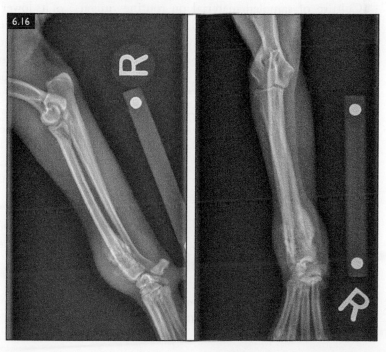

Fig. 6.16 Radiographs of the right forelimb of patient pictured in Fig. 6.15. Note the moderate amorphous periosteal proliferation on the cranial and medial aspects of the distal radial diaphysis and metaphysis, with mild multifocal lysis of the radial cortices at this level. There is also swelling of the soft tissues at the level of the distal radial diaphysis to the antebrachiocarpal joint. (Courtesy of Texas A&M Radiology service)

Cytology

Cytology (aspirates or smears) of body fluids, skin lesions, affected organs or tissues may reveal spherules or endospores together with granulomatous or pyogranulomatous inflammation (**Fig. 6.17**). However, this is an insensitive technique and organisms can be challenging to identify. In endemic regions, or with history of travel to these regions, this type of inflammation should raise the index of suspicion and encourage additional evaluation.

Serology

Given the low yield of organisms in cytologically sampled tissues, serology is commonly used. Serologic assays that detect IgG or IgM antibodies in serum are the initial serology-based test utilized; antibodies become positive within 2–5 weeks (IgM) or 8–12 weeks (IgG) after exposure. False-negative test results are possible but uncommon, and titers as low as 1:2 can be present in clinically affected pets. Level of titer is not believed to correlate with severity of disease.[44] Serologic assays performed on urine are not recommended, and nor are skin tests.[38]

Antigen or organism detection

Antigen-based and PCR testing are not currently advised, or commercially available.

Culture of sampled material on routine fungal culture media can result in isolation of *Coccidioides* spp., often within a period of days. Laboratory staff should be warned if coccidioidomycosis is suspected.

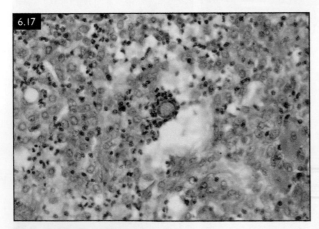

Fig. 6.17 *Coccidioides immitis* **pyogranulomatous cellulitis with central endospore. (Courtesy of Dr Ryan Jennings)**

Growing arthroconidia pose a human health risk, and culture should be attempted only by laboratories with suitable biocontainment.

Therapy

Pulmonary coccidioidomycosis may resolve spontaneously without therapy, leading to discussion of whether these cases should be treated. However, given the potential for dissemination, treatment is usually recommended. Debilitated patients, and those with evidence of dissemination or increasing titers, should always be treated.

Supportive care will vary depending on the patient (e.g. oxygen support, IV fluids). Long-term azole therapy is typically employed in dogs and cats, whether they have pulmonary or disseminated disease. Therapy is usually for no less than 6 months, and is often extended for years.[39] Ability to treat or proceed with extended therapy may be limited for many clients, owing to the cost of medications. The decision to stop therapy should be based on clinical and/or imaging resolution, and a serum antibody titer of 1:2 or less.[39]

Either itraconazole or fluconazole can be used (*Table 6.11*). Itraconazole is recommended for cases with bony involvement, and fluconazole is recommended in cases with CNS involvement or because of its lower cost.[39] Amphotericin B does not offer an advantage over the azoles, and the potential for renal toxicity and parenteral route of administration limit its use. However, amphotericin (lipid formulation) may be used in patients with advanced disseminated disease or when azole therapy is not tolerated.

Surgery is reserved for specific cases and often once medical treatment has failed. Examples include

Table 6.11 **Suggested azole doses for coccidioidomycosis therapy**		
ANTIFUNGAL	**SPECIES**	**DOSE**
Itraconazole	Dog	5 mg/kg PO q12h or q24h
	Cat	25–50 mg TOTAL DOSE PO q12–24h
Fluconazole	Dog	5–10 mg/kg PO q12h
	Cat	25–50 mg TOTAL DOSE PO q12–24h

amputation, enucleation, pericardectomy and spinal cord decompression. Antifungal drug therapy should be employed in all surgical cases.

Prognosis/complications

Prognosis can be good in animals presenting with pulmonary coccidioidomycosis; however, prognosis will vary according to disease severity at presentation. Prognosis is variable in the disseminated form, and involvement of the CNS imparts a poor prognosis. Relapse is common in cats once therapy has been discontinued, sometimes repeatedly.[38, 40]

COXIELLA BURNETII (Q FEVER)
Jason W Stull

Definition

Q fever, caused by the zoonotic bacterium *Coxiella burnetii*, is a rare cause of splenomegaly and neurologic and reproductive signs in dogs and cats. The main concern regarding *C. burnetii* in domestic animals is the health risk they pose to humans.

Etiology and pathogenesis

Coxiella burnetii is a gram-negative intracellular bacterium. Domestic animals become infected through inhalation or ingestion of organisms present in reproductive fluids/tissues (e.g. placenta), urine or milk from infected farm animals (e.g. small ruminants) or wildlife hosts, such as rodents, birds and rabbits. Ectoparasites (especially ticks) appear to be important in transmission of *C. burnetii* to wildlife and could serve as a source for domestic animals.[50]

Geography

Worldwide, with the exception of some geographically isolated countries (e.g. New Zealand).

Incidence and risk factors

The incidence of clinical disease is unknown, and it is likely rare. However, exposure may be relatively common in some locations (e.g. antibodies to *C. burnetii* found in 9% of cattery-confined breeding cats in Australia),[51] with a possible increased

Prevention

As no commercial vaccine is available, prevention is centered around avoidance of the organism where possible. Keeping pets indoors in endemic areas during periods of drought and wind, and avoiding digging behavior, are ways to reduce exposure.

Public health and infection control

Coccidioidomycosis is generally not directly transmissible from affected pets to humans. However, two cases of transmission from an infected patient to a veterinarian or veterinary staff member have been reported.[48, 49]

risk in stray populations.[52] Most canine and feline exposures likely follow direct contact with tissues/fluids from infected farm animals (especially following parturition).

Clinical signs

Most dogs and cats have subclinical infections. Splenomegaly is often the only clinical finding in dogs, whereas fever, inappetence and lethargy have been observed in experimentally infected cats. Abortion, premature birth, stillbirth and death shortly after delivery have been observed in dogs and cats.[53, 54] Neurologic signs (e.g. ataxia, seizures) can be observed in dogs with CNS manifestations.

Diagnosis

Serology (IgG), immunohistochemistry and PCR are the most frequently used methods for definitive diagnosis of *C. burnetii*. Given the highly infectious nature of reproductive tissues, the laboratory should be notified when planning to submit tissues if *C. burnetii* is suspected.

Serology

Paired acute and convalescent titers are needed (in humans, titers peak approximately 8 weeks after infection).[50] Cross-reaction (especially with *Bartonella* spp.) can complicate interpretation.[55]

Therapy

Clinically affected animals should be treated. It is unclear whether animals with subclinical infections, particularly non-pregnant animals, benefit from treatment or whether treatment alters zoonotic risk. At a minimum, owners of clinically and subclinically infected animals should be made aware of human health risks and encouraged to speak with their healthcare provider. Several antimicrobials, including tetracyclines and chloramphenicol, appear to be effective in treating clinically affected dogs and cats with *C. burnetii* (duration of therapy 2 weeks).[56]

Prognosis/complications

Animals with a positive test without clinical signs are likely to have an excellent prognosis as development of disease is rare. For clinically affected animals, the outcome is less clear owing to the rarity of disease and limited published reports. Pregnant animals with reproductive tract signs may be likely to suffer fetal consequences (e.g. abortion, premature birth, stillbirth, death shortly after delivery).

CRYPTOCOCCOSIS
Julie Armstrong

Definition

Cryptococcosis is an invasive mycosis caused by the yeasts *Cryptococcus neoformans* and *C. gattii*. This infection in cats commonly causes upper respiratory signs such as chronic nasal discharge and sneezing, and can cause dramatic nasal deformities. Dogs more often than cats develop neurologic signs and disseminated disease resulting in multisystemic signs.

Etiology and pathogenesis

The genus *Cryptococcus* includes over 37 species. The most important of the disease-producing encapsulated species are *C. neoformans* var. *neoformans*, *C. neoformans* var. *grubii* and *C. gattii*.

Cryptococcosis is acquired from the environment. The main infectious stage is thought to be the basidiospore (<2 μm yeast cell), which is inhaled and then may disseminate through the blood. The nasal cavity is thought to be the main site of infection, and

Prevention

In some regions, vaccines are available for livestock and humans; however, vaccines are not available for dogs or cats.

Reducing contact between dogs/cats and livestock or their environment (especially livestock with known or suspected *C. burnetii* infections or during parturition) is advised if practical. Dogs and cats should not be permitted to consume or have contact with placenta or uterine secretions. Reducing dog and cat predation of wildlife and use of tick control may reduce risk for *C. burnetii* exposure.

Public health and infection control

Q fever in humans is most commonly due to contact with infected livestock (e.g. sheep, goats, cattle) or surfaces contaminated with secretions from these animals. However, infected dogs and cats can be a source of infection for humans. Reports have described people becoming infected after exposure to aerosols or fomites contaminated by parturient infected dogs and cats, including an outbreak in a small animal veterinary hospital following a caesarean section in a queen.[53, 54, 57, 58]

disease may manifest as local osteomyelitis, including the orbits, or lysis of the cribiform plate.[59, 60] If hematogenous dissemination occurs, the CNS, skin, lymph nodes, eyes and lungs are commonly involved, although infection can occur in any organ (**Fig. 6.18**).[61, 62] Infrequent methods of infection are direct inoculation into a skin wound, or ingestion with subsequent primary intestinal lesions.[61]

The incubation period is potentially long but poorly understood. The time to onset of clinical disease after exposure in a British Columbia, Canada, outbreak of *C. gattii* ranged from 1 month to 12–13 months.[61] Pathogenesis of cryptococcosis is dependent on the amount of inhaled pathogen, the virulence of the strain and the status of host immune defenses. In most circumstances infected dogs and cats are immunocompetent; however, immunosuppression will play a role in clinical disease. Retroviral infection in cats has not been shown to affect disease

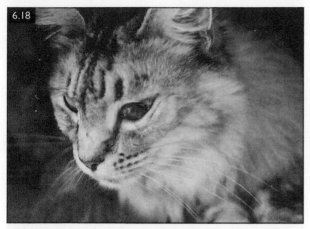

Fig. 6.18 Cryptococcosis involving the third eyelid of a cat. (Courtesy of Dr Margie Scherck)

risk, but concurrent viral infection may have a negative impact on response to therapy.

Geography

Cryptococcus spp. are disseminated worldwide, with regional variation in the presence of certain species. They are associated with environmental niches rich in avian guano, particularly pigeon excreta (*C. neoformans*), and decaying vegetation, especially in tree hollows and hardwood tree bark (*C. gatti* in eucalyptus trees in Australia). They have also been isolated from air, freshwater and seawater in the Pacific Northwest.[63, 64] Higher-risk geographic regions have mild winter temperatures, and there is an increased risk of *C. gatti* on southern Vancouver Island, and along the Pacific Northwest coast.

Incidence and risk factors

Risk factors vary based on the *Cryptococcus* spp. but often relate to environmental exposure, such as exposure to commercial soil disturbance/logging within 10 km of residence,[65] outdoor exposure/active lifestyle, exposure to pigeon guano/decaying vegetation and travel to endemic regions. The majority of dogs with cryptococcosis are purebred dogs younger than 6 years of age, but the disease can occur at any age.[60] The median age of affected cats is 6 years, and young adult cats appear to be at increased risk, although cats of any age may be affected.[64] Infection of strictly indoor animals can occur.[64]

Clinical signs

Clinical presentations of cryptococcosis are similar, although C. *gatti* appears more virulent and has a greater propensity to infect the CNS.[66] General complaints in cats include malaise/inappetence and may include changes in behavior with CNS involvement.[66] Common manifestations are outlined in *Table 6.12.*

Table 6.12 **Manifestations of cryptococcosis**	
Upper respiratory	Nasal discharge, sneezing, head shaking and stertor Facial or nasal bridge swelling Polyp-like mass may be visible in cats Sneezing, epistaxis and mucopurulent nasal discharge can be present in dogs
Dermatologic	Single/multiple (possibly ulcerated) lumps or nodules More common in cats than dogs Extensive cutaneous involvement should raise concern for possible disseminated disease
Neurologic	Variable neurologic signs in both cats and dogs CNS signs including seizures have been the most common clinical sign in dogs Given the propensity for CNS involvement or disseminated disease, lethargy, weight loss and inappetence are more common in dogs than in cats
Ocular	Blindness (cats more often than dogs), dilated/asymmetric pupils or red eye(s)
Lymph nodes	Hilar, mandibular (more common in cats) and mesenteric lymphadenopathy (more common in dogs)
Gastrointestinal	Gingival disease Intestinal/pancreatic mass detected or present with clinical signs of vomiting, diarrhea or abdominal pain (mainly dogs)
Renal	Lower urinary tract signs Polyuria/polydipsia Renal failure

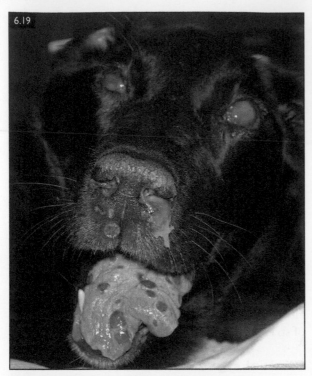

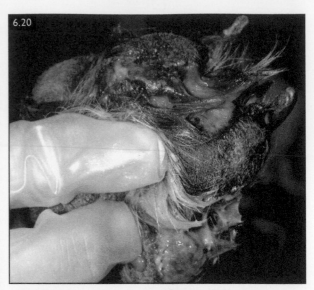

Fig. 6.20 Severe, mucopurulent, ulcerative, cryptococcal pododermatitis causing sloughing of the foot pads.

Fig. 6.19 Mature female spayed Labrador Retriever with disseminated cryptococcal disease. Note the numerous, variably sized ulcerated nodules on the tongue, lip philtrum and mucocutaneous junction of the nares. Mucopurulent discharge is present from the left nares.

Cryptococcus spp. can potentially affect any organ system and uncommon clinical signs will be variable and may include vomiting, diarrhea or lameness.

Fever is uncommon in cats and may be low grade in dogs. Lower respiratory signs can include cough, tachypnea or dyspnea. Swellings (firm to fluctuant) over the nasal, maxillary or frontal sinus area as well as a proliferative mass in the nares may be noted, especially in cats, along with mucopurulent nasal discharge and epistaxis. Local (head/neck) or generalized lymphadenopathy may be observed. Nodular and/or ulcerated skin lesions may be presented around the head and neck or be multifocal. Tongue, buccal mucosa, third eyelids and nail beds can be involved (**Figs. 6.19, 6.20**).

Fundic examination may reveal focal or multifocal chorioretinitis, exudative retinal detachment, signs consistent with optic neuritis, papilloedema and retinal hemorrhage (**Fig. 6.21**).[64]

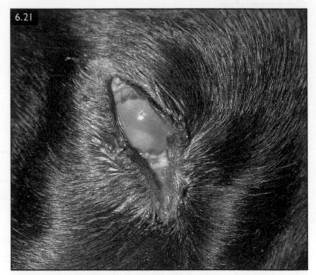

Fig. 6.21 Right eye of a dog with disseminated cryptococcosis. Note the episcleritis, corneal neovascularization, corneal edema and anterior lens luxation.

Abnormalities on neurologic examination may include obtundation, behavioral changes (cats), anisocoria, mydriasis, peripheral or central blindness, vestibular signs, twitching, tremors, ataxia, paraparesis and rarely paralysis, circling, neck pain (dogs) and spinal pain (cats).[64, 67]

Diagnosis

Diagnosis is typically made through cytology (or histopathology), culture or antigen detection with serology. Culture from the nasal cavity needs to be substantiated with additional testing.

Lab abnormalities

Changes in the CBC and serum biochemical profile are non-specific. Changes in the serum biochemical profile may include an increased globulin concentration with a polyclonal gammopathy and decreased albumin:globulin (A:G) ratio.[66] In dogs with disseminated disease, chemistry changes will reflect organ involvement. Urine sediment may show yeasts.

Cytology

Cytologic evaluation of tissue samples is a rapid, inexpensive and sensitive means of diagnosing cryptococcosis. Organisms can be found in aspirates, exudates, body fluids (e.g. urine, feces, CSF) or biopsy impression smears. In the patient they are identified as narrow-budding yeasts measuring 3–8 μm in diameter, surrounded by a variably sized capsule that does not take up stain (**Fig. 6.22**).[62] One cannot rule out cryptococcosis on the basis of negative cytology, and additional diagnostic testing

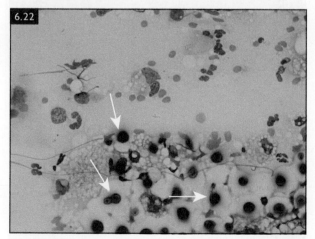

Fig. 6.22 *Cryptococcus* cytology. **In the lower half of the field, multiple yeasts with a thick clear capsule (halo effect) are present. The arrows point to organisms in variable stages of budding (narrow based).**

such as serology or culture should be performed in suspect cases.

Histology will identify the yeast in a similar manner to cytology. The capsule will not take up H&E stains and the yeast body is noted within this clear halo.[59]

Culture

Cryptococcus spp. can be easily cultured from the same specimens used for cytology/histologic examination. Antifungal susceptibility can also be determined once the organism is cultured if required (e.g. lack of response to current therapy). Subclinical colonization can occur within the nasal passage and concurrent histologic/cytologic evidence of cryptococcal infection is required to confirm diagnosis. Isolation from biopsy specimens is more definitive.[59]

Serology

Latex agglutination antigen assays are a fast and reliable means to detect cryptococcal capsular antigen of all known serotypes in serum, urine or CSF samples.[59] Diagnostic titers are usually high (>1:65,536); however, low titers (e.g. 1:2) can also be significant. False negatives are rare but can occur more often in dogs than cats. False negatives are more likely when disease is localized, such as with nasal, ocular or neurologic involvement.[64] False positives are similarly infrequent.

Titers are an important monitoring tool during therapy. It is common for titers to rise within the first month after therapy, due to dying organisms. Therefore, checking a titer at 6–8 weeks after initiation of therapy is advised to establish a monitoring baseline. From that point forward a declining antigen titer is associated with a good prognosis. The frequency of serologic testing may vary from monthly to every 3 months. The long term goal is to achieve a negative titer along with a positive clinical response.

Antigen testing

A variety of cryptococcal antigen test kits is available to laboratories. Interpretation of sequential titers is optimal, with consistent test methodology.

PCR

PCR assays are not commonly used diagnostically but, when available, they can permit identification of the species of *Cryptococcus*. Positive PCR should be paired with positive cytology, histology or culture.

Imaging

Radiographs may be normal or reflect pulmonary involvement (nodules, infiltrates), lymphadenopathy, or on rare occasions pleural effusion (**Fig. 6.23**).

CT imaging of cats with nasal cryptococcosis (**Figs. 6.24, 6.25**) may show soft tissue changes or

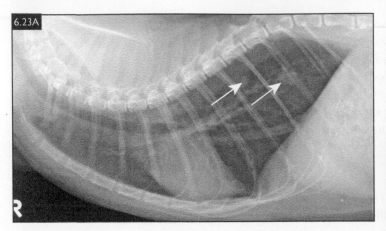

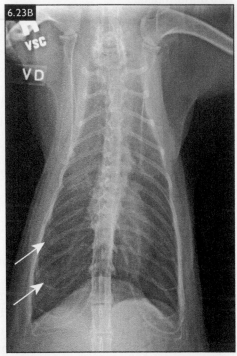

Fig. 6.23 Lateral (A) and ventrodorsal (B) radiographs of an adult cat. There are two somewhat poorly defined soft tissue nodules in the right caudal lobe (arrows). These were cryptococcal granulomas. (Courtesy of John Graham)

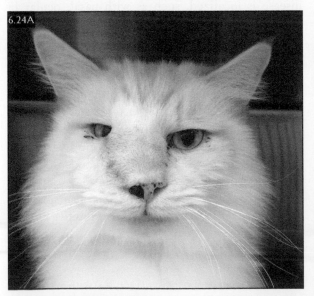

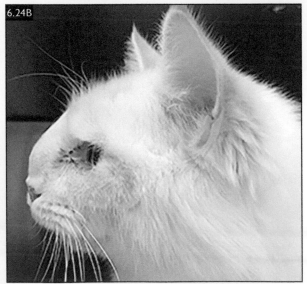

Fig. 6.24 A 1.5-year-old neutered male Ragdoll cat with nasal cryptococcosis caused by *C. gattii*. Differential diagnoses for facial distortion include other dimorphic mycoses, sino-orbital aspergillosis and nasal neoplasia. (Courtesy of Dr Joanna Whitney)

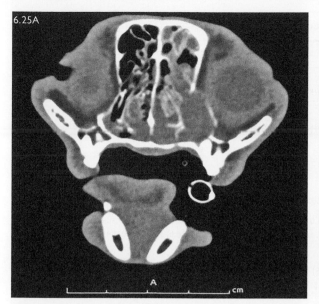
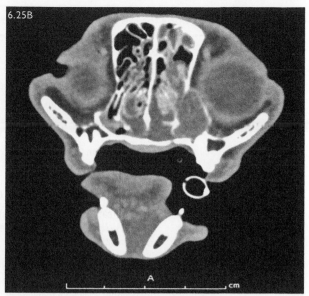

Fig. 6.25 Transverse CT of the cat in Fig. 6.24 with nasal cryptococcosis: soft tissue window, pre-contrast (A) and post-contrast (B). Note the mass effect extending from the left nasal cavity into the right orbit to cause dorsolateral displacement of the globe.

fluid opacification of the nasal cavity or frontal sinus, mass lesions and lysis of the nasal bones or cribriform plate. CT in dogs may reveal a mass effect in the frontal sinus, nasal cavity or nasopharynx along with variable degrees of local osteomyelitis, as noted in cats.

Ultrasound findings in dogs and cats depend on specific organ involvement; ultrasonography may reveal lymphadenopathy or abdominal masses.

Rhinoscopy may reveal nasal planum deformation and ulceration, ulcerated red turbinates or a mass. Mucosal or nasal biopsy can provide samples for cytology/culture or histopathology.

Therapy

Azole antifungal therapy is required for months to years and, even when continued for more than a year, does not preclude relapse, reinfection or development of subclinical colonization by the yeast in the nasal cavity. Therapy is continued until clinical signs have completely resolved and antigen titers are negative (*Table 6.13*).

It is advised that any animal with CNS involvement, including the majority of the animals infected with *C. gattii*, receive amphotericin B in addition to other antifungal agents to effect a cure. In cats (not dogs) one can consider flucytosine as an adjunctive therapy to amphotericin B.[59] If amphotericin B is not a clinical option despite CNS involvement, azole monotherapy (fluconazole/itraconazole), as for other clinical cryptococcal infections, can be used because clinical responses have been documented. Fluconazole is often considered the azole of choice as it penetrates well into the CNS, eye and urine, is less hepatotoxic and is readily absorbable with (or without) food. *C. gattii* isolates may be more susceptible to amphotericin B and ketoconazole than to itraconazole and fluconazole.

Large cryptococcal granulomas can respond to medical therapy alone; however, surgery may also be considered. Intestinal cryptococcosis has been reported to respond to terbinafine alone (dog); however, there are situations where surgical excision/debulking should be considered as an important part of ancillary therapy.

Cautious use of glucocorticoids to reduce inflammation from dying organisms in the CNS may be a consideration and improve outcome.[67] However, glucocorticoid use before diagnosis can lead to pathogen dissemination, CNS involvement and ultimately death.[66]

Table 6.13 **Drug options for the treatment of cryptococcosis**

DRUG	DOSING
Fluconazole	Cats: 50 mg/cat PO q12h Dogs: 5–10 mg/kg PO q12h or 10 mg/kg PO q24h
Ketoconazole	Cats: 5–10 mg/kg PO q12h Dogs: 10–15 mg/kg PO q12h Give with food
Itraconazole	3 mg/kg PO q24h (solution) 5 mg/kg PO q12–24h (capsules) Give with food Therapeutic drug monitoring can be considered
Amphotericin B: conventional formulation	0.5 mg/kg (cats) or 0.8 mg/kg (dogs) diluted to 5 mg/mL and then additionally diluted in 350–500 mL of 0.45% NaCl with 2.5% dextrose. Give SC 3 times a week. Abscess risk increases if drug concentration is >20 mg/L 0.25 mg/kg (cats) or 0.5 mg/kg (dogs) diluted in 5% dextrose in water (D5W) given slowly IV. Dilution volume depends on species, body size and fluid tolerance. Administered 3 times weekly. Cumulative dose limits should be considered
Amphotericin B: liposomal encapsulated	1 mg/kg (cats) or 3 mg/kg (dogs) diluted in D5W to 1 mg/mL and given as a slow infusion over 1–2 hours. Administered 3 times a week. Cumulative dose limits should be considered
Flucytosine	Cats only: 25–50 mg/kg PO q6–8h To be used in combination with amphotericin B
Terbinafine	30–40 mg/kg (dogs and cats) PO q24h. Consideration for intestinal disease in dogs or cases apparently resistant to azoles. Give with food
Voriconazole	Generally not recommended in cats owing to the very high likelihood of adverse effects (CNS, cardiac and gastrointestinal [GI]). Dogs may tolerate the drug but adverse side effects are possible (including GI, retinal and hepatic). This may be a consideration for CNS-associated disease in dogs because of good CNS penetration
Posaconazole	Good penetration into tissues but limited penetration into the CNS. CNS inflammation may allow better penetration. This drug has been tolerated in cats and could be considered for a patient refractory to other therapy

Prognosis/complications

Prognosis is variable and dependent on the severity of disease, early detection, underlying host immunocompetence, financial (and time) constraints and commitment of the owner. In cats, clinical signs typically improve within the first 1–2 weeks of treatment, and a favorable response with commitment to prolonged therapy and monitoring is possible. Prognosis with CNS infection is guarded, and altered mental status in dogs is a negative prognostic indicator.[67] Dogs with disseminated disease have a more guarded prognosis. It is important to communicate to clients that recurrence (or relapse) is possible after many years free of disease.

Prevention

There is no way to prevent infection completely and a vaccine is not available. General principles for prevention include avoidance of high-risk areas (and bird feces) if possible or practical, prudent use of immunosuppressive therapy and recognition of patients at higher risk of infection in order to allow early detection and appropriate therapy.

Public health and infection control

Cryptococcosis is not a zoonotic disease. Dogs, cats and humans acquire the infection from similar environments, and therefore dogs and cats may serve as sentinels.

CYTAUXZOON FELIS (CYTAUXZOONOSIS)
Michelle Evason

Definition

Cytauxzoonosis is an emerging protozoal infection of cats transmitted primarily by the tick-borne vector *Ambylomma americanum* (lone star tick) (**Fig. 6.26**). Disease is typically severe and prompt therapy is essential (**Fig. 6.27**). Domestic and wild cats (bobcats, pumas, etc.) are the reservoir hosts.

Etiology and pathogenesis

Cytauxzoon felis is a hemoprotozoan parasite that relies on host ticks *A. americanum* (the predominant vector) and *Dermacentor variabilis* (American dog tick) for transmission. Seasonal patterns of feline infection reflect peak tick-feeding periods, such as April through September in North America.[68] After 36–48 hours of tick attachment, the sporozoite form of the parasite enters the cat.[69] Infected mononuclear cells underdo schizogony at approximately 2 weeks post-infection. Distended monocytes

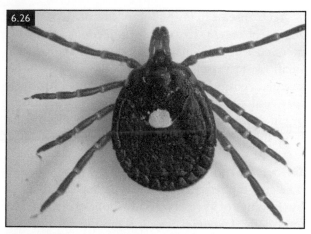

Fig. 6.26 Adult lone star tick (*Amblyomma americanum*). The tick is 3–4 mm in length. (Courtesy of Dr Katie Clow)

rupture and release merozoites, which become piroplasms within red blood cells. Both schizont and piroplasm forms may exist within infected cats. Ticks are infected after ingestion of piroplasms from wild or domestic cats.

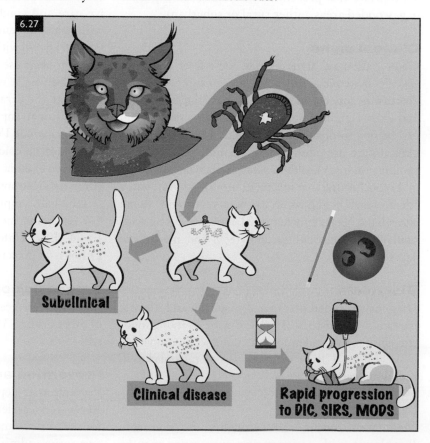

Fig. 6.27 Tick transmission of the sporozoite form of *Cytauxzoon felis* in a cat, leading to either subclinical or rapidly progressive and severe clinical disease.

Subclinical

Clinical disease

Rapid progression to DIC, SIRS, MODS

Acute disease manifests clinically, due to the schizogony phase (13–16 days post-infection). Distended mononuclear cells may act as thrombi and occlude small blood vessels, leading to disseminated intravascular coagulation (DIC), systemic inflammatory response syndrome (SIRS), sepsis and multiple organ dysfunction syndrome (MODS). The spleen, lung, liver and lymph nodes are most often affected.

Geography
The geographic location of this pathogen is dictated by the range of its reservoirs (e.g. bobcats) and vectors (especially *A. americanum)*. It is most common in the south central, southeastern and mid-Atlantic regions of the USA, as well as South America and parts of Europe (France, Portugal, Italy, Spain).[68, 70, 71]

Risk factors
Risk factors are predominantly those that predispose to tick exposure, such as younger age, outdoor lifestyle, strays, rural area, together with lack of appropriate tick prevention and increased exposure (e.g. wooded areas, either rural or suburban).[70]

Clinical signs
Common clinical signs include acute fever and non-specific systemic signs such as lethargy, weakness, decrease in appetite and gastrointestinal signs.[70] Anemia and icterus are common. Dyspnea may be present and can be due to pleural effusion. Although non-specific, clinical signs are often very severe and there is a rapid progression from health to severe disease or death.

Hypothermia may occur in moribund cats, and a "death yowl" vocalization has been reported.[68] Renal signs have been reported in 23% of cats, along with ocular (9%), musculoskeletal (8%) and neurologic signs (3%).[70]

Diagnosis
Diagnosis is based on clinical suspicion and history, particularly a history of tick exposure or living in (or traveling to) an endemic area, along with compatible clinical signs, CBC changes, cytology (piroplasms in red blood cells) and PCR.

Lab abnormalities
Moderate-to-severe pancytopenia is common. Piroplasms with a signet-ring appearance may be

detected in affected cats.[68, 72] Elevated bilirubin, alkaline phosphatase and alanine aminotransferase can be noted.[68] Urinalysis may be normal, or reveal bilirubinuria or mild glucosuria.

Cytology of whole blood smears, lymph node, spleen, liver or lung aspirates may reveal piroplasms in blood cells or merozoites in mononuclear cells within organ aspirates. This is most commonly how infection is confirmed. However, negative findings do not rule out infection and repeat (multiple) samples may improve diagnoses. False positives may occur in carrier states. A skilled interpreter is needed to differentiate hemoplasmosis, precipitates or Howell–Jolly bodies.

Currently, PCR of whole blood is considered the most sensitive and specific route of diagnosis, particularly for screening of carrier cats.

Therapy
Although this was once considered a hopeless disease for which prompt euthanasia was recommended, survival is possible. Therapy consists of supportive care and combination oral therapy for 10 days with azithromycin (10 mg/kg q24h) and atovaquone (15 mg/kg q8h with a fatty meal).[68, 71] This treatment has also been used to reduce parasitemia in carrier cats; however, it is not curative, because it may not eliminate the parasite.

Additional supportive therapy for critically ill cats can include IV fluid support with supplemented potassium chloride, analgesics, blood transfusions for severe anemia, or plasma in DIC, and anticoagulation medications (e.g. heparin).

Clinical improvement typically occurs in 4–7 days, and most cats have disease resolution by 10–14 days. Unfortunately, many cats die within 24 hours of presentation owing to severe illness.

Prognosis/complications
Most untreated cats die within 24 hours of the onset of overt disease. With treatment, mortality rates are still ~50%.

Prevention and infection control
Prevention is dependent on effective tick control. Recovered (carrier) cats can be a source of infection for naïve ticks and should be kept indoors and tick preventives administered.

DIROFILARIA IMMITIS (HEARTWORM)
Darcy B Adin

Definition
Heartworm disease is caused by *Dirofilaria immitis*, a filarial parasitic nematode spread by mosquitoes. The worm lives in the lungs, heart and associated vasculature of the host animal (**Fig. 6.28**).

Species affected
Canids are the natural host for *D. immitis*; however, cats and ferrets can be infected.

Etiology and pathogenesis
Infected canids are the reservoir hosts. Microfilaria are produced by a mature infection of male and female worms in a host animal and are taken up by mosquitoes during a blood meal from the host. Their development into L1, L2 and L3 larvae within the mosquito is temperature dependent, requiring 6 weeks at a minimum of 57°F (14°C) and as little as 2 weeks at higher temperatures. After migrating to the salivary glands, L3 larvae are injected under the skin of a dog (or other potential host) while the mosquito feeds. Larvae mature over 1–2 weeks into L4 larvae, which migrate to abdominal and thoracic muscles to mature into juvenile adults (also known as L5 larvae). These penetrate systemic veins and travel to the pulmonary vasculature, where they mature into adult heartworms. The prepatent period (L3 infection to maturation into adult worms with subsequent microfilaria production) is typically 6–7 months in the dog; however, immature worms (L5) reach the pulmonary vasculature as early as 67 days after infection. Adult heartworms can live for 5–7 years, and microfilaria for up to 30 months, in the dog. Aberrant migration to other sites occasionally occurs during worm development.

Blood flow carries heartworms distally in the pulmonary arterial tree where they induce pulmonary arterial damage (endothelial villous proliferation, arterial dilation and tortuosity) and thromboembolism. Rarely, dogs can develop allergic pneumonitis secondary to heartworm infestation. Pulmonary hypertension and right-sided congestive heart failure (CHF) are possible sequelae to worm-induced arterial damage, particularly with large worm burdens.

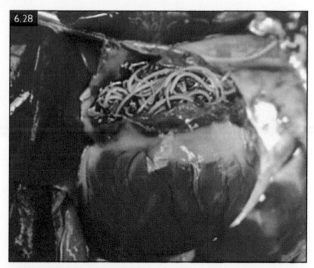

Fig. 6.28 Heartworms are visualized in the right atrium of a dog at necropsy. (Courtesy of Dary Adin)

Although cats can be infected with heartworms, the larvae are less likely to reach maturity, and therefore patent infections in cats are uncommon. When mature infections occur in the cat, the worm burden is low, and the heartworm lifespan is shorter (3–4 years) than in the dog. Juvenile heartworms can cause significant lung disease and asthma-like signs in cats even if they do not mature to adult heartworms (i.e. "heartworm-associated respiratory disease").[73]

Geography
Dirofilaria immitis is widely disseminated in tropical, sub-tropical and temperate regions of the world, where mosquitoes live and temperatures rise above 57°F (14°C).

Incidence and risk factors
The prevalence of infection and incidence of heartworm disease vary greatly among regions. In the USA, heartworm disease is endemic, with an overall prevalence in dogs estimated at 1.3%, with higher levels in the southeast (2.9% overall, but much higher in certain areas).[74] Cats are less susceptible to patent infections than dogs (<25% of the canine rate);[73] however, antibody prevalence estimates (indicating exposure) range from 4% to 16% in some regions.[75,76] Climate, mosquito populations and the number of reservoir hosts (wild, feral or domestic) influence heartworm exposure risk.

Because mosquitoes can enter houses, indoor pets are at risk for heartworm infection.

Clinical signs

Dogs with heartworm infection may not have overt abnormalities on physical examination. However, possible cardiac abnormalities include right-sided systolic heart murmur of tricuspid regurgitation, a split S2 heart sound due to pulmonary hypertension or, rarely, signs of right-sided CHF (including hepatomegaly, ascites and jugular venous distension or pulsation). Pulmonary auscultation may reveal crackles, increased bronchovesicular sounds and tachypnea. Fever and hemoptysis may accompany recent heartworm-associated pulmonary thrombo-embolism. High worm burdens and chronic infections are more likely to result in clinical signs related to the presence of worm-induced pulmonary arterial pathology. Cough, tachypnea, dyspnea and exercise intolerance are the most commonly reported signs, but severely affected dogs may also show signs of right-sided CHF, hemoptysis or renal failure.

Caval syndrome is an uncommon, severe complication of a heavy worm burden.[77] Many dogs with caval syndrome have some degree of pulmonary hypertension and it is thought that this, in combination with a drop in cardiac output, allows the worms to fall back into the right ventricle and right atrium. Once the worms are within the heart, they can become entangled in the tricuspid valve, interfering with valve function and causing shear stress on red blood cells. Clinical findings in dogs with caval syndrome include anorexia, lethargy, right-sided CHF, hemolytic anemia, hemoglobinemia, hemoglobinuria, hepatic dysfunction and renal dysfunction, in addition to respiratory signs.

Cats may not have clinical signs, may have respiratory signs that resemble asthma or have non-specific signs (vomiting, diarrhea, neurologic abnormalities). Sudden death has been associated with heartworm disease in cats and is thought to be due to heartworm pulmonary embolism.[73, 75]

Diagnosis

Antigen testing

Detection of heartworm antigen in the blood of dogs is the diagnostic cornerstone. Antigen tests are highly specific and sensitive; however, false-negative and false-positive tests can occasionally occur, depending on prevalence and worm number. For this reason, confirmatory testing of positive results is recommended using a different antigen test or microfilaria test.

Microfilaria testing

Observation of microfilariae on a blood smear or concentration test confirms the presence of a patent heartworm infection, if the microfilariae are confirmed to be *D. immitis*. The absence of microfilariae in a heartworm-infected (antigen-positive) dog indicates an occult infection and may be due to prepatency (immature adults), single sex infection, or elimination of microfilariae by recent treatment with macrocyclic lactones used for prevention.

Radiography

Thoracic radiographs should be performed on heartworm-positive dogs to assess disease severity. Abnormal findings that support a diagnosis of heartworm disease include main pulmonary artery enlargement, right ventricular enlargement, pulmonary interstitial changes, and distal pulmonary arterial enlargement, tortuosity and truncation (**Fig. 6.29**).

Echocardiography

Because heartworms reside in the distal pulmonary arteries in most dogs, echocardiography is relatively insensitive as a diagnostic tool. In dogs with heavy worm burdens or caval syndrome, worms may be visualized within the main pulmonary artery, right ventricle or right atrium. Worm echoes appear as parallel hyperechoic lines of varying length (**Fig. 6.30**). Echocardiography may also be used to diagnose pulmonary hypertension and evaluate right heart size and function.

Therapy

Adulticide therapy

Definitive treatment for heartworm disease in dogs requires elimination of adult heartworms to prevent ongoing pulmonary arterial damage. Before adulticidal therapy, dogs should be started on monthly heartworm prevention and

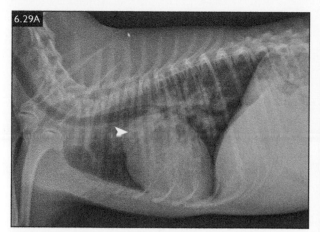

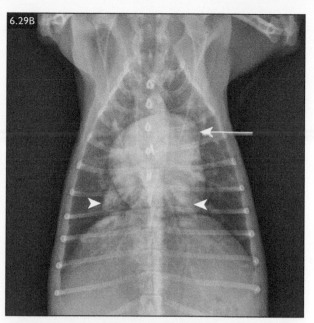

Fig. 6.29 Right lateral (A) and dorsoventral (B) thoracic radiographs from a dog with advanced heartworm disease. Right-sided cardiomegaly is present. The main pulmonary artery is enlarged (arrow) and the distal pulmonary arteries are enlarged, truncated and tortuous (arrowhead).

given a 4-week course of doxycycline (10 mg/kg PO q12h) to eliminate *Wolbachia* spp. Dogs with clinical heartworm disease should be treated with prednisone before adulticide treatment (0.5 mg/kg PO q12h tapering over 4 weeks). Melarsomine (2.5 mg/kg) is administered as a deep IM injection followed 1 month later by two additional 2.5 mg/kg doses IM, 24 hours apart. The first dose kills some worms (males) whereas the two doses 24 hours apart kill the remaining worms (females) with a 99% efficacy. Exercise restriction is very important to reduce the chance of thromboembolism in the 4–6 weeks following adulticide therapy. Additional courses of tapering prednisone can be administered after each injection. Antigen testing can be repeated in 6 months to verify successful adulticide therapy.

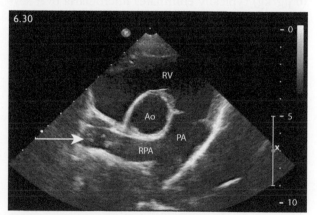

Fig. 6.30 Right-sided, parasternal, short-axis echocardiogram at the heart base. Heartworm echoes are visualized in the enlarged right pulmonary artery as parallel hyperechoic lines (arrow). Ao, aorta; PA, pulmonary artery; RPA, right pulmonary artery; RV, right ventricle.

Heartworm extraction

Dogs with caval syndrome require immediate removal of the heartworms from the right heart. Extraction is performed under general anesthesia or heavy sedation, and forceps are passed into the right atrium through a jugular vein after surgical cutdown, to grasp and remove worms (**Fig. 6.31**). Flexible alligator forceps (Ishihara forceps) allow the removal of worms from the right ventricle and pulmonary artery; this may also benefit dogs that

do not have caval syndrome but are at high risk for thromboembolic complications with adulticide therapy owing to their heavy worm burden. Extraction should be followed by melarsomine treatment.

Microfilaricidal treatment

Dogs with circulating microfilaria should receive heartworm prevention, which acts as a microfilaricide. The preventive dose of ivermectin

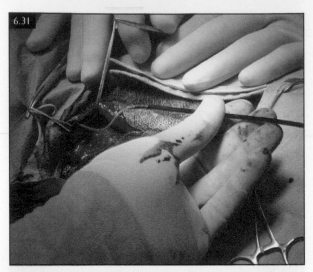

Fig. 6.31 Heartworms being removed from the right jugular vein using Ishihara forceps.

(6 µg/kg) typically eliminates microfilaria over several months, whereas the preventive dose of milbemycin (500 µg/kg) rapidly clears microfilaria. The latter method necessitates close observation for an anaphylactic reaction and treatment with corticosteroids and antihistamines if necessary.

Cats
Adulticide therapy is not recommended for treatment of heartworm disease in cats because of the unacceptable mortality and low efficacy associated with the arsenical. Surgical removal can be pursued if worms are present in the right atrium. Monthly preventive administration is recommended to

control disease. Short-term corticosteroid therapy may help manage respiratory complications.

Prognosis/complications
Pulmonary thromboembolism is the most common complication following adulticide therapy and can be minimized by strict exercise restriction after treatment. Chronic heartworm disease results in pulmonary pathology, glomerulonephritis, CHF and sometimes death. Caval syndrome and aberrant worm migration are rare.

The prognosis for dogs without clinical signs of heartworm disease is good after treatment. The prognosis is guarded for dogs that are symptomatic or have caval syndrome. However, recovery is possible with closely managed treatment and caval extraction of worms if indicated.[77]

Prevention
Macrocyclic lactones, including ivermectin, milbemycin oxime, moxidectin and selamectin, are used to prevent heartworm disease. Most products are administered monthly, either orally or topically; however, some injectable formulations provide slow release over 6–12 months. The macrolides most effectively kill larvae within 1–2 months of infestation (L3 and L4 stages) and therefore must be administered monthly if the formulation is not slow release. Prevention should be started at the first puppy examination and continued year-round or during periods when disease transmission is possible, depending on the epidemiology of *D. immitis* in the area.

EHRLICHIOSIS AND ANAPLASMOSIS
Michelle Evason

Definition
Ehrlichiosis and anaplasmosis are tick-borne infections of dogs, and less commonly cats. A variety of species may be involved, including *Ehrlichia canis*, *E. ewingii*, *E. chaffeensis*, *E. muris*, *E. ruminantium*, *Anaplasma phagocytophilum* and *A. platys*.

Species affected
Dogs can develop clinical disease after infection with *E. canis*, *E. ewingii*, *A. phagocytophilum* or *A. platys*. It is

less certain whether other species (e.g. *E. chaffeensis* and *E. muris*) cause clinical disease. Clinical illness in cats due to *A. phagocytophilum* and *E. canis* (or *E. canis*-like *Ehrlichia* spp.) has been described.[78–80]

Etiology and pathogenesis
Ehrlichia and *Anaplasma* spp. are intracellular, gram-negative bacteria that rely on host ticks for transmission (*Table 6.14*). It is thought that 2–48 hours of tick attachment must occur for bacterial transmission;

Table 6.14 **Pathogen, preferred cell type, and tick vectors for ehrlichiosis and anaplasmosis**

PATHOGEN	PREFERRED CELL TYPE	TICK VECTOR
Ehrlichia canis	Monocytes, macrophages	*Rhipicephalus sanguineus* *Dermacentor variabilis*
E. ewingii	Granulocytes, neutrophils	*Amblyomma americanum*
E. chaffeensis	Monocytes, macrophages, neutrophils, lymphocytes	*Amblyomma americanum* *Dermacentor variabilis*
Anaplasma platys	Platelets	*Rhipicephalus sanguineus*
A. phagocytophilum	Granulocytes, neutrophils, eosinophils	*Ixodes scapularis* *Ixodes pacificus*

however, true attachment time is unknown for most infections. After tick attachment/bite, the bacteria migrate to their preferred leukocyte cell types. Replication occurs within cells, and this may be visualized cytologically as a morula (mulberry) appearance.

Canine monocytic ehrlichiosis (or *E. canis* infection) has been divided into three disease states: acute, subclinical and chronic.[81] Clinically, there are no clear markers between disease states because onset and length of infection are typically unknown.[81, 82] The acute phase of *E. canis* infection can last 1–4 weeks. Clinical disease usually occurs between 8 and 10 days post-infection. After that time, appropriately treated dogs may recover completely. However, inappropriately treated dogs (or untreated dogs) may appear to recover but then develop subclinical (or persistent) infection. Persistently infected dogs may develop chronic infection, which lasts for months to years, or go on to recover completely.

Infection with *A. phagocytophilum* and *A. platys* is both acute and rapid, with incubation periods of 14–20 and 8–15 days, respectively. Infections are thought to be self-limiting.[83, 84] Cyclic parasitemia and thrombocytopenia occur with *A. platys* at 1- to 2-week intervals, but this may resolve over time.

Geography

Worldwide but more likely in tropical and subtropical regions.

Incidence and risk factors

In dogs, seropositivity rates for *A. phagocytophilum* have ranged from 0% to 50% depending on region,

study and whether healthy or clinically ill dogs were sampled.[83] A similar study in south central USA reported the seroprevalence of *E. chaffeensis* (17.5%), *E. canis* (1.4%), *E. ewingii* (45%) and *Anaplasma* spp. (5.6%).[85]

Risk factors for seropositivity and clinical disease include lack of appropriate tick prevention, increased tick exposure, time spent outside, season, co-infection with other tick-borne pathogens, and living in forested or urban wooded areas.[83, 85, 86] Older dogs are more likely to be seropositive owing to increased risk of exposure over time.

Similar to dogs, seroprevalence and risk factors in cats appear dependent on region and tick exposure.[79]

Common clinical signs
Dogs

Given the infected cell type(s) and the ability of the bacteria to travel throughout the body, both ehrlichiosis and anaplasmosis are considered multisystem diseases (*Table 6.15*). Common clinical signs include acute fever (39.5–40.5°C, 103.1–104.9°F) and nonspecific systemic signs (e.g. lethargy, weakness and decrease in appetite). Bleeding tendencies are common, with petechiation (**Fig. 6.32**), ecchymoses and pallor noted most frequently. However, dogs with *A. phagocytophilum* infection appear less likely to show these signs.[83] Epistaxis, lymphadenopathy and an enlarged spleen and/or liver have been reported.[81, 82, 86] Icterus (**Fig. 6.33**) may be present but is uncommon.

Ocular signs due to bleeding tendencies or systemic disease such as hypertension or thromboembolism can occur (e.g. uveitis, subretinal bleeding, hyphema).[87] Neuromuscular signs secondary to

Table 6.15 **Common clinical signs associated with ehrlichiosis and anaplasmosis**

PATHOGEN	FEVER/LETHARGY	POLYARTHRITIS	MUCOSAL HEMORRHAGE	INAPPETENCE
E. canis	X		X	X
E. ewingii	X	X		X
A. phagocytophilum	X	X		X
A. platys	X			

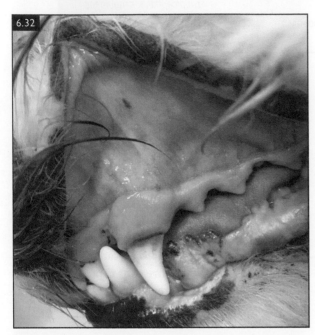

Fig. 6.32 Petechial hemorrhage in the oral mucous membranes of a dog with anaplasmosis. (Courtesy of Atlantic Veterinary College)

bleeding or meningitis may result in seizures, ataxia, stupor, tremors or additional CNS signs. Polyarthritis and joint swelling, stiffness and generalized muscle pain are common with *E. ewingii* and *A. phagocytophilum* and may occur with *E. canis* also.

Infection with *A. platys* typically results in subclinical disease in the USA. However, more severe clinical disease has been reported outside of North America, and infection may result in fever, lethargy, petechiation and lymphadenopathy.[84]

Cats

It is uncommon for cats to develop clinical illness with *A. phagocytophilum*. However, fever, anorexia and lethargy have been described in PCR-positive cats in endemic regions.[79, 80]

Fever, non-specific systemic signs (e.g. lethargy, inappetence, weight loss) and joint pain, together with irritable behavior, have all been reported in cats with suspected *E. canis*.[80] Rapid clinical improvement was noted after doxycycline therapy.

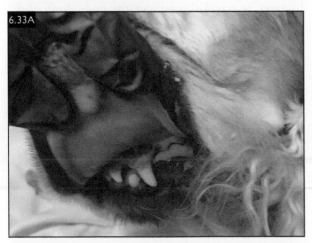 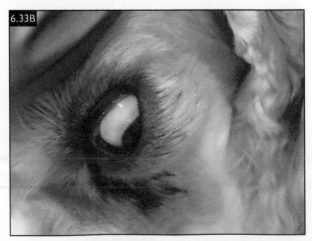

Fig. 6.33 Icterus of (A) the oral mucous membranes and (B) the sclera in a dog with anaplasmosis. (Courtesy of Atlantic Veterinary College)

Diagnosis

Diagnosis is based on clinical suspicion and history (e.g. tick exposure, living in or travelling to an endemic area), taken together with compatible clinical signs, CBC changes, serology and PCR (*Table 6.16*). Co-infections are common and should be investigated. Clinical diagnosis of anaplasmosis or ehrlichiosis may be based on:

- Endemic area exposure.
- Consistent acute clinical and lab (CBC) findings, e.g. fever, polyarthropathy, thrombocytopenia.
- Detection of morulae combined with a positive test result, e.g. serology, PCR.
- Rise (and subsequent decrease) in antibody titer (acute and convalescent) within 4 weeks.
- Positive PCR using specific primers or isolation from the blood.
- Rapid response/resolution of illness with doxycycline therapy.

Lab abnormalities

Moderate-to-severe thrombocytopenia occurs in most clinically affected dogs; mild anemia and leukopenia may also be noted. Dogs with subacute or persistent *E. canis* infection may have a mild thrombocytopenia. In chronic *E. canis* infection, anemia of inflammatory disease (normocytic, normochromic and non-regenerative), thrombocytopenia or pancytopenia can be present.

In cats, thrombocytopenia is less common with anaplasmosis. Ehrlichiosis is thought to be similar to dogs.[79]

Morulae (**Fig. 6.34**) may (or may not) be detected in affected dogs or cats. A monoclonal or polyclonal gammopathy can occur; monoclonal gammopathy should raise suspicion for *E. canis*.[86]

Urinalysis may be normal, indicate inflammation or be consistent with protein-losing nephropathy. Urine protein:creatinine ratios >5 (or higher) have been observed in some dogs with chronic ehrlichiosis

Cytology may show morulae located within preferred cell types, CSF or joint fluid. Joint (synovial) fluid may be normal or consistent with suppurative inflammation. CSF analysis may be normal or consistent with subacute-to-chronic inflammation. Bone marrow from dogs with chronic ehrlichiosis may reveal hypoplasia or aplasia, decreased iron levels and marrow plasmacytosis. Some dogs may have normal to hypercellular marrow.

Detection of serum antibodies is the basis of current testing methods, and the main route for confirmation of clinical illness, together with PCR.[78, 81, 82, 88]

Table 6.16 **Laboratory assays for ehrlichiosis and anaplasmosis**

DIAGNOSTIC	SAMPLE	TARGET	OUTCOME/UTILITY
IFA	Serum	Antibodies to *E. canis*, *A. phagocytophilum*	Acute and convalescent (taken 2–3 weeks later) titers are required for diagnosis. Limitations: initial (early) results can be negative owing to lack of antibody development, and positive results may represent exposure vs. true clinical disease. Cross-reaction between *Ehrlichia* spp. and *Anaplasma* spp. can occur, in addition to cross-reaction with different types of ehrlichiosis or anaplasmosis
ELISA serology	Serum, plasma	Antibodies to *E. canis* or *E. ewingii* antigens, and *A. phagocytophilum*, *A. platys*	Can be performed "in-house", inexpensive and rapid. Lack of quantification of antibody titer, and similar limitations to those above
PCR	Whole blood, aspirates from lymph node, spleen/liver, bone marrow or tissue specimens	DNA	Confirms active infection. Limitations: lab variability, may not be sensitive for chronic *E. canis* infection and techniques (and results) can vary for both *Anaplasma* spp. and *Ehrlichia* spp.

Abbreviations: ELISA, enzyme-linked immunosorbent assay; IFA, immunofluorescent antibody

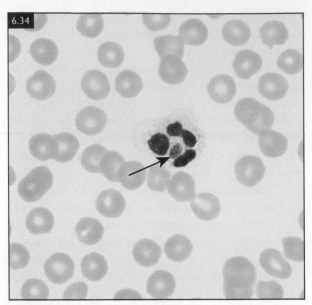

Fig. 6.34 *Anasplasma phagocytophilum* morula (arrow) (Wright–Giemsa stain, 1,000× magnification). (Courtesy of Dr Noel Clancy)

Therapy

Rapid clinical improvement (within 24–48 hours after antimicrobial therapy) is typical and supports the diagnosis. Platelet counts should return to reference range after 10–14 days of therapy for both ehrlichiosis and anaplasmosis.

Treatment consists of supportive care and antimicrobial therapy for 28 days. Doxycycline (10 mg/kg PO q24h) is the drug of choice, in part owing to its efficacy against possible co-infecting pathogens.[78] Chronic *E. canis* infections may also respond well (and quickly) to antimicrobial therapy; however, treatment for up to a year may be required.[81]

Ongoing monitoring of CBC (e.g. platelet counts) at 1 and 3 months is indicated after recovery, because of concerns regarding reinfection or persistent infection with *E. canis*. It is important to note that many dogs will remain seropositive (for months to years) despite effective antimicrobial therapy and resolution of clinical signs. Continued seropositive status should not be used to guide further (or ongoing) therapy. PCR assessment may be helpful for determining ongoing active infection, along with clinical status and platelet counts.

Controversy and debate surround the topic of empiric therapy for clinically normal seropositive dogs, particularly those in kennel situations. However, in the typical companion dog population there is no evidence that treatment of seropositive but clinically normal individuals is effective for preventing subsequent disease.

Cats infected with *E. canis* or *A. phagocytophilum* have been successfully treated with doxycycline (10 mg/kg PO q24h for 28 days), but some cats remained PCR positive after months of therapy.

Prognosis/complications

Most dogs respond completely and rapidly with appropriate therapy and have an excellent prognosis. Unfortunately, dogs in the chronic state of *E. canis* infection have a guarded-to-poor prognosis.[81, 82, 86]

Prevention

Blood products may be a source of infection. Screening of blood donors for *E. canis* by immunofluorescent antibodies is recommended, whereas screening for *E. chaffeensis*, *E. ewingii*, *A. phagocytophilum* and *A. platys* should be considered in high-risk areas.

Prevention efforts should focus on reducing tick exposure and prevention of tick bite/attachment, along with prompt (and safe) tick removal, particularly in endemic areas.

ENVIRONMENTAL AND OPPORTUNISTIC FUNGAL PATHOGENS
Vanessa Barrs and Michelle Evason

Definition

In dogs and cats, fungal pathogens may cause specific focal (e.g. sinus or nasal) or multisystemic disease. Fungal infections may be opportunistic in patients with underlying immunosuppression (e.g. feline leukemia virus) during immunosuppressive drug therapy (e.g. prednisone) or with concurrent disease. Additionally, infection with fungal pathogens should always be considered in endemic geographic regions and in patients with lack of the anticipated disease resolution with antimicrobial therapy (e.g. non-healing wounds, urinary tract infection).

Dimorphic systemic mycoses

These include ascomycetes (*Histoplasma capsulatum* complex, *Blastomyces dermatitidis*, *Coccidioides immitis*, *C. posadasii*, *Sporothrix schenkii*, *S. brasiliensis*) and basidiomycetes (*Cryptococcus gattii* species complex).

Risk factors for dimorphic systemic mycoses are listed in *Table 6.17*. Although young age and outdoor activities are common risk factors for these infections, animals of any age and animals with no outdoor access can be affected. Knowledge of whether an animal is located in or has travelled to an endemic area is essential for ranking of differential systemic mycoses.

Diagnosis

Clinical presentation and diagnostic tests for systemic mycoses are listed in *Tables 6.18* and *6.19* (**Figs. 6.35, 6.36**). Serologic assays should be performed only in animals with consistent clinical signs. Antibody assays should mainly be used as confirmatory tests because of the inability to differentiate among subclinical infection, exposure or recovered infection, and active infection.

Therapy

Antifungal drugs for treatment of mycoses are listed in *Table 6.20*. Itraconazole is used as first-line treatment for sporotrichosis, histoplasmosis, coccidioidomycosis and blastomycosis. In animals with refractory, severe or disseminated disease, amphotericin B (AMB) should be used in combination with itraconazole, either parenterally or, in the case of refractory cutaneous lesions caused by sporotrichosis, intralesionally.[89] Treatment duration is usually a minimum of 4–6 months, but is often longer, sometimes years.

Fluconazole is used as first-line treatment for cryptococcosis, and itraconazole as second line. Where there is CNS involvement or disseminated disease, AMB should be given parenterally 2–3 times weekly for 4 weeks in combination with fluconazole (dogs) or flucytosine (cats), after which fluconazole monotherapy is continued.

Prognosis/complications

The prognosis for systemic dimorphic mycoses depends on the severity of disease and the degree of dissemination. The prognosis is generally good for animals with localized disease, although long treatment periods are often required. With coccidioidomycosis, animals with only pulmonary involvement are most likely to recover. However, those with multifocal bone involvement are least likely to recover and may require lifelong treatment. Neurologic involvement is a negative prognostic factor in cryptococcosis

---

Table 6.17 Risk factors for systemic dimorphic mycoses

RISK FACTORS	SPOROTRICHOSIS	COCCIDIOIDOMYCOSIS	HISTOPLASMOSIS	BLASTOMYCOSIS	CRYPTOCOCCOSIS
Host species susceptibility	Cats > dogs	Dogs > cats	Cats > dogs	Dogs > cats	Cats > dogs
Sex	✓ (Male cats)	✗	✓ (Female dogs)	✓ (Male dogs)	✗
Breeds	✗	Large breeds Sporting breeds Working breeds	Persian cats Sporting breeds Working breeds	Large breeds Sporting breeds	Ragdoll Birman Siamese American Cocker Spaniels Large breeds
Age	✓ (Cats ≤4 years)	✓ (Dogs ≤4 years)	✓ (Dogs ≤7 years)	✓ (Dogs ≤4 years)	✓ (Dogs)
Travel to endemic area	✓	✓	✓	✓	✓
History of fighting	✓ (Cats)	✗	✗	✗	✗
Free roaming or active outdoors	✓ (Cats)	✓ (Dogs)	✓ (Dogs)	✓ (Dogs)	✗

Table 6.18 Clinical signs and presentations of dimorphic mycoses

SIGN	SPOROTRICHOSIS	COCCIDIOIDOMYCOSIS	HISTOPLASMOSIS	BLASTOMYCOSIS	CRYPTOCOCCOSIS
Localized or multifocal cutaneous lesions (may include nodules, ulcers, crusts, draining tracts)	✓ Especially nose, eyelids, pinnae and limbs (most common presentation in cats). Solitary lesions (more common in dogs)	✓ Especially on trunk.[86] Infection route: hematogenous (common) or cutaneous inoculation (uncommon)	✓ Single or multifocal (more common in cats)	✓ Multifocal (50% dogs at presentation), especially trunk, limbs, digits, muzzle. Also tongue. Infection route: hematogenous (common) or cutaneous inoculation (uncommon)	✓ Usually multifocal. More common in cats than dogs. Infection route: hematogenous
Nasal mucosal involvement: (sneezing, nasal discharge, epistaxis, stertor, spread to adjacent tissues, e.g. nasal bridge, facial distortion)	✓(Common)	✓(Uncommon)	✓(Common)	✓(Common)	✓(Common, cats) More often subclinical in dogs
Pulmonary involvement: (may include cough, dyspnea, tachypnea, harsh lung sounds)	✓(Common)	✓ (Localized infections with pulmonary involvement most common presentation)	✓ (Common: 40% cats)	✓ (50% dogs)	✓ (Uncommon in cats, common in dogs but often subclinical)
Single or multi-organ extrapulmonary involvement (disseminated)	✓ Hematogenous dissemination. Common organs affected (cats): liver, spleen, kidney, lymph nodes, testicles. Bone/joint involvement (rare, dogs); lameness, joint effusion	✓ Hematogenous dissemination. Especially bones and joints (lameness, swelling, draining tracts in overlying skin, focal pain especially neck or back – vertebral osteomyelitis common), CNS (seizures common, ataxia, paresis, paralysis), skin, lymph nodes, eyes (e.g. chorioretinitis, uveitis, panophthalmitis, retinal detachment), testes, prostate, myocardium (sudden death, syncope, arrhythmia), pericardium (right-sided heart failure)[87]	✓ Hematogenous dissemination. Multiple organ involvement common at presentation (cats) especially eyes (25%) – as for coccidioidomycosis plus glaucoma; bone (20%) (lameness, swelling, focal pain); lymph nodes, skin, liver, spleen, bone marrow. Gastrointestinal (chronic diarrhea, melena/hematochezia, tenesmus); bone marrow, liver, spleen involvement common in dogs	✓ Hematogenous dissemination. Especially skin, eyes, bone, CNS, prostate, testes. Ocular signs as for histoplasmosis	✓(Common) Hematogenous dissemination or direct extension from nasal cavity or lungs. Especially CNS (decreased mentation/coma, behavioral change, vestibular signs, cranial nerve deficits, ataxia, paresis, tremors, seizures, cervical pain) and eyes (as for histoplasmosis, optic neuritis with mydriasis and chorioretinitis common), also lymph nodes and skin. Other widespread organ involvement common in dogs: gastrointestinal, bones, joints, pancreas, adrenal glands
Other systemic signs	✓ Fever, lethargy inappetence, lymphadenopathy, weight loss, vomiting	✓ Fever (50%), lethargy, inappetence, lymphadenopathy, weight loss/muscle wasting; other signs referable to specific organ involvement, e.g. CNS signs	✓ Fever, lethargy (70%), inappetence, lymphadenopathy, weight loss (50%), pale mucous membranes (>40%), other signs referable to specific organ involvement, e.g. jaundice	✓ Fever, lethargy, inappetence, lymphadenopathy, weight loss, other signs referable to specific organ involvement	✓ Fever is uncommon. Weight loss, lethargy, inappetence common (dogs), other signs referable to specific organ involvement

Table 6.19 Diagnostic tests for dimorphic systemic mycoses

TESTS	SPOROTRICHOSIS	COCCIDIOIDOMYCOSIS	HISTOPLASMOSIS	BLASTOMYCOSIS	CRYPTOCOCCOSIS
Serology: antibody	✓ Serum ELISA: >90% Se & Sp, but limited commercial availability[88]	✓ Serum or CSF AGID (IgG) or (IgM) qualitative assay; AGID (IgG) quantitative assay (titer) High Se (>90%) and moderate–high Sp[87, 89] FP: subclinical infections in endemic areas (titers ≤1:16, confirmatory tests recommended)	✗ Serum AGID or CF: low Se & Sp, no rigorous studies in dogs and cats	✓ Serum AGID, RIA or EIA: AGID has lowest Se, no longer recommended. RIA & EIA highest sensitivity (76–93%)[90, 91]	✗
Serology: antigen	✗	✓ Blood, urine Low Se (<20%) and Sp, not clinically useful[92]	✓(First line) Urine, serum, BAL fluid Detects *H. capsulatum* antigen EIA: >90% Se and Sp (urine) compared with organism detection (cytology, histology)[93, 94] FN: Se is lower with blood, antigen tests may be negative in focal or localized infections, e.g. ocular histoplasmosis[95] FP: cross-reacts with other fungi, e.g. *Blastomyces, Coccidioides, Sporothrix* Perform organism detection tests in positive cases	✓(First line) Urine, serum Detects the fungal cell wall antigen galactomannan EIA: 87% Se (serum); 94% Se (urine) Sp is low because of cross-reactivity with other fungal infections, especially histoplasmosis, since other fungi possess galactomannan	✓ Sample: blood, CSF High Se & Sp FN: more likely in dogs and focal infections FP: more likely at low titers
Cytology: FNA, fluid analysis, impression smear	✓ Moderate Se cats (80% compared with culture)[96] Low Se dogs (30–40%)[97] FN: scant organisms or misidentified as other fungi, e.g. *Cryptococcus, Histoplasma* spp. FP: Other fungi misidentified as *Sporothrix* spp.	✓ Low Se FN: low organism numbers in some cases and sample types, especially BAL fluid	✓ High Se and Sp: organisms usually abundant FN: chronic, fibrotic infections, fewer organisms; misidentified as other fungi, e.g. *Sporothrix* spp. FP: other fungi misidentified as *Histoplasma* spp.	✓ Moderate Se (~75%)[98, 99] Organisms often abundant Appropriate samples include BAL, TTA and FNA of lung tissue, nodules, etc. FN: organisms not present in sample	✓ Moderate-to-high Se and Sp FN: in CSF (CNS granulomas) and nasal secretions (caudal nasal/nasopharyngeal infections); misidentified as other fungi, e.g. *Sporothrix* spp. FP: Other fungi misidentified as *Cryptococcus* spp.

(Continued)

Table 6.19 Continued

TESTS	SPOROTRICHOSIS	COCCIDIOIDOMYCOSIS	HISTOPLASMOSIS	BLASTOMYCOSIS	CRYPTOCOCCOSIS
Fungal culture (notify laboratory if dimorphic mycoses suspected)	✓ Moderate-to-high Se & high Sp (Skin biopsies or secretions, nasal swabs if no skin lesions) Slow growing (days to weeks)	✗ (First line) ✓ (Second line) High Se & Sp Not recommended for 1st line diagnosis - high risk of zoonotic infection in laboratory workers. Performed only in accredited laboratories after notification	✓ High Se & Sp (Biopsies, FNA, blood, body fluids) Slow growing (days to weeks)	✗ (First line) ✓ (Second line) High Se & Sp Not recommended for first-line diagnosis – high risk of zoonotic infection in laboratory workers. Performed only in accredited laboratories after notification	✓ High Se FN: focal infections not sampled FP: subclinical nasal colonization, confirmatory test required, e.g. serology
Histopathology	✓ Low-to-high Se with Grocott's silver stain (60–95% compared with culture)[100,101]	✓ Low Se FN: low organism numbers hamper detection. Multiple biopsies increase chance of detection	✓ High Se & Sp	✓ High Se & Sp	✓ High Se & Sp
PCR: fresh/frozen tissue, body fluids or fungal culture material	✓ Se & Sp data lacking in cats and dogs	✓ High Se & Sp in a qPCR using BAL fluid, sputum, CSF, pleural fluid (humans).[102] Data lacking for dogs and cats	✓ Se & Sp data lacking in cats and dogs	✓ Se & Sp data lacking in cats and dogs	✓ High Se & Sp in a multiplex PCR using CSF (humans) (Filmarray™).[103] Data lacking for dogs and cats Molecular testing C. gattii vs. C. neoformans
Diagnostic imaging	✓ Thoracic radiographs: changes not well described. Appendicular radiographs: osteopenia if bone involvement (rare). CT: nasal/sinus involvement: turbinate and paranasal bone lysis, soft tissue attenuation, mass effect	✓ Thoracic radiographs: changes common, especially hilar lymphadenopathy and/or pulmonary infiltrates (interstitial, nodular–interstitial, alveolar), pleural effusion. Appendicular radiographs: lytic and proliferative bone lesions, joint effusion. CT/MRI for CNS signs: solitary granulomas[89]	✓ Thoracic radiographs: changes common (>50%), especially interstitial infiltrates – diffuse, linear or nodular (cats).[104] Alveolar, bronchial or mixed patterns, pleural effusion, tracheobronchial lymphadenopathy, calcified nodules or lymph nodes (especially dogs)[105]. Appendicular radiographs: lytic and proliferative bone lesions below elbows and stifles; pathologic fractures[106]. Abdominal ultrasound: visceral changes	✓ Thoracic radiographs: changes present in most – alveolar infiltrates in ≥1 lung lobe (alveolar masses or interstitial nodules); miliary interstitial or diffuse interstitial; pulmonary bullae; tracheobronchial lymphadenopathy in 25%; pleural effusion uncommon[99]. Appendicular radiographs: multifocal lytic and proliferative bone lesions, pathologic fractures	✓ Thoracic radiographs: changes uncommon in cats with C. neoformans infection, more common in C. gattii infection. Changes present in ~20% dogs[107]. CT: nasal/sinus involvement – turbinate and paranasal bone lysis, soft tissue attenuation, mass effect. MRI for CNS disease: solitary or multifocal lesions or meningeal enhancement alone (dogs)

Abbreviations: AGID, agar gel immunodiffusion assay; BAL, bronchoalveolar lavage; CF, complement fixation; EIA, enzyme immunoassay; FFPE, formalin-fixed, paraffin-embedded histologic samples; FNA, fine-needle aspirate; FN, false negatives; FP, false positives; qPCR, quantitative PCR; RIA, radioimmunoassay; Se, sensitivity; Sp, specificity; TTA, transtracheal aspirate

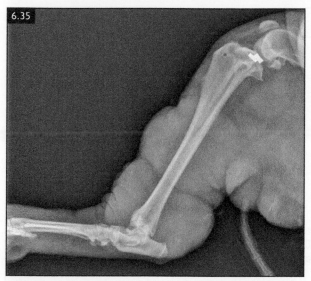

Fig. 6.35 Radiograph showing a dog with hindlimb swelling due to systemic mycosis (sporotrichosis). (Courtesy of Atlantic Veterinary College)

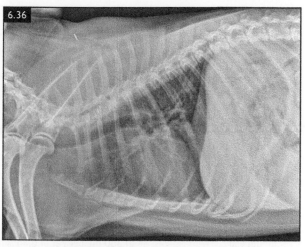

Fig. 6.36 Lateral thoracic radiograph of a dog with disseminated systemic mycosis (sporotrichosis). (Courtesy of Atlantic Veterinary College)

Table 6.20 **Dosage of antifungals used in the treatment of mycoses caused by environmental pathogens**

DRUG/FORMULATION	DOSAGE/ROUTE OF ADMINISTRATION	SPECIES	INDICATIONS FOR THERAPY	ADVERSE EFFECTS
Fluconazole 50 mg capsules 10 or 40 mg/mL oral suspension	2.5–10 mg/kg q12h or 50 mg per cat PO q12–24h	C	Crypto (first line), Histo (second line)	Gastrointestinal: inappetence Hepatotoxicity (rare)
Fluconazole 50–100 mg capsules	5 mg/kg PO q 12 h	D	Cocci (first line)	
Itraconazole 100 mg capsules	5 mg/kg PO q12–24h Administer with food	D	Cocci (first line), Crypto, Blasto, Phaeo, Zygo	
Itraconazole 100 mg capsules 10 mg/mL oral suspension (Sporanox)	Capsules: 5 mg/kg PO q12h or 10 mg/kg PO q24h Administer with food Oral suspension: 3 mg/kg PO q24h PO	C	Crypto, Sporo, Blasto, Phaeo, Zygo	Gastrointestinal: anorexia, vomiting Hepatotoxicity: elevated liver enzyme levels, jaundice. Monitor ALP/ ALT monthly. If hepatotoxicity occurs, reduce dosage to 5 mg/ kg PO q24h or 10 mg/ kg PO q48h (capsules)
Posaconazole 100 mg delayed-release tablet	5 mg/kg PO q48h (delayed-release tablet)	D	DIA, SOA, DH, Phaeo Crypto (second line), Zygo	
Posaconazole 40 mg/mL oral suspension	15 mg/kg PO loading dose then 7.5 mg/kg PO q24h with food	C		

(Continued)

Table 6.20 Continued

DRUG/FORMULATION	DOSAGE/ROUTE OF ADMINISTRATION	SPECIES	INDICATIONS FOR THERAPY	ADVERSE EFFECTS
Voriconazole 50 mg tablets 40 mg/mL powder for oral suspension (Vfend)	6 mg/kg PO q24h	D	DIA, Phaeo, Zygo	Gastrointestinal: anorexia, diarrhea Neurologic problems: blindness, ataxia, stupor Can cause irreversible hindlimb paralysis in cats
Clotrimazole	1% solution in polyethylene glycol, intranasal infusion UGA	C, D	SOA	
Enilconazole	1% solution UGA	C, D		
Amphotericin B deoxycholate 50 mg vial	0.5 mg/kg of 5 mg/mL stock solution in 350 mL per cat of 0.45% NaCl + 2.5% dextrose 2 or 3 times weekly to a cumulative dose of 10–15 mg/kg	C	Crypto, Histo, DIA, SOA, Blasto, Cocci, Phaeo, Zygo	Nephrotoxicity: monitor urea/creatinine every 2 weeks. Discontinue for 2–3 weeks if azotemic
Amphotericin B Liposomal (AmBisome)	1–1.5 mg/kg IV q48h to a cumulative dose of 12–15 mg/kg Give as a 1–2 mg/mL solution in 5% dextrose by IV infusion over 1–2 h	C		
Amphotericin B lipid complex (Abelcet)	C: 1 mg/kg IV, D: 3 mg/kg IV 3 x weekly Give as a 1 mg/mL solution in 5% dextrose by IV infusion over 1–2 hours	C, D		
Terbinafine 250 mg tablets (Lamisil)	30 mg/kg PO q24h	C, D	DIA, DH, SNA, SOA, Phaeo	Gastrointestinal: anorexia, vomiting, diarrhea
Flucytosine 250 mg capsules 75 mg/mL oral suspension	50 mg/kg PO q8h or 75 mg/kg PO q12h	C	Crypto	Gastrointestinal: anorexia, vomiting, diarrhea Not recommended in dogs because of severe cutaneous reactions

Abbreviations: ALP, alkaline phosphatase; ALT, alanine aminotransferase; Blasto, blastomycosis; C, cat; Cocci, coccidioidomycosis; Crypto, cryptococcosis; D, dog; DIA, disseminated invasive aspergillosis; DH, disseminated hyalohyphomycoses; Histo, histoplasmosis; Phaeo, phaeohyphomycoses; SNA, sinonasal aspergillosis; SOA, sino-orbital aspergillosis; UGA, under general anesthesia; Zygo, zygomycoses

and blastomycosis, and the prognosis for cryptococcosis is better overall for cats than for dogs.

Relapse rates of 15–20% are not uncommon after apparent cure of systemic dimorphic mycoses and cessation of treatment.

Prevention
In endemic areas exposure to systemic dimorphic fungal species is common. These mycoses can even occur in indoor-housed animals, due to dissemination of fungal spores in air, water, or by contact with soil on shoes etc.

Public health and infection control
Most dimorphic fungal species that cause disease in cats and dogs also infect humans. However, with the exception of *S. brasiliensis*, direct transmission from animals to humans does not occur.

Filamentous ascomycetes, non-pigmented (aspergillosis)

Michelle Evason and Vanessa Barrs

Definition

Aspergillus is the most clinically important of this fungal group, although others include *Penicillium*, *Scedosporium/Lomentospora*, *Paecilomyces*, *Talaromyces*, *Fusarium*, *Acremonium* and *Geosmithia* spp.

In dogs and cats, *Aspergillus* spp. can be the cause of localized sinonasal aspergillosis (SNA) and sino-orbital aspergillosis (SOA) or, less commonly, disseminated disease. The fungus is an environmental contaminant and can be an opportunistic pathogen.

Etiology and pathogenesis

Aspergillus spp. are saprophytic fungi (molds) that grow on organic environmental debris and are found in soil, water and air. Infections occur when the animal's immune system fails to clear inhaled fungal spores (conidia) (**Fig. 6.37**).

Immunocompetent animals may have focal upper respiratory tract (URT) disease after infection with *Aspergillus fumigatus*. There are two forms of URT aspergillosis. SNA accounts for almost all cases in dogs, and a third of feline cases. Infection is usually non-invasive and caused by *A. fumigatus*.[90, 91] SOA is rare in dogs, but accounts for two-thirds of feline

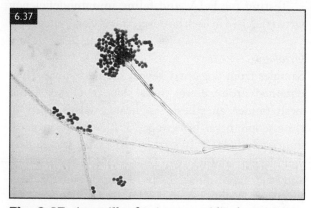

Fig. 6.37 *Aspergillus fumigatus* **conidiophore with clusters of conidia (spores) that grow outward from a phialide, as well as free conidia that have broken away. (Courtesy of US Centers for Disease Control and Prevention)**

cases. Infection is typically aggressive, invasive and caused by *A. felis* or *A. udagawae*.[92] In SNA, fungal plaques attach to but do not penetrate the respiratory epithelium. The host inflammatory response contributes to nasal turbinate destruction. In severe disease, lysis of the cribriform plate and orbit can occur, occasionally leading to meningitis. In SOA, infection extends from the nasal cavity or sinuses through the orbital or frontal bones to form a retrobulbar fungal granuloma in the ventromedial orbit. Orbital granulomas can extend into the oral cavity, paranasal soft tissues and brain.

In immune-compromised animals, hematogenous spread may lead to disseminated invasive aspergillosis (DIA). In dogs, DIA is most commonly caused by *A. terreus*, *A. deflectus* or *A. niger*.[93] Embolic fungal foci may lodge in the intervertebral disks, renal pelvis, uvea, long bones and muscles, liver, spleen and lymph nodes; however, any organ (or several) may be affected. German Shepherd Dogs are most frequently infected, and a breed-related immune defect is considered likely.[93]

Geography

Worldwide; ubiquitous in the environment.

Incidence and risk factors

See *Table 6.21*. Incidence is unknown for SNA, SOA and DIA; however, in cats the incidence of SOA appears to be increasing.[91] Disseminated aspergillosis is rare in cats, and is associated with concurrent immune disease (e.g. panleukopenia, feline infectious peritonitis, feline leukemia virus [FeLV]) or glucocorticoid therapy.[91]

A risk factor for canine SNA may be concurrent nasal disease (e.g. nasal tumor or nasal foreign body), likely due to decreased local immunity.[94, 95]

Clinical signs

SNA

Mucopurulent nasal discharge and sneezing, together with depigmentation, crusting or ulceration of the nares (unilateral or bilateral), are most common. Nasal discomfort (pain and face pawing), epistaxis, lethargy and decreased appetite may occur. Unilateral signs often progress to bilateral after

Table 6.21 **Risk factors for aspergillosis**

RISK FACTORS	SNA	SOA	DIA
Host species susceptibility	Dogs > cats	Cats > dogs	Dogs > cats
Sex	✓ (Male dogs)	✗	✓ (Female dogs)
Breeds	✓ Dolichocephalic and mesatocephalic breeds (dogs) Brachycephalic breeds (cats)	Brachycephalic breeds (cats), e.g. Persian Exotic shorthair British shorthair	German Shepherd Dog Rhodesian Ridgeback
Age	✓ (Mostly young to middle aged)		✓ (Dogs ≤7 years)
Immunosuppressive drugs	✗	✗	✓

Abbreviations: DIA, disseminated invasive aspergillosis; SNA, sinonasal aspergillosis; SOA, sino-orbital aspergillosis

deterioration of the nasal septum. Clinical signs may be subtle in early disease.

SOA

Most cats have a history of sneezing and nasal discharge; however, these signs may have resolved up to 6 months before presentation. Clinical signs are related to a fungal lesion ("mass effect") in the orbit and can include unilateral exophthalmos and third eyelid prolapse/hyperemia, corneal ulceration (exposure keratitis) and conjunctivitis, and in severe disease facial distortion. Disease is typically unilateral but can be bilateral. A mass or ulcer in the palatine fossa, together with stertor, submandibular lymphadenopathy and fever, may also be present.[91]

DIA

Clinical signs vary with affected body system(s). The most commonly reported signs include: weight loss (40%), fever (27%), progressive spinal/vertebral pain (17–27%), neurologic signs of paresis or paralysis (20%), weakness and inappetence (20%) or lameness (13%) with swelling and fistula formation.[93] Uveitis may present before other signs.

Diagnosis

Focal aspergillosis infection is diagnosed based on location (e.g. nasal involvement in SNA) of clinical signs. A lack of or incomplete response to antimicrobials may be part of the patient's history.

A combination of diagnostics may be needed to confirm local or disseminated disease. These typically include cytology, serology (antibody or antigen), PCR and imaging (e.g. CT). Negative tests do not rule out infection.

Lab abnormalities

CBC, serum chemistry and urinalysis may be normal or reveal changes consistent with inflammation or infection (e.g. lymphocytosis, elevated globulins). Eosinophilia or anemia (e.g. blood loss with epistaxis or chronic infection) may be present. Urinalysis may reveal fungal hyphae in DIA, but sensitivity is low.

Testing for FeLV and feline immunodeficiency virus is advised in cats; however, this is usually negative.

Cytology

Samples from dogs may reveal fungal hyphae when obtained from direct nasal smear (13%), blind swab (under anesthesia or heavy sedation; 20%), rhinoscopic nasal brushing (93%) or biopsy squash imprints (100%).[96] In cats, nasal cavity lavage may yield larger samples than endoscopic biopsies alone, and the nasal flush helps with debridement of plaques.[91] Wright's stain is effective for identification of hyphae. Inflammatory cells and bacteria will also be present on slides.

Fungal hyphae may be noted on cytology of blood, synovial fluid, aspirates of lymph node, bone, organs (e.g. kidneys) and intervertebral disks (**Fig. 6.38**).

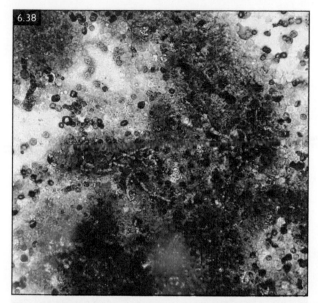

Fig. 6.38 Renal aspirate revealing systemic aspergillosis in a dog with disseminated disease. (Courtesy of Christine Rutter)

Radiology/imaging

In SNA, either unilateral or bilateral loss of nasal turbinates, radiolucency (destruction) and caudal radiopacities (fluid/mass) can be seen on nasal and frontal sinus radiographs. Both CT and MRI are preferred over radiology for assessment of the nasal cavity, sinus and cribriform plate.[97] CT or MRI is always advised before therapy in order to assess the patency of the cribriform plate and select an appropriate therapy protocol (**Fig. 6.39**).

Cats with SOA may have an orbital mass and lytic orbital bone lesions noted on CT. Concurrent nasal involvement can usually be detected.[91] There is some overlap of the CT findings seen with neoplasia, aspergillosis and cryptococcosis. CT can be used to guide biopsy of orbital lesions if more accessible lesions are not present (e.g. palatine fossa mass).

With DIA, MRI and CT can be normal. Long bone lesions (e.g. lysis, proliferation) in multiple sites and diskospondylitis are common; these were

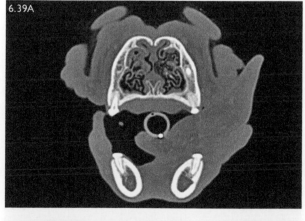

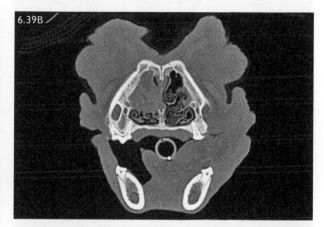

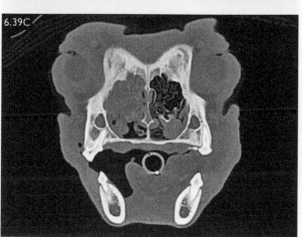

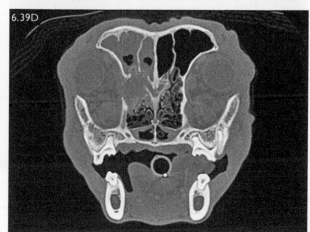

Fig. 6.39 Series of CT images (A–J) of a dog with an osteodestructive sinonasal aspergillosis granuloma.

(Continued)

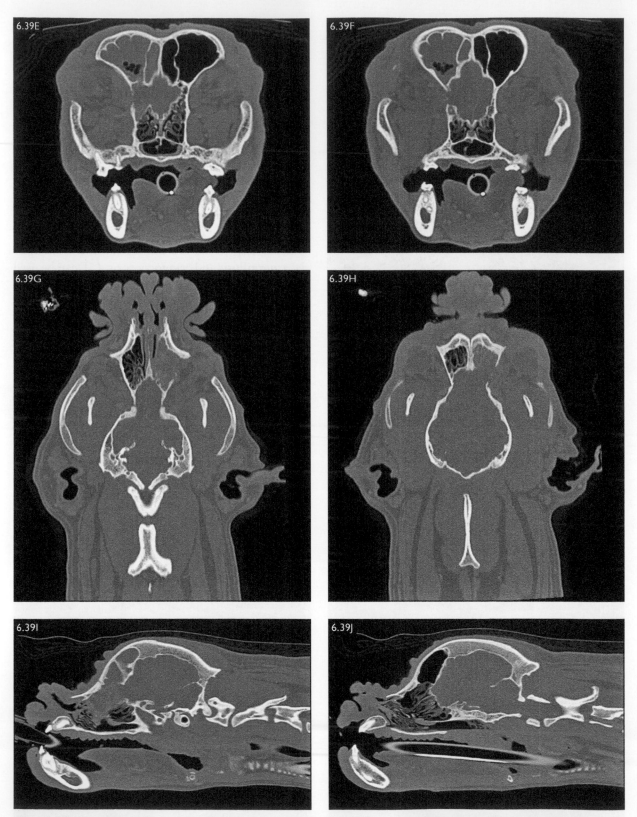

Fig. 6.39 (Continued) Series of CT images (A–J) of a dog with an osteodestructive sinonasal aspergillosis granuloma.

observed in 50% of dogs in one study.[93] Dogs with bronchopulmonary aspergillosis may have lung lobe consolidation and a bronchial pattern.

Culture

Given that *Aspergillus* spp. are ubiquitous in the environment and part of the normal nasal microbiota, culture results should be interpreted cautiously.

Most clinical isolates of *A. fumigatus* from dogs and cats with SNA are susceptible to azoles, but antifungal susceptibility testing should be performed when there has been poor response to initial therapy and when DIA is present. Antifungal susceptibility testing is recommended in all cases of SOA in cats, because the infecting fungi are often resistant to commonly used antifungals. Positive nasal cultures obtained from fungal plaque biopsies, together with classic SNA presentation and fungal hyphae on cytology or histology, provide a definitive diagnosis.[98]

With SOA, histologic or cytologic identification of fungal hyphae in orbital mass/nasal lesions obtained via the nasal cavity (endoscopy), oral cavity palatine mass biopsy or orbital mass with CT guidance and positive fungal culture provides definitive diagnosis.

In cases of DIA, culture of *A. terreus* or *A. deflectus*, together with systemic disease, is strongly suggestive of diagnosis, particularly when samples are obtained from sites that are usually sterile (e.g. urine, blood, lymph node, bone).

Serology

The sensitivity (Se) of serological tests to detect the fungal antigen galactomannan (GM) or *Aspergillus*-specific antibodies depends on systemic immunocompetence.[99] In immunocompetent animals with SNA, IgG enzyme-linked immunosorbent assay (ELISA) has moderate-to-high Se and high specificity (Sp).[100, 101] Agar gel double immunodiffusion (AGID) has moderate Se and high Sp in canine SNA, but has low Se for diagnosis of feline SNA and canine DIA. Therefore, a negative serology result does not rule out infection, and further diagnostic investigations (e.g. culture) should be pursued. In DIA, detection of GM in serum or urine has high Se and Sp for diagnosis.[102]

However, serum GM has low Se for diagnosis of canine SNA and feline URT infection and is generally not clinically useful. False positives can occur with other systemic mycoses, Plasmalyte use and certain antimicrobials.[102] Serology should be used to support diagnosis, rather than relied on as sole confirmation.

PCR

PCR of tissue biopsies is not as sensitive as serology for SNA and DIA.[103] PCR can be used for confirmation and speciation. Species identification is important to guide therapy, especially in SOA.

Rhinoscopy and sinoscopy

Rhinoscopy and sinuscopy performed under general anesthesia are considered the optimum diagnostics for SNA. Endoscopy allows visualization of fungal plaques, effective cytology and biopsy sampling, and therapeutic plaque debridement. Intranasal infusion therapy can often be performed under the same anesthesia. Abnormalities include turbinate destruction, mucopurulent secretions and fluffy off-white to greenish-yellow fungal plaques. Ideally the frontal sinus is explored to determine the extent of involvement, need for therapeutic debridement and effective topical therapy. Trephination or surgical exploration may be needed to assess and treat the sinus. In SOA, fungal plaques may not be visible because lesions may be submucosal. Optimal sites for biopsy include palatine fossa mass lesions or other paranasal mass lesions identified on CT.

Therapy

Dogs with SNA

Topical infusion of an antimycotic (after extensive fungal plaque debridement and lavage) under general anesthesia during rhinoscopy and sinuscopy is advised. SNA may be challenging to treat effectively, and conversations with clients about outcome, expectations and cost are needed. Treatments that incorporate extensive debridement and direct administration of antifungals to the frontal sinuses appear most successful.[104] Systemic therapy is far less likely to provide clinical cure than topical or combined topical and systemic therapy.[91]

Cats with SNA

Protocols for topical infusion, plaque debridement and systemic therapy are similar to those for dogs (**Fig. 6.40**). Therapy with systemic antifungals (itraconazole, posaconazole or combined with amphotericin B [AMB]) may be successful when used in conjunction with topical debridement.

Cats with SOA

Optimal treatment regimens are unknown. Posaconazole monotherapy or combined with AMB and/or terbinafine may be used. Many isolates of *A. felis* have high minimal inhibitory concentrations of itraconazole and this is no longer recommended for first-line therapy. Unfortunately, relapse is common, and therapy may be needed for more than 6 months.

DIA

Systemic antimycotics will be required if there is evidence of cribriform plate involvement, DIA or pulmonary disease. Ideally, treatment of DIA is based on the infecting fungal species. Antifungal susceptibility testing is recommended because isolates of *A. terreus* are often intrinsically resistant to AMB. Azole drugs used to treat DIA in dogs include itraconazole, posaconazole and voriconazole as monotherapy, or in combination with AMB or terbinafine (see *Table 6.20*).[93, 105] Individual dogs have

also responded to treatment with echinocandin or caspofungin.

Surgical therapy

In cases of SNA with no response to the above methods, or where topical therapy is not possible (e.g. compromise of the cribriform plate), aggressive surgical debridement and sinusotomy may be considered. It is unknown whether concurrent therapy with systemic antimycotics improves outcome. This may be considered on an individual case basis in both cats and dogs. Consultation and referral to a specialist are indicated before this is attempted.

Surgical debridement of orbital granulomas has not been demonstrated to be beneficial over medical treatment alone for SOA.[94]

The bronchopulmonary form of the disease (without systemic signs) may have complete remission after surgical resection.

Prognosis/complications
Dogs with SNA

Long-term prognosis is considered good with topical therapy (5–24 months). Rapid clinical response to treatment is considered the best prognostic indicator. A mild persistence of serous nasal discharge (>1 week) may indicate ongoing rhinitis. However, this may also indicate unresolved fungal plaques and the need for additional infusion treatments.

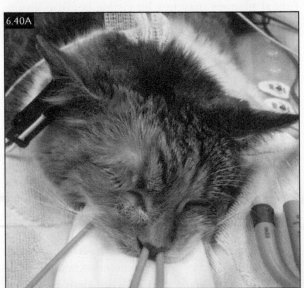
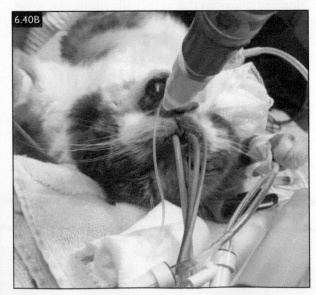

Fig. 6.40 Nasal lavage in a cat with fungal rhinitis. (Courtesy of Jinelle Webb)

The best way to prevent relapse is to repeat endo-scopic examination and azole infusion every 4 weeks until all fungal plaques are resolved. Another study found that 50% of dogs had continued mild nasal signs.[104]

Serology is not helpful in determining ongoing treatment need or prognostic response, as ELISA titers may vary or persist for >2 years.[106]

Dogs with DIA

Prognosis is guarded to poor in these dogs, particu-larly with advanced disease. One study found that 57% of 30 dogs with systemic illness were eutha-nized within 1 week of examination.[93] Another prospective study of 10 dogs on oral posaconazole monotherapy found a mean survival time of 241 days, and survival >1 year in four dogs.[105] It should be noted that, in cases with improved survival rates, relapse was common and cost of therapy may limit treatment.

Prognosis with localized bronchopulmonary dis-ease can be excellent. Cure has been obtained with systemic antifungals or lung lobectomy.[93, 105]

Cats with SNA

Prognosis is favorable to guarded with debride-ment and topical or systemic therapy.[94] In cats that have not responded to a single azole infusion, systemic azole drugs can be added and may be helpful.

Cats with SOA

This has a poor prognosis,[91] and only 20% resolve with treatment. In non-responders, disease usually progresses slowly over several months until fatal CNS involvement occurs.

The endpoint of therapy is difficult to determine because resolution of changes on CT may not corre-late with mycologic cure. Cats should be rechecked frequently and monitored for recurrent clinical signs.

Prevention

Aspergillus spp. is an environmental contaminant. Routine disinfection procedures and removal of gross debris are indicated.

Dematiaceous (pigmented) fungi (phaeohyphomycoses)
Vanessa Barrs

Etiology and pathogenesis

Phaeohyphomycoses in humans and animals are caused by over 100 species of dematiaceous fungi. The most common causes are *Cladophialophora* (syn. *Cladosporium*) spp., especially *C. bantiana* in cats and dogs and *Alternaria* spp. in cats. These are the most common fungi identified in the microbiota of canine and feline skin.[107]

Immunocompetent and -compromised animals are susceptible to infection. Routes of infection include traumatic cutaneous or ocular inoculation, or inhalation with subsequent hematogenous dis-semination. *Alternaria* spp. typically cause focal skin and nasal lesions and do not disseminate,[108] whereas *Cladophialophora* spp. are neurotropic and more likely to disseminate even in immunocom-petent animals. Predilection sites for CNS lesions, which can be solitary or multifocal, include the cerebrum and cerebellum. Other organs may or may not be involved.

Geography

The dematiaceous fungi that cause infections in dogs and cats have worldwide distribution and are ubiquitous environmental molds found in soil, air, plants and organic debris. To date, *Alternaria* spp. infections have only been described in cats and dogs in the northern hemisphere. By contrast, *Cladophialophora* spp. infections have been reported in many geographically diverse regions.

Incidence and risk factors

Although phaeohyphomycoses are uncommon overall, their incidence is increasing in humans and companion animals because of immune sup-pression from disease (e.g. diabetes mellitus[109]) and drugs including immunomodulating agents (e.g. prednisolone,[110] ciclosporin) and chemotherapeutic agents. Infections are more common in cats than dogs. Male and outdoor roaming cats are more at risk of cutaneous inoculation by dematiaceous fungi, although infections can occur in indoor only cats.[108]

Clinical signs and physical examination

Skin lesions are focal or multifocal nodules, plaques or draining tracts and are poorly circumscribed and slow growing (**Fig. 6.41**). Predilection sites are the nasal planum, digits and pinnae. Dark pigmentation may be apparent in some cases due to melanin. CNS signs are often referable to cerebral or cerebellar disease, e.g. seizures, circling, obtundation, ataxia and tremors.

Diagnosis

Serologic tests are not available. A definitive diagnosis is made by identification of fungal hyphae in cytologic and histologic specimens, and fungal culture. Culture should be performed only in accredited laboratories with appropriate biosecurity to prevent inhalation of fungal spores. Molecular testing (PCR) is often required for species identification.

Therapy

Single lesions (e.g. cutaneous, pulmonary, cerebral) have been cured by radical surgical excision with wide margins where possible, and adjunctive therapy with oral itraconazole or posaconazole (cats and dogs), or voriconazole (dogs only), for several months to prevent recurrence at the surgical site.[109, 111, 112] These drugs are also indicated for non-surgical lesions. In severe disease, combination therapy with other drugs including terbinafine or amphotericin B (AMB) may be indicated (see *Table 6.20*). Antifungal susceptibility testing is recommended to guide therapy. Minimal inhibitory concentrations (MICs) of posaconazole and voriconazole are often lower than those of itraconazole. Fluconazole has little activity against *C. bantiana* and AMB MICs may be high for some isolates.[113]

Prognosis/complications

The prognosis for single cutaneous lesions is good if wide excision can be achieved. The prognosis for cases with disseminated or CNS involvement is generally poor, although individual patients have been cured. Relapse is common if surgery is incomplete or if antifungal therapy is not given for an adequate duration.[114]

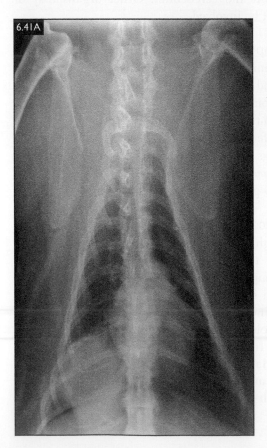

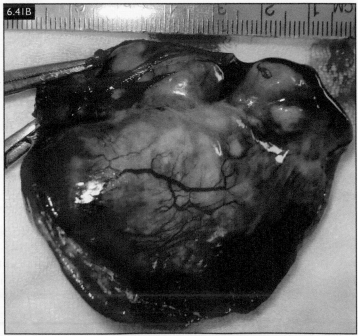

Fig. 6.41 Phaeohyphomycosis: *Cladophialophora bantiana* infection in a cat resulting in a pulmonary granuloma in the left caudal lung lobe, seen on thoracic radiography. Black pigmentation within the lung lesion is caused by melanin in the fungal cell walls, a feature of dematiaceous fungi.

FELINE IMMUNODEFICIENCY VIRUS
Lisa Carioto

Definition

Feline immunodeficiency virus (FIV) is a retrovirus that can cause chronic, persistent infection that may lead to immunodeficiency. Subclinical, systemic, neoplastic, neurologic and opportunistic infection due to immunosuppression are all recognized presentations of the disease. However, while often compared with human immunodeficiency virus (HIV) infection, the degree of immunosuppression in infected cats is typically much less and survival time does not appear to differ between infected (seropositive) and uninfected cats.

Etiology and pathogenesis

FIV is an enveloped RNA virus belonging to the *Lentivirus* genus of the Retroviridae. The virus invades cells and becomes integrated into the host genome. Transcription of DNA leads to synthesis of new viral components, and virus assembly and budding occur at the cell surface. Depending on the cat's cellular environment, viral DNA may become either latent (and evade the immune system) or active.

Infected cats can shed virus via various mucosal sites.[115–117] Bites are the major mode of transmission, owing to high viral concentration in saliva.[117] Transmission may also occur through blood donation.[37] Vertical transmission (via the placenta, during parturition, and via lactation) and viral presence in semen have been documented experimentally, but this has not been found in naturally infected cats.[115, 118–121] Unlike HIV, sexual transmission is uncommon.

Following bite inoculation and transmission, virus replication occurs in the lymphoid tissues, with the main target being the CD4+ T cell. High blood concentrations of virus are present 2 weeks after infection, with peak viremia occurring at 8–12 weeks post-infection. This may be associated with acute transient illness lasting 3–6 months. After this stage, cats may progress to subclinical or terminally infected (sick) status depending on the effect of the virus on the immune system (i.e. either activation or immunosuppression).

Geography

Worldwide.

Incidence and risk factors

Prevalence of FIV varies among studies from 1% to 31% in healthy cats, and is generally higher in sick cats.[116, 122–124] Systemic illness, feral, free-range or male cats, and having a history of bite wounds or feline leukemia virus (FeLV) infection have been associated with seropositivity.[115–118, 120, 121, 124] The majority of cats (80–90%) are 2 years of age or older when diagnosed (mean 6–8 years). FIV is associated with a higher risk of FeLV, and vice versa.

Clinical signs

Three phases of disease have been described, based on an individual cat's immune response to the virus and presence of co-infection (*Table 6.22*). The terminal stage is most frequently recognized and diagnosed clinically. Common clinical signs during the terminal phase of infection include: oral disease

Table 6.22 **Stages of feline immunodeficiency virus infection**

STAGE	DESCRIPTION
Acute	Fever, anorexia, diarrhea, stomatitis, lethargy, weight los and/or lymphadenomegaly may be observed, although this is transient and often unrecognized by owners
Subclinical	Cats may remain subclinically infected for years, or even for life, or may progress to the terminal (sick) stage
Terminal	Clinical signs occurring in the terminal phase of FIV vary widely, and reflect clinical disease seen with opportunistic bacterial, viral or parasitic/protozoal infections, neoplastic disease, myelosuppression, neurologic and ophthalmic disease. Many infected cats never develop FIV-related clinical signs, and instead die from other causes. Infections in FIV-positive cats may be less responsive to treatment, and exaggerated, when compared with those in immunocompetent cats

(e.g. periodontal disease, gingivitis, lymphoplasma-cytic stomatitis and feline odontoclastic resorptive lesions), acute or chronic dermatologic manifestations (e.g. otitis externa, pyoderma, dermatophytosis, or mycobacterial and fungal infections [e.g. crypto-coccosis and sporotrichosis]), parasitic infestations (e.g. demodicosis), multisystemic diseases (e.g. myco-plasmosis, toxoplasmosis), neoplasia (particularly lymphoma [**Fig. 6.42**]), ocular abnormalities (e.g. uveitis, hyphema, chorioretinitis, glaucoma), myelo-dysplasia, neurologic abnormalities (e.g. aggression or cognitive dysfunction, tremors, seizures, delayed reflexes or abnormal cranial nerve function, and possibly urinary and fecal incontinence) and various immune-mediated and inflammatory disorders (e.g. immune-mediated glomerulonephritis, inflamma-tory cardiac and other myopathies), chronic diarrhea, weight loss and poor body condition.

Diagnosis

Cases are frequently diagnosed incidentally through screening serology that detects antibodies against FIV. Serology (enzyme-linked immunosorbent assay, ELISA) is the method of choice for initial diagno-sis in a cat that has not been vaccinated and is over 6 months of age (*Table 6.23*).[125, 126] Testing should also be performed before being vaccinated against FIV and before becoming blood or tissue (e.g. kidney) donors. Cats that are seronegative and have a recent risk of exposure should be retested 2–3 months later to allow time for possible seroconversion.

Diagnostic test information below refers to cases with terminal infections.

Laboratory abnormalities

The most common hematologic abnormalities are neutropenia (leukopenia), mild anemia and lym-phopenia. Severe anemia, thrombocytopenia or thrombocytosis may also occur. Hyperproteinemia is common, and other abnormalities may be pres-ent depending on co-infection or concurrent disease.

Urinalysis

Proteinuria may be present with glomerulonephritis.

Serology (antibody) tests

Highly sensitive and specific point-of-care ELISA tests detect antibodies to FIV core proteins in serum, plasma or whole blood.[127] Most cats produce anti-bodies within 60 days of virus exposure, although it may take up to 12 months if exposure is low. Severe immunosuppression and inability to mount an anti-body response may also lead to false-negative results. False negatives are uncommon in kittens less than 6 months old.

Any positive result discovered during screen-ing of a healthy cat should be confirmed using an ELISA from a different manufacturer, PCR or western blotting. False-positive results due to the presence of antibodies can occur in cats vaccin-ated against FIV or in kittens less than 6 months

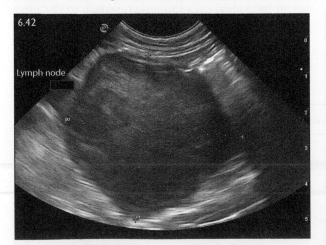

Fig. 6.42 Abdominal ultrasound image of an enlarged lymph node associated with lymphoma in an FIV-positive cat. (Courtesy of Lisa Carioto)

Table 6.23 **Recommendations for when FIV testing should be performed**
Sick cats, regardless of a previous negative result
Outdoor, free-roaming cats
Cats with bite wounds, abscesses or oral disease
Cats with known exposure to an FIV-positive cat
Cats and kittens housed in multi-cat households or group settings, particularly if the status of every cat is unknown
Cats with ongoing risk of infection (e.g. access to outdoors or living with an infected individual) should be tested annually, if not FIV vaccinated
Newly adopted cats or kittens, with retesting of kittens 60 days later if negative

of age.[125, 128, 129] Kittens with positive ELISA results should be retested after 6 months of age.[125, 128, 129] Cats previously vaccinated against FIV may remain antibody positive for 1 year and possibly more than 4 years.

PCR

A variety of PCR assays is available. Sensitivities and specificities vary depending upon the laboratory used and can range from 40% to 100%. It is important to combine interpretation of results with serology. Currently, molecular testing with PCR assays is required to identify infection in previously vaccinated cats; however, some infected cats test PCR negative, thereby complicating the diagnosis. Molecular testing may also be used to confirm infection in kittens less than 6 months of age who test positive on serology.

Therapy

Clinically normal patients do not require treatment.

Any underlying disease or opportunistic infection should, ideally, be identified and treated in cats demonstrating clinical signs. In some cases, supportive care, such as intravenous fluids and nutritional support, may be required. Empiric therapy with feline interferon-omega at 10[6] U/kg SC once a day may be administered, where available.[130] Other treatment approaches may be required depending on concurrent diseases that are present (e.g. stomatitis).

Prognosis/complications

FIV-infected cats can have an excellent quality of life for many years; however, once terminal disease occurs the prognosis may decline.[128] Prognosis is largely dependent on owner commitment to therapy of opportunistic infections in cats showing clinical signs, and management capability in multi-cat households, breeding or shelter scenarios. Very young and geriatric cats may have a more severe and progressive disease course, and consequently a decreased prognosis.

Prevention

Transmission of FIV is reduced when cats are kept indoors. If a positive cat is identified in a multi-cat household, all other cats should be tested, and new cats should not be introduced.

Vaccination against FIV is controversial for a number of reasons. Vaccination provides only partial protection from infection. Existing serologic assays cannot differentiate between natural infection and vaccination. This may lead to euthanasia of healthy (vaccinated) cats. PCR results cannot be relied on in vaccinated cats. Given the interference with diagnostic tests, less than 100% efficacy and the increased risk of sarcoma formation associated with adjuvanted vaccines, the FIV vaccine is considered a non-core vaccine, and should be used only in high-risk cats. It should be administered only to cats with negative FIV ELISA results.

FIV is susceptible to all disinfectants, including soap; therefore, routine cleaning procedures should prevent transmission of the virus within a hospital. FIV-positive status does not justify hospitalization of a cat in an infectious disease or isolation ward, because this will increase the risk of contracting secondary (opportunistic) diseases.

FELINE INFECTIOUS PERITONITIS
Lisa Carioto

Definition

Feline infectious peritonitis (FIP) is an invariably fatal disease of cats, which is characterized by body cavity effusions, neurologic and/or ocular signs. FIP is caused by a feline coronavirus (FCoV) that has spontaneously mutated from a benign, minimally pathogenic virus to one that causes systemic pyogranulomatous or granulomatous disease that progresses over a period of weeks to months. In addition to cats and wild felids, ferrets can be affected.[131]

Etiology and pathogenesis

Feline coronaviruses are large, enveloped, single-stranded RNA viruses that are ubiquitous in nature.

The mode of transmission is primarily fecal–oral.[132] The most widely accepted theory for the development of FIP is that cats are initially infected with a low-pathogenicity coronavirus after oronasal exposure, which may or may not cause mild enteric signs. That strain then mutates to a virulent strain that multiplies within macrophages and causes systemic pyogranulomatous vasculitis.[133] Cat-to-cat transmission of FIP is not a concern because effective replication of virulent strains within the gastrointestinal tract does not occur.[134] Multiple gene mutations may be involved, predominantly in the spike protein gene, membrane protein gene, and the non-structural 3c and 7b genes.[135, 136]

Geography
Worldwide.

Incidence and risk factors
The majority of domestic cats that develop FIP range between 3 months and 3 years of age, and at least 50% of affected cats are 12 months old or younger.[137] Kittens in the post-weaning period appear to be most susceptible. However, cats of any age may be affected and a secondary peak of incidence in geriatric cats (>10 years of age) may occur.[137] There may be a predisposition in males and sexually intact cats,[137–139] and a disease peak in the fall and winter.[140] Although all breeds are affected, purebred cats are more susceptible.[137–141]

Any factor leading to increased gastrointestinal (GI) replication of FCoV increases the risk for the mutation to occur, and subsequent development of FIP (e.g. cats living in multi-cat households, hoarding situations, catteries and shelters). Examples of stressors include vaccinations, surgery, rehoming, inter-animal conflict, young age and immunosuppression due to concurrent disease, e.g. feline leukemia virus infection. Cats in households with a history of FIP (that are not littermates) are as likely to develop FIP as cats in households without FIP.[142]

Clinical signs
Historically, two clinical forms of FIP were said to exist, the effusive (wet) and non-effusive (dry) forms. However, this classification is no longer clinically relevant, because microgranulomas are present in cats with body cavity effusion, and cats with the "dry form" will commonly develop effusion. Therefore, these classifications represent different stages or manifestations of the same disease. Treatment options and prognosis are equally poor. Identification of effusion is still important for diagnostic purposes, because tests performed on the effusion tend to be more sensitive than those performed on blood.

Clients report clinical signs of lethargy, decreased appetite, weight loss, vague poor health and stunted growth in kittens. Abdominal distension, due to ascites, may be misinterpreted by owners as weight gain or pregnancy. In addition, a chronic, fluctuating fever that is unresponsive to antibiotics commonly occurs, and polydipsia and polyuria may occur secondary to pyrexia. Pleural effusion or severe ascites may be associated with tachypnea, or dyspnea, and diarrhea may be present due to intestinal granulomas (*Table 6.24*, **Fig. 6.43**).

Table 6.24 **Physical examination abnormalities that may be found with feline infectious peritonitis**

ABDOMINAL	CARDIORESPIRATORY	NEUROLOGIC	OCULAR	OTHER
Abdominal effusion	Pleural effusion	Behavioral changes	Conjunctivitis	Icterus
Lymphadenomegaly	Dyspnea	Cranial nerve deficits	Mucopurulent discharge	
Intestinal thickening	Muffled heart and lung sounds	Head tilt	Thickening/hyperemia of the nictitans	
Intestinal masses		Ataxia	Uveitis	
Hepatomegaly		Peripheral neuropathy	Anisocoria	
Enlarged kidneys		Paresis/paralysis	Hypopyon	
Abdominal distension		Urinary incontinence	Hyphema	
Abdominal fluid wave			Chorioretinitis	
			Blindness	

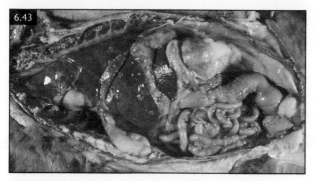

Fig. 6.43 Intestinal granuloma lesions associated with FIP in a cat. (Courtesy of Dr Ryan Jennings)

Diagnosis

Laboratory abnormalities

Complete blood count may be normal, or a stress leukogram may be present. Mild non-regenerative anemia due to chronic inflammation may occur, although occasionally a severe anemia, usually non- or poorly regenerative, may be observed. Microcytosis, schistocytes or agglutination may be present. In some cats, a left shift and toxic neutrophils are seen. Mild-to-moderate thrombocytopenia is common in cats with non-effusive disease, which may represent disseminated intravascular coagulation or immune-mediated platelet destruction. However, thrombocytosis can also occur.

Hyperproteinemia (sometimes profound) due to hyperglobulinemia, resulting from a polyclonal gammopathy, is common. Hypoalbuminemia due to liver involvement, vasculitis, glomerulonephritis or inflammation (i.e. albumin is a negative acute-phase reactant protein) may be observed.

Serum α_1-acid glycoprotein, an acute phase protein, often exceeds 1,500 μg/mL in cats with FIP;[132] however, concentrations may also increase with other inflammatory diseases.

Table 6.25 **Rivalta test**
Add one drop of 98% acetic acid to 7–8 mL distilled water in a transparent 10 mL tube
Mix thoroughly
Add one drop of effusion
Positive result (exudate): the drop retains its shape and stays attached to the surface of the tube, moving slowly down the solution

Urinalysis may be unremarkable or contain protein due to immune-mediated glomerulonephritis. FIP should be considered in cats with protein-losing nephropathy, which is otherwise rare in cats. Hematuria and, less commonly, pyuria and cylinduria may be present. Bilirubinuria may be detected with liver involvement.

Thrombocytopenia, prolonged prothrombin and partial thromboplastin times, and increased fibrin degradation products or D-dimer concentrations may occur as a result of severe liver injury.

Fluid analysis (ascites, pleural and pericardial)

The "classic" effusion in cats with FIP is straw to golden yellow in colour, viscous, clear to slightly cloudy, and becomes frothy when shaken. It is characterized as a non-septic exudate with protein concentration >35 g/L, and often 50–120 g/L and a high specific gravity (1.017–1.047); it contains a low-to-moderate number of nucleated cells (<5,000 cells/μL), usually non-degenerate to mildly degenerate neutrophils and macrophages. Erythrophagocytosis, leukophagia and reactive mesothelial cells can be observed in the fluid from some cats. An effusion albumin:globulin ratio >0.8 almost certainly excludes FIP, whereas it remains a possibility between 0.45 and 0.8.

Rivalta test

The Rivalta test can help differentiate between transudates and exudates and is an inexpensive point-of-care test (*Table 6.25*, **Fig. 6.44**). Positive test

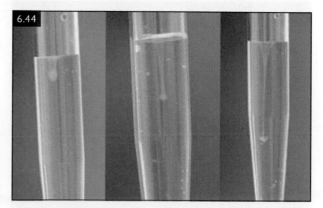

Fig. 6.44 Rivalta test for differentiation of exudates and transudates. As in this image, when the drop of effusion stays together and slowly moves down the tube, it is an exudate. (Courtesy of Lisa Carioto)

results indicate the presence only of an exudate, therefore cytologic examination of the fluid must still be performed.

Diagnostic imaging

Pleural effusion and ascites may be observed radiographically. Sonographic changes may include ascites, pleural effusion (**Fig. 6.45**), lymphadenomegaly, abnormal hepatic and renal architecture due to the presence of granulomas, as well as omental or mesenteric masses. Focal masses affecting the ileum, ileocecocolic junction or colon may be observed.

Serology

A positive FCoV antibody titer is not diagnostic for FIP, as the presence of antibodies only represents exposure to FCoV strains or other related coronaviruses. Similarly, a negative antibody titer does not rule out FIP. Approximately 10% of cats with advanced disease either fail to produce antibodies, due to severe immunosuppression, or possibly have a virus load so high that it complexes with antibodies, yielding a low or negative titer.[143] The test may also be performed too soon after exposure to the virus, as antibodies to FCoV appear 18–21 days after infection. Antibody presence without infection may be observed early in the neonatal period, and maternal antibodies disappear by 5–6 weeks of age. In addition, increasing antibody titers do not indicate that a cat is going to develop FIP, because the majority of cats with increasing FCoV antibody titers tend to eliminate the virus and become seronegative.

PCR

PCR targeting FCoV cannot differentiate between benign FCoV strains and FIP, because cats with enteric FCoV infection may also be viremic.[132] A real-time PCR assay for messenger RNA has been developed to detect a specific mutation in the spike protein which leads to inability of the virus to replicate in enterocytes, and the test should detect only the mutated virus. Testing of effusions is more sensitive than blood.

Immunostaining of FCoV antigen

FCoV antigen may be detected in effusion or tissue macrophages in biopsy samples. A positive test confirms a diagnosis of FIP.

Histopathology

Histopathology remains the gold standard for diagnosis of FIP, which is characterized by perivascular pyogranulomatous inflammation.[132]

Therapy

FIP is currently incurable, and the goal of treatment is to improve the quality of life and prolong the patient's survival time. This is achieved by decreasing inflammation and providing supportive care. Acute treatment may consist of thoraco- and abdominocentesis if effusions are present, oxygen, intravenous or subcutaneous fluids, and nutritional support. Prednisolone (1–2 mg/kg PO q24h, decreasing to the minimally effective dose) or chlorambucil (2 mg/cat PO q48–72h) have been used for their anti-inflammatory and immunosuppressive effects. Antiviral drugs tend to be ineffective and may cause severe side effects. Immunomodulating drugs may also be used (*Table 6.26*) but convincing data are lacking.[144-146] A 3C-like protease inhibitor (GC376) showed promise in decreasing virus replication and inducing remission of clinical signs in cats with naturally occurring, non-neurologic presentations of FIP but is not yet available commercially.[147]

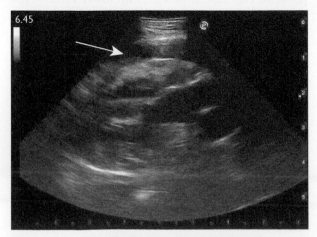

Fig. 6.45 Ultrasound image showing pleural effusion (arrow) in a cat with feline infectious peritonitis. (Courtesy of Lisa Carioto)

Table 6.26 Immunomodulating drugs that may be used for the treatment of feline infectious peritonitis

DRUG	DOSE
Human interferon alfa-2b	30 units/cat PO q24h on alternating weeks
Feline interferon-omega	Non-effusive form: 50,000 U/cat PO q24h until albumin, globulins, hematocrit and lymphocyte count return to within normal limits and there is improvement in clinical signs Effusive form: 1 mega-unit/kg injected into the cavity site of effusion. If the latter is not possible, SC administration every other day, then once a week, once in clinical remission
Polyprenyl immunostimulant	3 mg/kg PO 2–3 times a week for non-effusive FIP

Prognosis/complications

Prognosis is grave, and most cats are euthanized or die within a few days to weeks of diagnosis. Cats without effusion tend to survive for longer periods (weeks to months), whereas clinical deterioration tends to occur rapidly once neurologic signs develop.

Prevention

An intranasal live attenuated vaccine is available; however, its efficacy is controversial, it is ineffective in cats previously exposed to FCoV and it is not recommended by the American Association of Feline Practitioners vaccination advisory panel.[148]

FELINE LEUKEMIA VIRUS
Lisa Carioto

Definition

Feline leukemia virus (FeLV) is a feline retroviral pathogen that causes immunosuppression, bone marrow disorders, neoplasia, and reproductive and neurologic disorders. Although the prevalence has decreased in the last 20 years, it remains an important cause of mortality in domestic cats.

Etiology and pathogenesis

FeLV is an enveloped RNA retrovirus. Three main subtypes of FeLV exist: FeLV-A, FeLV-B and FeLV-C. Only FeLV-A is transmitted between animals, whereas subgroups B and C are derived from mutations and recombinations of subtype A with host DNA within an FeLV-A infected cat. Subtype B is commonly associated with neoplasia and FeLV-C is associated with non-regenerative anemia.[149–151]

Transmission of FeLV-A primarily results from close contact with salivary secretions, such as through playing, mutual grooming, and shared food and water dishes. Transmission may also occur via other routes, such as biting, blood transfusion, transplacentally and during lactation. Fleas may also be a source of transmission.[152–154]

The outcome of FeLV infection is extremely variable and depends on the virus strain involved, the challenge dose, the route of inoculation, and factors that influence host immune function, such as age, genetics, co-infections, stress and treatment with immunosuppressive drugs.

Virus replication occurs in oral lymphoid tissue following oronasal exposure. The virus is shed primarily in saliva, whereas low virus loads are shed in urine and feces.

The response to exposure is variable and various types of infection are described (*Table 6.27*).[155, 156] Cats with progressive infections have clinical signs and positive antigen test results (*Table 6.28*). Regressive infections can persist for life and may be reactivated with immunosuppression. Due to integration of viral DNA within host cellular oncogenes, cats with regressive infections may develop FeLV-negative malignancies later in life. However, most cats with regressive infection never develop clinical signs related to FeLV infection.

Geography
Worldwide.

Table 6.27 **Classification of feline leukemia virus infection**

INFECTION TYPE	DESCRIPTION
Regressive	Immune system is able to suppress viral replication within a few weeks of infection, before significant bone marrow infection can occur. Proviral DNA is present in the host cell genome, but virus production and shedding no longer occur. This may occur after the initial period of viremia; however, viremia may never be detectable
Abortive	Cats are exposed to low doses of FeLV, and develop antibodies to the virus. However, they fail to develop viremia, thus although antibody testing may be positive, virus cannot be detected using any antigen testing method
Focal	Proviral DNA becomes latently sequestered within selected tissues or organs (e.g. kidney, gastrointestinal tract, bone marrow), but not in blood or bone marrow. As with abortive infections, focal infections never test antigen positive
Progressive	Cats have persistent viremia, and develop a rapid onset of clinical signs due to FeLV-related disease. Progressive infection occurs once the virus becomes established in the bone marrow and the host's immune system is unable to suppress viral replication and cellular destruction

Table 6.28 **Clinical outcomes of progressive feline leukemia virus infection**

- Neoplasia, particularly lymphoma, leukemia and fibrosarcoma (with feline sarcoma virus)
- Opportunistic infections
- Bone marrow disease
  - pure red cell aplasia
  - aplastic anemia
  - myelodysplasia
  - myelofibrosis
- Immune-mediated diseases
  - immune-mediated hemolytic anemia
  - thrombocytopenia
  - glomerulonephritis
  - polyarthritis
  - uveitis
- Neurologic signs
  - anisocoria
  - urinary incontinence
- Reproductive disorders
  - abortion and infertility in infected queens
- "Fading kitten syndrome"
- Gastrointestinal or renal lymphoma
- Other
  - osteochondromatosis
  - cutaneous horns

Incidence and risk factors

The prevalence of FeLV infection in cats has decreased worldwide in the last 20 years, mainly due to increased testing and removal programs, as well as vaccination. Rates of 1–6% are commonly reported.[134, 140, 142] Cats with outdoor access and those in contact with other cats are at increased risk of FeLV infection. Cats co-infected with feline immunodeficiency virus (FIV) are also at increased risk of clinical FeLV infection.[134, 142, 157] Young cats (<1 year of age) are more likely to become progressively infected, although adult cats may also become infected, particularly when exposed to high virus loads or if immunocompromised.

Clinical signs

Clinical findings in cats with progressive FeLV infection vary depending upon the stage of infection and secondary disease processes; however, some cats do not show any clinical signs, whereas others may show vague signs such as fever, lethargy, weight loss, peripheral lymphadenomegaly, stomatitis, subcutaneous abscesses and upper respiratory tract signs (e.g. ocular, nasal discharge).

Cats suffering from anemia may demonstrate pale mucous membranes, tachypnea and tachycardia. Hemic murmurs may be audible on auscultation and splenomegaly may be palpated. If thoracic neoplasia and secondary pleural effusion are present, decreased lung sounds and displaced cardiac sounds may be noted on auscultation, as well as decreased compressibility of the cranial thorax.

Lymphoma may cause abdominal or generalized organomegaly and lymphadenomegaly (**Fig. 6.46**). Neurologic signs such as anisocoria or ataxia may also occur, although not as commonly as with feline

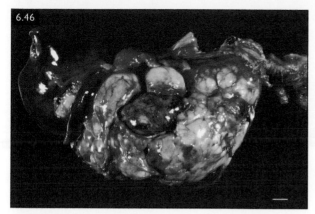

Fig. 6.46 Mediastinal mass in a cat with FeLV-associated lymphoma. (Courtesy of Dr Ryan Jennings)

infectious peritonitis. Uveitis may also be present on physical exam but is often associated with ocular lymphoma or co-infections with other pathogens.

Diagnosis

Screening of all cats using an enzyme-linked immunosorbent assay (ELISA) or a similar immuno-chromatographic in-house assay that detects free FeLV antigen in the serum is recommended (*Table 6.29*). These assays are sensitive, specific, rapid and widely available. A negative ELISA result is highly reliable in excluding a progressive infection (when living in a low prevalence area). Diagnosis of a regressive infection requires PCR to detect integrated provirus in white blood cells, whereas detection of abortive infection requires identification of antibodies against FeLV.

Laboratory abnormalities

CBC results may be within normal limits, or may show a regenerative or non-regenerative anemia. Agglutination may be evident if immune-mediated hemolytic anemia (IMHA) is present, whereas circulating blasts, megakaryocytes or dysplastic cells may be seen in cats with leukemia or myelodysplastic syndromes. Serum biochemical profile and urinalysis results are often within normal limits or non-specific.

Diagnostic imaging

Radiographs and ultrasonography may show mass lesions, which may be aspirated or biopsied for cytologic evaluation of FeLV-associated neoplasia. Thymic lymphoma should be considered when thoracic radiographs show a mediastinal mass. Abdominal ultrasonography findings suggestive of lymphoma include hypoechoic and enlarged abdominal lymph nodes, splenomegaly with a "lace-like" echotexture, and a hypo- or hyperechoic liver, which

---

Table 6.29 Feline leukemia virus testing recommendations

All cats should be antigen tested as a baseline, even if cats are kept indoors and live in a single-cat household

Sick cats, even if they previously tested negative, should be tested

Newly acquired cats and kittens, or cats with known recent exposure to an FeLV-infected cat or to a cat with unknown status, should be tested. Cats that have a negative test for FeLV (and FIV) should, ideally, have confirmatory testing performed to ensure negative status. However, if funds are limited, confirmatory testing should be focused on sick cats and cats with other risk factors (e.g. bite wounds). Healthy cats may otherwise forgo confirmatory testing, providing clients are informed of the small risk of a false-negative result in a healthy cat. Although FeLV retesting alone can be performed a minimum of 30 days later, it is more practical and cost-effective to retest for both FeLV and FIV a minimum of 60 days later using a patient-side or referral laboratory ELISA

Unless isolated, cats living in multi-cat households with FeLV-infected cats (or cats of unknown FeLV status) should be tested on an annual basis

"High-risk cats", including those with access to outdoors, evidence of fighting (e.g. abscesses, bite wounds) or those that roam in cat-dense neighborhoods, should be retested annually

Cats should be tested before initial vaccination against FeLV

Cats used for blood or tissue donation should have a negative screening test for FeLV, and a negative real-time PCR. The antigen test should be performed yearly

Pooled serum should NOT be used to perform screening tests. Individual tests are required for each patient

may be normal or increased in size. Splenomegaly and hepatomegaly may be present with IMHA.

Bone marrow cytology and histopathology

Cats with pancytopenia or non-regenerative anemia should have bone marrow aspirates collected. Bone marrow findings in FeLV-infected cats include: evidence of neoplastic lymphoid, erythroid or myeloid cells; myelodysplasia; hypoplasia or aplasia of one or all cell lines; or hyperplasia of one or all cell lines, despite peripheral cytopenias.

Antigen assays

An ELISA or similar immunochromatographic assay is the initial assay of choice for the diagnosis, and detects the p27 capsid protein antigen. Whole blood, serum or plasma may be used; however, serum is the preferred specimen.[158]

Immunofluorescent antibody (IFA) tests are occasionally used to detect intracellular FeLV antigen in neutrophils and platelets in blood and bone marrow smears; however, ELISA is more sensitive and detects progressive infection earlier than IFA.

Regressive FeLV infections are diagnosed using PCR, which detects integrated provirus. PCR tests may be used in cats with a clinical suspicion of FeLV infection, despite negative antigen test results, as some clinical syndromes such as lymphoma or myelosuppression can be caused by both progressive and regressive infections. PCR assays may be performed on blood, buffy coat, bone marrow or tissues of cats that test negatively for FeLV antigen. PCR may also be used to confirm a positive antigen test result. PCR on bone marrow aspirates is the most sensitive test to rule out regressive FeLV infection.[155]

Antibody assays

Antibody assays are not readily available but may be used to detect abortive infections. The detection of antibodies may help predict whether a cat is protected from new infection. Detecting antibodies may act as an additional screening test to decide whether a cat should be vaccinated.

Therapy

Cats without clinical signs do not require treatment. However, cats with progressive infection should always be kept indoors, not only to prevent the spread of infection to other cats, but also to decrease the risk of exposing infected cats to opportunistic infections.

FeLV infection cannot be eradicated but opportunistic infections and lymphoma can be managed. Cats with opportunistic infections may require longer treatment periods or, in some cases, lifelong treatment. Glucocorticoids should be avoided, if possible. If they are required (e.g. because of immune-mediated cytopenia), they should be used judiciously and at the minimum effective dose.

Discordant results have been published regarding the benefit of antiviral agents and immunomodulators in cats with FeLV infections.[159–161] Treatment may include feline recombinant interferon-omega (IFN-ω; 1 million U/kg SC q24h) administered for 5 days for 3 cycles for a total of 15 doses over 9 weeks (e.g. given on days 1–5, 14–19, 60–65) or low-dose oral human recombinant IFN-α (30–50 U/cat PO q24h for 7 days), discontinued for 7 days and then resumed (i.e. "7 days on 7 days off"). Zidovudine (azidothymidine, AZT) is not as effective in FeLV-infected cats as in those with FIV, although some studies have shown improvements in oral cavity inflammation, reduced antigenemia and prolonged survival times in both naturally and experimentally infected cats with FeLV.

Prognosis/complications

Considerable variation exists in the survival of infected cats, depending on the stage of infection, host immunity and FeLV strain involved. Virtually all progressively infected cats develop FeLV-related disease within 5 years of diagnosis.[162] Many progressively infected cats, especially adults, may live for several years with an excellent quality of life; therefore, euthanasia should not be recommended on the basis of a positive result alone.

Many cats with FeLV-associated lymphoma may have long-term remission when treated with standard chemotherapy protocols, and a negative prognosis should not necessarily be given. Cats with leukemia tend to have the least favorable prognosis, surviving less than a few weeks.[163]

Prevention

Infected cats should be spayed or neutered and always kept indoors, not only to prevent the spread of infection to other cats but also to decrease the risk of exposing infected cats to opportunistic infections. When a cat from a multi-cat household tests antigen positive, all cats in the household should be tested and, if possible, any positive cats should be separated from negative cats. Infected and uninfected cats should not share food and water bowls or litter boxes. Individuals who obtain cats with an unknown retrovirus status should be educated regarding the need to quarantine and test following (or, ideally, before) addition of the cat to the household. Euthanasia of sick FeLV-positive cats that enter shelters may be considered.[164]

FeLV lives outside the host for only a few minutes and is susceptible to all disinfectants, including soap; therefore, routine cleaning procedures should prevent virus transmission within the hospital.

Immunity and vaccination

Vaccination against FeLV is efficacious in cats at risk of virus exposure; however, the degree of protection is insufficient with very high infectious pressures, such as a naïve cat living with a FeLV-shedding cat. Acutely ill cats should not be vaccinated, and cats that have been potentially exposed to virus between "boosters" should be retested before being revaccinated. There is no value in administering vaccine to FeLV antigen-positive cats, because it will not offer protection and may contribute to further immunosuppression. Vaccination is usually reserved for cats with a realistic risk of exposure.

HEMOTROPIC MYCOPLASMAS
Julie Armstrong

Definition

Previously known as *Haemobartonella* and *Eperythrozoon* spp., hemotropic mycoplasmas are small, wall-less, pleomorphic bacteria that parasitize the surfaces of red blood cells in a variety of mammals. These organisms cannot be cultured, making diagnosis difficult. Clinical signs relate to the onset and severity of anemia, and include weakness, pallor, lethargy and decreased appetite.

Etiology and pathogenesis

The species of significance in cats are *Mycoplasma haemofelis* (formerly known as *Haemobartonella felis*), *Candidatus Mycoplasma haemominutum* and *Candidatus Mycoplasma turicensis*. *Hemoplasma* spp. as well as host factors can greatly impact clinical disease. *M. haemofelis* often causes hemolytic anemia (feline infectious anemia) in acute infection and is considered the most pathogenic species. Experimentally a drop in PCV is noted with *M. minutominutium* and *Ca. M. turicensis*; however, clinically significant anemia is not typical unless there is concurrent disease such as feline leukemia virus (FeLV).[165] Subclinical carriage can occur, particularly with *M. haemominutium*.

After infection with *M. haemofelis* clinical signs of acute anemia are believed to occur within 2–34 days, and severity and duration of disease vary among cats. Most of the hemolysis is associated with extravascular hemolysis, occurring primarily within the liver and spleen, which is followed by a regenerative response. Parasitemia with *M. hemofelis* is episodic, with decreasing hematocrits at times of parasitemia. After initial recovery from the acute illness, recurrence of clinical signs may occur during times of stress or corticosteroid administration, pregnancy, concurrent infection or neoplasia, although this is uncommon.[166] Spontaneous recovery and clearance are possible.

In dogs, the two most commonly reported species are *M. haemocanis* (previously *Haemobartonella canis*) and *Candidatus M. haematoparvum*.[167–169] In immunocompetent dogs, infections are usually chronic and subclinical.[170] Clinical hemolytic anemia occurs following splenectomy, or in association with concurrent infections or immunosuppression.[167]

Transmission is believed to be vector borne (e.g. ticks or primarily fleas in cats) but is also thought to occur through dog or cat bites (ingesting infected blood), subcutaneous inoculation, fresh blood transfusion and possibly other means.[166, 171]

Experimental transmission by the brown dog tick *Rhipicephalus sanguineus* has been identified;[172] however, the relevance of this is not clear.

Geography
Worldwide.

Incidence and risk factors
In cats, *M. haemominutum* is most prevalent (10–32.1%), although highly variable rates have been identified for the three main species in different regions.[173–175] Risk factors for cats include being male and having outdoor access, and vary depending on the infecting species: younger age (*M. hemofelis*), older age (*M. haemominutium*), feline immunodeficiency virus (FIV) and FeLV positivity (*M. hemofelis*), FIV positivity (*M. haemominutium*) and steroid exposure (*M. turicensis*).

In dogs, the prevalence varies with study population and geography; however, reported values are 0–45% for *M. haemocanis* and 0–33% for *Candidatus M. haematoparvum*.[167, 168, 170, 171] Risk factors for dogs may include history of splenectomy, immunosuppression or tick exposure (*R. sanguineus*), being in a kennel and concurrent infection with *Babesia* or *Ehrlichia* spp.[170, 176]

Clinical signs
Clinical disease most commonly consists of lethargy, weakness, fatigue, or infrequently collapse or moribund state, depending on the degree of anemia. Clinical disease in dogs is uncommon.

Pyrexia is present in the majority of cats with *M. haemofelis*, along with increased respiratory and heart rates secondary to anemia. With cats, vague client concerns such as decreased social interaction, decreased appetite, pica, mild weight loss or "not right" behavior may be noted. Mucous membranes will demonstrate variable degrees of pallor and mild jaundice. Pulses may be bounding, and a cardiac murmur may be auscultated. Abdominal palpation may reveal a palpably enlarged spleen.

Diagnosis
Diagnosis of *M. haemofelis* in cats and *M. haemocanis* in dogs is typically made through clinical signs, evidence of regenerative anemia on CBC and confirmation through PCR assays. In many cases diagnosis is made incidentally. PCR assays must be interpreted together with clinical signs and degree of anemia.

Laboratory abnormalities
In cats, moderate-to-severe macrocytic regenerative anemia may be present. The Coombs test may be positive.[177, 178] Non-regenerative anemia is possible in cases of peracute hemolysis or when there is concurrent disease. Autoagglutination may be noted. Chemistry results may include alanine aminotransferase elevation secondary to hypoxia, azotemia secondary to dehydration and mild hyperbilirubinemia.[165] Bilirubin elevation is noted in severe hemolysis, and bilirubinuria may be seen.

In dogs, spherocytes may be seen in addition to the changes seen in cats.

Cytology
Fresh blood smears are best. In both dogs and cats, the pleomorphic mycoplasmas can be seen in chains or in ring forms (**Fig. 6.47**). Detection of *M. haemominutum* is rare. Overall, the sensitivity of cytology is low, and hemoplasmas cannot be ruled out on the basis of negative slide review. False positives are also possible due to misidentification of stain precipitate, basophilic stippling, siderocytes, Pappenheimer bodies or Howell–Jolly bodies. Importantly, the organisms are non-refractile.

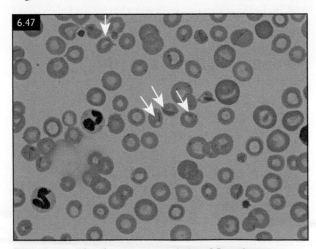

Fig. 6.47 Blood smear containing *Mycoplasma haemocanis*. Note the non-refractile darker staining organisms, both singly and in chains (arrows) (100× magnification). (Courtesy of Dr Sally Lester)

Culture
Culture is low yield.

Imaging
Splenomegaly may be noted on plain radiographs or ultrasound examination.

DNA testing
PCR testing of blood is the diagnostic method of choice. Quantitative PCR techniques allow monitoring of the copy number during therapy (keeping in mind cyclical parasitemia). PCR results must be interpreted together with clinical signs, because not all hemotropic mycoplasmas are associated with severe anemia.

Therapy
Treatment options for *M. haemofelis* in cats are outlined in *Table 6.30*.[178-181] Fluoroquinolones appear to offer a better chance for clearance. Signs of improvement occur rapidly, typically within 48–72 hours with appropriate therapy. Treatment options for dogs are presented in *Table 6.31*.[169]

Glucocorticoids may not always be indicated, and immediate use in conjunction with antibiotics is controversial. Immunosuppressive steroid treatment (2 mg/kg per day) is a consideration in patients that are not responding after appropriate duration of therapy, clinically deteriorating, have a positive Coombs test or slide agglutination, and when concurrent differential diagnoses have been carefully considered and ruled out. Transfusion support and intensive monitoring may be required in severe cases.

Prognosis/complications
Cats with regenerative anemia have a good prognosis for clinical recovery. The prognosis may be guarded for cats with non-responsive anemia or concurrent disease, such as co-infection with FeLV or underlying neoplasia.

In dogs, most infections are subclinical. Prognosis is guarded when clinically significant anemia develops.

Prevention
Vaccination is unavailable, and prior infection (with any species) does not provide future protection. Screening of blood donors by PCR is recommended.[182] Flea and tick prevention along with management of inter-cat and -dog aggression will reduce risk.

Table 6.30 Treatment options for *M. haemofelis* in cats

DRUG	DOSE	COMMENTS
Pradofloxacin	5–10 mg/kg PO q24h for 14 days	Experimental studies suggest this drug may offer a better chance for long-term clearance than doxycycline; 5 mg/kg per day may be as effective as 10 mg/kg per day
Marbofloxacin	2.75 mg/kg PO q24h for 14–28 days	Hematologic improvement but may not consistently eliminate infection as detected by PCR
Enrofloxacin	5 mg/kg PO q24h for 14 days	Use of other veterinary fluoroquinolones is preferred
Doxycycline	10 mg/kg PO q24h or divided into 2 doses, for 14–28 days	Use appropriate pilling techniques to minimize risk of esophagitis

Table 6.31 Treatment options for hemotropic *Mycoplasma* spp. in dogs

DRUG	DOSE	COMMENTS
Doxycycline	10 mg/kg PO q24h for 14–28 days	
Pradofloxacin	3–4.5 mg/kg PO q24h for 14–28 days	Not licensed for use in dogs in all regions. Higher doses (5–10 mg/kg) have also been used
Enrofloxacin	5–10 mg/kg PO q24h for 14 days	

HEPATOZOON AMERICANUM (AMERICAN CANINE HEPATOZOONOSIS)
Johanna Heseltine

Definition
American canine hepatozoonosis is a chronic protozoal infection resulting in muscle pain, weight loss, lethargy and a marked leukocytosis. Untreated infections are fatal.

Etiology and pathogenesis
Hepatozoon americanum infection occurs following ingestion of infected nymphal or adult Gulf Coast ticks (*Amblyomma maculatum*). Infection by ingestion of an infected paratenic host (rodent or rabbit) has been demonstrated experimentally, and vertical transmission is suspected.[183]

After tick ingestion, mature oocysts release sporozoites into the intestinal wall, which are phagocytized by mononuclear cells and disseminate via blood or lymph. Meronts form between myocytes of striated muscle, where they subsequently rupture and release merozoites. Severe pyogranulomatous inflammation and myositis result. Cysts are found in muscle as early as 2 weeks post-infection. Clinical signs develop as early as 3–5 weeks post-infection. Proliferation on the surface of long bones may develop, through an unclear mechanism. Chronic inflammation can also lead to glomerulonephritis or amyloidosis. Merozoites enter the bloodstream and form gamonts, which can infect other ticks.

Before 1997, canine hepatozoonosis was attributed to *H. canis*. *H. americanum* has since been recognized as a separate species, responsible for most canine infections in the United States, whereas *H. canis* accounts for a small number of canine infections in the United States and infections in other countries. *H. americanum* causes severe illness in dogs. In contrast to *H. americanum*, *H. canis* infection is often subclinical or associated with mild disease. High parasite burdens can cause more severe illness with lethargy, anorexia, pallor and, rarely, bone pain. Whereas *H. americanum* infects striated muscle, *H. canis* infects primarily hemolymphatic tissues (*Table 6.32*).[183]

Geography
The disease is most common in the southern United States, with cases also reported in Washington, California, Nebraska, Vermont and Virginia.[184]

Incidence and risk factors
Disease is most often reported in young adult dogs, but dogs of any age can be infected. It is diagnosed most often in dogs in rural areas, especially those kenneled outdoors or allowed to roam.

Clinical signs
Clinical signs are often waxing and waning and include lethargy, marked weight loss despite a normal appetite, and a stiff gait with reluctance to walk or stand. Muscle, bone, spinal or paraspinal pain is common. Muscle atrophy, especially of temporal muscles, is often present. Mucopurulent ocular discharge (due to myositis of extraocular muscles or decreased tear production) is common. Ocular examination may reveal uveitis, retinal scarring or hyperpigmentation, or papilledema. Lymphadenopathy is sometimes present.

Diagnosis
H. americanum infection should be suspected when a dog in an endemic area is presented with non-antibiotic-responsive fever, hyperesthesia and muscle wasting, coupled with a marked leukocytosis and sometimes periosteal proliferation. Diagnosis is confirmed with PCR testing of ethylenediaminetetraacetic acid (EDTA) whole blood or via muscle biopsies.

Laboratory abnormalities
Leukocytosis is the most consistent abnormality and is predominantly due to a mature neutrophilia, although a left shift may be present. Normocytic, normochromic anemia is common. Rarely, gamonts may be found in peripheral blood monocytes (≤0.1% of cells) as early as 32 days post-infection (**Fig. 6.48**). If numerous gamonts are seen, infection is likely *H. canis*. Platelet count is normal to high; however, thrombocytopenia occurs with concurrent rickettsial infection. Hypoalbuminemia, but not hyperglobulinemia, is common. Unless there is renal failure, urea is often low. Elevated alkaline phosphatase, hypoalbuminemia, hypoglycemia and low urea can be mistaken for liver failure, but pre- and post-prandial bile acids

Table 6.32 **Comparison of *Hepatozoon americanum*, *Hepatozoon canis* and *Hepatozoon felis***

DIAGNOSTIC CRITERION	H. AMERICANUM	H. CANIS	H. FELIS
Species	Dog	Dog, cat	Cat
Geographic distribution	Southern United States	Africa, Asia, South America, Europe, Middle East, Grenada, Cape Verde Islands, United States	India, Thailand, South Africa, Nigeria, Brazil, Israel, southeastern Europe, United States
Primary tick vector	*Amblyomma maculatum*	*Rhipicephalus sanguineus*	Unknown
Common clinical signs	Severe disease: fever, lameness, lethargy, mucopurulent ocular discharge, generalized hyperesthesia	Subclinical or mild disease: fever, lethargy, weight loss	Subclinical or mild disease
Common laboratory findings	Anemia, marked leukocytosis, elevated serum alkaline phosphatase, hypoalbuminemia	Rare: anemia, thrombocytopenia, leukocytosis	Rare: anemia, thrombocytopenia
Radiographic lesions	Periosteal proliferation	Non-specific, bone lesions uncommon	Non-specific
Major target organs	Skeletal muscle, myocardium	Spleen, bone marrow, lymph nodes	Skeletal muscle, myocardium
Unique morphologic features	"Onion-skin" cysts in muscle, myositis, pyogranulomatous inflammation	"Wheel-spoke" meronts in spleen	Meronts surrounded by a thick membrane in muscle without inflammation
Primary diagnostic procedures	PCR, muscle biopsy	PCR, blood smear	PCR, blood smear
Visualization of gamonts	Rare; found in <0.1% of peripheral leukocytes	Common; found in 1–100% of neutrophils	Rare; found in <0.1% of peripheral leukocytes
Treatment (note treatment controls clinical signs but is not curative)	Trimethoprim sulfadiazine, clindamycin, pyrimethamine, decoquinate *or* ponazuril, decoquinate	Imidocarb dipropionate, doxycycline	Doxycycline *or* oxytetracycline, primaquine

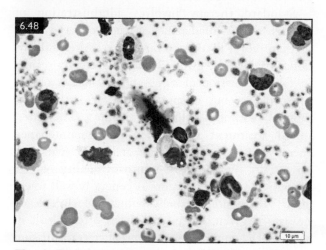

Fig. 6.48 *H. americanum* gamont (pale-blue staining ellipsoid bodies [8.8 × 3.9 μm] with faintly staining nuclei) in a peripheral monocyte. (Courtesy of Dr Gwen Levine)

are normal or only mildly increased. Creatine kinase is normal, despite myositis. Proteinuria may be present as a result of protein-losing nephropathy.

Imaging
Periosteal proliferation that resembles hypertrophic osteopathy may be found on radiographs, especially of affected dogs less than 1 year of age (**Fig. 6.49**). Lesions are most common on proximal long bones, but may also occur on distal long bones and other sites, including scapulae, vertebrae and pelvis.[185]

Histopathology
Biopsies of the biceps femoris or semitendinosus muscle can confirm the diagnosis, and false negatives are uncommon. The pathognomonic lesion is

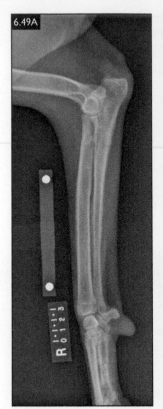
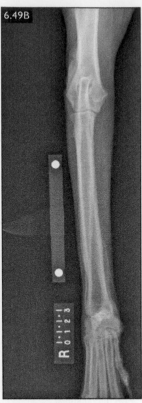

Fig. 6.49 Lateral (A) and anteroposterior (B) radiographs showing periosteal proliferation on the radius and ulna of a dog with *H. americanum* infection. (Courtesy of Texas A&M Radiology, College Station, TX)

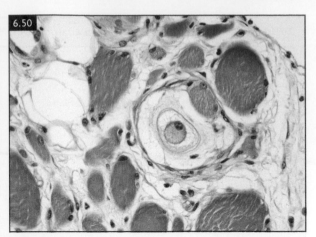

Fig. 6.50 "Onion-skin" cyst in the muscle of a dog infected with *H. americanum*. (Courtesy of Brian Porter)

Table 6.33 **Treatment for *Hepatozoon americanum* infection**

DRUG COMBINATIONS	DOSAGE
Trimethoprim sulfadiazine	15 mg/kg PO q12h for 14 days
Clindamycin	10 mg/kg PO q8h for 14 days
Pyrimethamine	0.25 mg/kg PO q24h for 14 days
Decoquinate	10–20 mg/kg PO q12h for 2 years
Ponazuril	10 mg/kg PO q12h
Decoquinate	10–20 mg/kg PO q12h for 2 years

an "onion-skin" cyst between myocytes, caused by secretion of mucopolysaccharides in response to infected mononuclear cells in muscle (**Fig. 6.50**). The cyst results in pyogranulomatous inflammation and myositis.[183]

PCR

Real-time PCR on EDTA whole blood can confirm the diagnosis. PCR can be positive from approximately 42 days post-infection. False negatives are uncommon but can occur with a low parasite burden or chronic infection. Muscle biopsy should be performed in cases in which PCR is negative and disease is suspected. PCR can differentiate *H. americanum* from *H. canis* infection.

Therapy

Treatment is aimed at resolving parasitemia (*Table 6.33*); PCR testing will remain positive.[186]

Treatment can result in remission but is not curative, and encysted organisms remain in muscles for years.

Standard therapy involves administration of trimethoprim sulfadiazine, clindamycin and pyrimethamine (TCP combination). Alternatively, ponazuril may be given. Treatment usually results in rapid remission of signs and resolution of the neutrophilia, but relapse will occur within 2–6 months without additional therapy. Therefore, initial treatment is followed with maintenance therapy with decoquinate for at least 2 years and potentially lifelong, as it improves quality of life, extends life expectancy and is generally well tolerated.[187] Remission is usually maintained while decoquinate is given, but missed doses often result in relapse. Decoquinate may also reduce transmission to susceptible ticks and, therefore, other dogs. An alternative maintenance approach is to repeat PCR testing every 3–6 months, discontinuing treatment when the test is negative, and restarting treatment when the test becomes positive. However, this could result in relapse of signs and the need to repeat TCP combination therapy. Relapses can usually be controlled with TCP combination therapy. Supportive therapies, such as analgesia, non-steroidal anti-inflammatory drugs, fluids and nutritional support, are given as needed.

Prognosis/complications

With TCP combination and decoquinate, a 2-year survival rate of >84% has been reported.[187] Acutely ill patients often respond well. Prognosis is more guarded with chronic infections, as complications such as glomerulonephritis or amyloidosis may not resolve. Proteinuria should be monitored and managed, if it persists. All infected patients should be considered to have lifelong disease and be monitored.

Untreated dogs will die (or be euthanized) within 1 year.

Prevention

Tick prevention and removal can minimize the risk of tick ingestion during self-grooming. Dogs should not be allowed to eat carcasses that may harbor ticks.

HISTOPLASMOSIS
Johanna Heseltine

Definition

Histoplasmosis is a systemic disease that occurs in dogs, cats or humans when spores (microconidia) are inhaled. Infection may be subclinical or cause acute or chronic respiratory, gastrointestinal (GI) or ocular signs.

Etiology and pathogenesis

Histoplasma capsulatum is a dimorphic fungus. The mycelial phase is widely present in soil and forms spores (macroconidia and microconidia). Transmission occurs when spores are inhaled into the lower respiratory tract and convert to the yeast phase. Infection may be limited to granulomatous inflammation of the pulmonary tract. However, more commonly yeast organisms disseminate throughout the animal, causing acute or chronic disease. Incubation periods may be a few weeks to several years.

Geography

Endemic areas include Latin America and parts of the USA (Ohio and south-central river valleys), but cases have been reported elsewhere. In warm climates, the organism is widely found in soil, especially in areas rich in bird or bat guano.

Incidence and risk factors

Most cases have been reported in young to middle-aged cats and dogs, but it can occur at any age. Sporting and hunting dogs may have increased risk.

Common clinical signs

Clinical signs may be non-specific or reflect infected body systems. Inappetence, weight loss and fever are common. Respiratory signs may be absent or include tachypnea/dyspnea and cough in dogs. Anecdotally, dogs appear more susceptible than cats to GI tract signs such as large bowel diarrhea and protein-losing enteropathy, often without respiratory signs. Cough is uncommon in cats, but ocular involvement may occur (e.g. chorioretinitis, uveitis, optic neuritis). Many infections are believed to be subclinical.

Physical examination

Infected animals are often febrile, thin and may have pale mucous membranes. Abnormalities may involve one or more body systems. Increased bronchovesicular lung sounds are often present. Hepatomegaly (± icterus), splenomegaly and visceral lymphadenopathy are common. The rectal wall may be thickened on palpation in dogs.

Diagnosis

Diagnosis is based on clinical signs and identification of the organism on cytology (or histopathology), or positive urine *Histoplasma* antigen testing. Urine antigen assay is recommended before more invasive diagnostic testing, particularly in endemic areas.

Laboratory abnormalities

Anemia is common (anemia of chronic disease, bone marrow infection or GI hemorrhage). An inflammatory leukogram is typical and thrombocytopenia may occur. Pancytopenia occurs with bone marrow infection. The yeast form may be found on stained blood or buffy coat smears, usually in monocytes or neutrophils.

Hypoalbuminemia and hyperglobulinemia are common. Elevated liver enzymes and bilirubin reflect hepatic involvement. Most cats are feline leukemia virus and feline immunodeficiency virus negative.

Culture of samples from suspected histoplasmosis cases must be done only by specialized laboratories because of the biosafety risks associated with growth of this zoonotic pathogen. Samples should never be cultured in clinics.

Imaging

Thoracic radiographs often show a diffuse interstitial lung pattern that may be miliary, nodular or coalescing (**Fig. 6.51**). Hilar lymphadenopathy is common in dogs and may be severe. Pleural effusion is uncommon. Joint swelling and bony lesions are reported, mainly in cats. Radiographs may be normal.

Abdominal imaging often shows hepatomegaly, splenomegaly, lymphadenopathy and sometimes ascites. Thickening of the intestines with or without loss of normal layering is common in dogs with GI involvement.

Endoscopy

At endoscopy (duodenoscopy or colonoscopy), the internal mucosa may be thickened, irregular and friable (**Fig. 6.52**). Ulceration may be present in the colon.

Cytology

Numerous organisms are typically found in tissues, and cytology is often diagnostic. Yeast may be found in cytology of rectal scrapings, liver, spleen, lymph node, bone marrow, lung aspirates, bronchoalveolar lavage fluid, scrapings of oral ulcers, joint fluid, impressions of skin lesions, impressions of intestinal biopsies and, rarely, body cavity effusions (**Fig. 6.53**).

Histopathology

The yeast form may be found in tissues, often associated with pyogranulomatous inflammation. Special stains may aid in identification and should be requested based on index of suspicion.

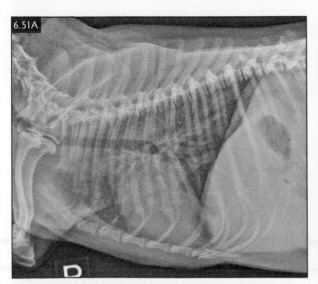

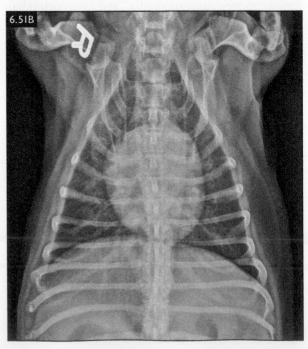

Fig. 6.51 Thoracic radiographs from a dog with histoplasmosis, showing a diffuse interstitial-to-nodular pattern, sternal lymphadenopathy and hepatomegaly. (Courtesy of Texas A&M Radiology Department, College Station, TX)

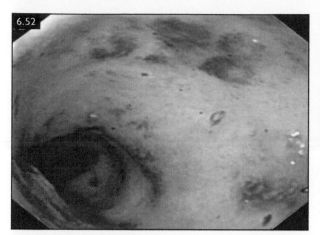

Fig. 6.52 Colonoscopy of a dog with histoplasmosis showing ulceration of the colonic mucosa. (Courtesy of Dr Michael Willard)

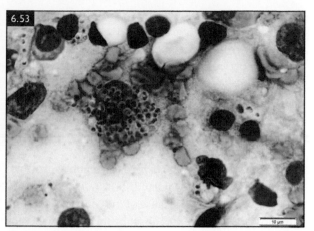

Fig. 6.53 *Histoplasma capsulatum* in a liver aspirate from a cat with histoplasmosis (100× magnification). (Courtesy of Dr Gwendolyn Levine)

Hyphae are rarely found in tissue; however, they have been reported on heart valves and in GI biopsies.[188]

Serology and antigen testing:

Histoplasma antigen detection by enzyme-linked immunosorbent assay (ELISA) has the highest sensitivity when performed on urine (dogs: sensitivity 89.5%, specificity 100%, negative predictive value 95.4%).[189] In cats this test may be similarly effective. The test can also be performed on serum, airway lavage fluid or CSF. Cross-reaction with *Blastomyces dermatitidis* (and other fungal pathogens) can occur and interpretation should be based on geographic risk factors and travel history.

Serum antibody titers lack sensitivity and specificity and cannot differentiate between exposure and clinical disease.

Therapy

Therapy (*Table 6.34*) consists of supportive care based on severity of clinical signs and appropriate antifungal treatment. Itraconazole or fluconazole has been advised, with typical therapy duration of 6 months or longer depending on disease severity and chronicity.[190] The itraconazole oral solution is recommended because it has more consistent absorption than capsules. Other antifungals may be used in specific cases or presentations. Fluconazole has better penetration into the eye and CNS; it may be less expensive and may be used if hepatotoxicity develops with itraconazole. Similarly, amphotericin B may be initially given to patients with GI histoplasmosis or more severe infections and then followed by itraconazole, as this may provide more rapid control of disease. More extensive monitoring is required with

Table 6.34 **Drug therapy for histoplasmosis**		
DRUG	**DOSAGE**	**POTENTIAL ADVERSE EFFECTS**
Itraconazole	Dog/cat: 5–10 mg/kg PO q12–24h Food improves absorption	GI upset, hepatotoxicity, cutaneous vasculitis
Fluconazole	Dog: 5–10 mg/kg PO q12–24h Cat: 50–100 mg per cat PO q24h	GI upset uncommon, mild increases in liver enzymes
Amphotericin B deoxycholate	Dog: 0.5–1 mg/kg IV 3 times/week to a cumulative dose of 4–8 mg/kg Cat: 0.25 mg/kg IV 3 times/week to a cumulative dose of 4–6 mg/kg	Nephrotoxicity (discontinue if azotemia develops), infusion reaction (trembling, fever, nausea)
Amphotericin B lipid complex	Dog: 1–3 mg/kg IV 3 times/week to a cumulative dose of 12–36 mg/kg Cat: 1 mg/kg IV 3 times/week to a cumulative dose of 12 mg/kg	Nephrotoxic (less than deoxycholate), infusion reaction

this drug owing to concerns with nephrotoxicity and the need for amphotericin B to be given as an IV infusion over >2 hours and diluted in 5% dextrose.

Glucocorticoids have been used in therapy for some dogs,[190] and have been specifically used to decrease hilar lymphadenopathy in dogs with respiratory signs (cough) and positive titers, and without detectable organisms, disseminated disease or evidence of active infection.[191]

Spontaneous recovery from canine pulmonary histoplasmosis is rarely reported; however, treatment is always recommended because of the concern regarding infection dissemination. Discontinuation of therapy is considered after 4–6 months. Treatment is usually continued 1–2 months beyond resolution of clinical signs and changes on diagnostic imaging. Urine antigen levels typically decline and may be negative with effective therapy; however, further assessment of serial titers as a monitoring tool is needed. Urine antigen level increases with relapse, so should be monitored 3 and 6 months after discontinuing therapy.

Prognosis/complications
Prognosis for pulmonary histoplasmosis is fair to excellent and depends on the client's financial and monitoring commitment, particularly when longer duration of therapy is required (12 months or longer). Prognosis for disseminated histoplasmosis is fair to good. The most difficult sites to treat are the CNS, eye, bone and epididymis (requires neutering).

The overall survival rate in cats has been reported as 55–100%,[192–194] with recrudescence in 40% of cats after discontinuation of therapy.[194] Immunosuppression can reactivate latent infection. Immunosuppression should be avoided in patients with prior histoplasmosis if possible.

Prevention
Prevention consists of avoiding exposure to known contaminated environments if possible or practical.

Public health and infection control
Direct transmission from animals to humans has not been reported; infected cats and dogs may serve as sentinels for human risk. Fungal cultures contain mycelia and are highly infectious and require care in handling. If skin lesions are bandaged to reduce environmental contamination, dressings should be changed frequently and discarded promptly.

LEISHMANIA SPP. (LEISHMANIOSIS)
Michelle Evason

Definition
Infection with the vector-borne protozoan *Leishmania infantum* may cause a wide range of clinical signs in dogs. Visceral (severe loss of weight and muscle mass, lymphadenopathy and renal failure), dermatologic (cutaneous) and mucocutaneous manifestations are diagnosed most commonly. Clinical signs may not appear until months to years post-infection.

Dogs are an important reservoir for human infection. Infection in cats occurs; however, clinical disease appears less common, particularly in the absence of dermatologic signs.[195]

Etiology and pathogenesis
Leishmania infantum is the cause of canine and feline visceral leishmaniosis. In South America, *L. braziliensis* is the cause of localized cutaneous lesions referred to as American tegumentary leishmaniosis.

Transmission is typically through the sandfly vectors *Phlebotomus* spp. (Africa, Europe and Asia) (**Fig. 6.54**) and *Lutzomyia* spp. (South and North America). Vertical transmission (hunting dogs) and transmission through blood transfusion may occur.

Infected female sandflies (**Fig. 6.55**) carry the promastigote form of *Leishmania* spp. in their guts (**Fig. 6.56**). Once the sandfly bites, the flagellated promastigote enters the dog's skin and is taken up by macrophages, after which it changes into a nonmotile, round amastigote. Replication and eventual cell rupture occur, resulting in release of amastigotes and further macrophage infection. If the dog's immune system is unable to control the infection,

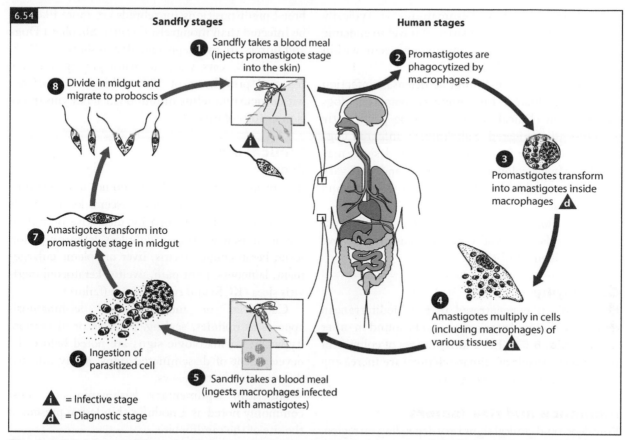

Fig. 6.54 *Leishmania* life cycle. (Courtesy of the Centers for Disease Control and Prevention, https://www.cdc.gov/dpdx/leishmaniasis/index.html)

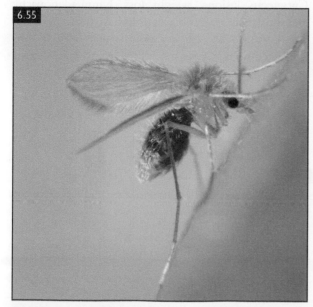

Fig. 6.55 *Phlebotomus papatasi* sandfly. (Courtesy of Professor Frank Hadley Collins)

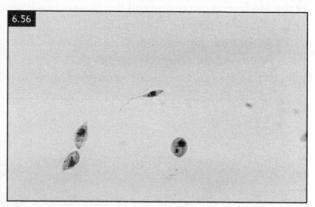

Fig. 6.56 *Leishmania* sp. promastigote. (Courtesy of Dr Mae Melvin)

amastigotes spread hematogenously (lymphatics and blood). Feeding female sandflies ingest the intracellular amastigotes and are converted back to promastigotes in the sandfly over 1 week. Multiplication within the sandfly completes the life cycle.

In North America, leishmaniosis is typically diagnosed in dogs with a history of travel to endemic areas; cases of endemic transmission occur within certain breeds, notably foxhounds.[196]

In dogs with normal immune defenses, infection is often eliminated. Less immunocompetent dogs may develop clinical signs or become persistently (subclinically) infected. Subclinically infected dogs act as a reservoir for infection. Clinical signs may develop after prolonged incubation and can vary widely from mild dermatitis to severe immune and renal disease.

Dog-to-dog transmission (without sandfly vectors), transplacental and venereal transmission have been described.[196, 197]

Geography
Leishmania is concentrated in the Mediterranean region and South America but can be found in other regions (**Fig. 6.57**). Expanding ranges of competent vectors (as a result of climate change) are increasing parasite infection in these areas.

Incidence and risk factors
Prevalence and clinical signs vary depending on region, infecting species, sandfly vector and canine response to infection (i.e. clinical or subclinical disease). In parts of the Mediterranean region and Brazil, seroprevalence or PCR positive rates may be as high as 70%.[198]

Risk factors for canine infection have been described as outdoor lifestyle, greater than 2 years of age, lack of topical insecticide protection, potential breed predispositions (purebreds are more likely to be infected than mongrels; German Shepherd Dogs and Boxers are overrepresented) and short fur.[199, 200]

In Brazil, cats with dermatologic signs had a reported prevalence of 50%. This was associated with concurrent feline immunodeficiency vius infection in 10% of cats.[195]

Clinical signs
Dogs
The majority of infected dogs do not develop clinical signs.[198] Clinical signs of visceral leishmaniosis can include lymphadenopathy, ulcerative or scaling lesions, muscle wasting, weight loss, lethargy, pallor, fever, keratoconjunctivitis, liver or splenic enlargement, lameness, joint pain, uveitis, keratoconjunctivitis sicca (KCS) and renal disease (failure).

Cutaneous or mucocutaneous leishmaniosis appears as nodules, scaling, alopecia or ulceration. Typically, dermatologic signs are noted before the development of disseminated signs. Many infected dogs develop brittle claws.

American tegumentary leishmaniosis is most commonly noted as a nodular skin lesion present at the site of the sandfly bite.

Cats
Cutaneous lesions, weight loss, lymphadenopathy and similar signs to those in dogs have been reported. In one study, 70% of cats with dermatologic lesions had disseminated disease.[195] Skin lesions may be pruritic or non-pruritic.

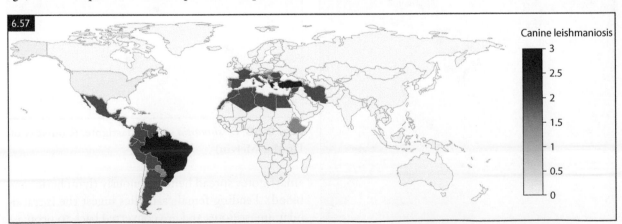

Fig. 6.57 Approximate geographic range of leishmaniasis. (Available at https://www.wormsandgermsblog.com/2018/07/articles/animals/dogs/canine-leishmania-map)

Diagnosis

Diagnosis may be challenging, particularly in endemic areas where subclinical infections and sero-prevalence can cloud interpretation of positive test results. In non-endemic regions, an awareness of infection risk based on clinical history, breed and canine importation is critical.

Diagnosis is typically made through direct cytologic or histologic detection, or through a combination of direct and indirect (serology or PCR) identification taken together with clinical signs. Following algorithms in consensus guidelines will aid diagnosis.[198]

Lab abnormalities

Mild-to-moderate non-regenerative anemia, thrombocytopenia and lymphopenia are common. Most dogs have hyperglobulinemia and hypoalbuminemia; azotemia may also be present. Urinalyses may show proteinuria, or reduced urine specific gravity with renal disease (or failure).

Joint fluid may be inflammatory and sometimes reveal organisms (amastigotes). Bone marrow exam can be abnormal, although amastigotes may be present (**Fig. 6.58**).

Cytology (fine-needle) or histopathologic exam (biopsy [**Fig. 6.59**]) may allow identification of amastigotes in the skin, lymph nodes, bone marrow or spleen. Organism identification is regarded as diagnostic, and obtaining specimens is strongly encouraged. An experienced clinical pathologist (particularly in non-endemic regions) is required to avoid misidentification or confusion with other pathogens.

Radiology/imaging

Radiology and ultrasound (abdominal) may show non-specific spleen, liver or lymph node enlargement. Radiographs may show bone or joint abnormalities (e.g. proliferation, opacities, and/or erosive or non-erosive joint changes).

Serology

Immunofluorescent antibody testing (IFA) or enzyme-linked immunosorbent assay (ELISA) can be helpful in diagnosis, particularly when cytology is negative.[200] IFA and ELISA may help identify and differentiate reservoirs or subclinical infection (lower titers) from sick (higher titers) dogs.[200]

False-negative results (due to the extensive incubation period) can occur. False-positive results due to cross-reaction with vaccine or *Trypanosoma cruzi* infection (USA and South America), and high rates of subclinically infected dogs in endemic regions may confuse diagnosis. Lab variation in titer interpretation may occur.

PCR is advised in cases where there is a strong clinical suspicion and negative cytology.[200] In dogs without dermatologic lesions, performing PCR on bone marrow or lymph nodes is considered optimum for DNA detection.[200] As with serology, subclinically infected dogs will be positive despite the lack of clinical disease.

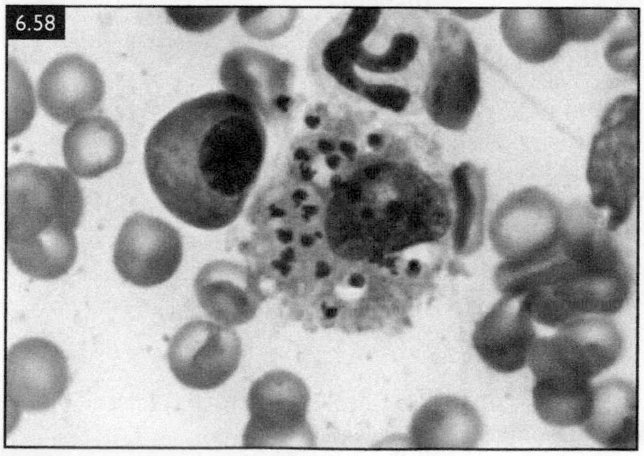

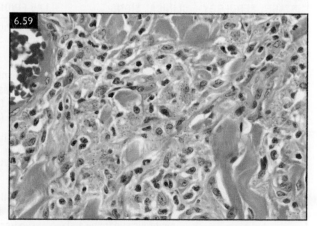

Fig. 6.58 *Leishmania* sp. within a histiocyte. (Courtesy of Dr Francis Chandler)

Fig. 6.59 Histology of a lesion of cutaneous leishmaniasis from a dog (Giemsa stain). (Courtesy of Dr Ryan Jennings)

Therapy

Clinical classification following consensus guidelines is recommended in order to target optimum therapy and diagnosis, predict progression and assist with prognosis.

Dogs

"Clinical cure" of leishmaniosis can occur; however, "parasitologic cure" (i.e. eradication of the organism) is highly unlikely. Many (most) dogs will require long-term therapy, and relapses are common.

Staging and therapy guidelines are summarized in *Table 6.35*. A combination of allopurinol (10 mg/kg PO q12h) and meglumine antimoniate (100 mg/kg SC q24h for 4–8 weeks) is typically advised as first-line therapy.[198] Other recommended treatments and protocols in dogs have been grouped as second- and third-line therapies based on disease stages. These have included allopurinol as a sole agent, sodium stibogluconate, amphotericin B, miltefosine and allopurinol, metronidazole and spiramycin, and marbofloxacin.[198] Additional therapy needs are based on patient assessment, International Renal Interest Society (IRIS) staging (dietary and medication) and management of concurrent infection.

Treatment is continued until there is resolution of clinical signs and negative serology.[198] Typically, 6–12 months of therapy is required.

Monitoring of lab and urine parameters is advised during treatment, and frequency of diagnostics will vary depending on clinical signs and disease progression. Dogs on chronic allopurinol therapy are at risk for development of xanthinuria.[201]

Monitoring of serology (or PCR) may help to determine when to discontinue therapy. Discontinuation of allopurinol should be based on complete clinical and clinical pathologic recovery at 1 year and decrease in antibody levels (e.g. negative or borderline low serology).[198]

Cats

There is little information regarding therapy in cats. Surgical removal of skin lesions may be curative, and long-term therapy may result in clinical improvement.[195]

Prognosis/complications

Prognosis is highly dependent on clinical staging and concurrent renal disease. Dogs with advanced IRIS stage renal disease have a poor prognosis, whereas dogs at earlier IRIS stages (or with no renal compromise) can do very well. Most dogs will show clinical improvement within their first month of therapy.[198]

It is important to educate owners that therapy is directed at control of clinical signs and

Table 6.35 **Clinical staging and therapy of leishmaniosis in dogs**					
STAGE	SEROLOGY	CLINICAL SIGNS	LAB FINDINGS	THERAPY	PROGNOSIS
I	Negative to low titers	Mild: lymphadenopathy, papular dermatitis	None, UP:C <0.5	None Meglumine and allopurinol Allopurinol	Good
II	Low to high titers	Moderate: as for stage I, ± cutaneous lesions, fever, weight loss, anorexia, epistaxis	Mild anemia, hyperglobulinemia, hyperviscosity syndrome Substage (a) UP:C <0.5 Substage (b) UP:C 0.5–1.0	Allopurinol and meglumine Miltefosine and allopurinol	Good to guarded
III	Medium to high titers	Severe: as for stage I, II and immune complex disease, e.g. glomerulonephritis, uveitis, arthritis, vasculitis	As stage II, and chronic kidney disease (CKD) IRIS I with UP:C >1 or IRIS II	As stage II, and IRIS guideline-directed therapy for CKD	Guarded to poor
IV	Medium to high titers	Very severe: as for stage III, and thromboembolism, nephrotic syndrome and end-stage renal disease	As stage III, and advanced IRIS stages and nephrotic syndrome	Allopurinol as sole agent IRIS guideline-directed therapy for CKD	Poor

Abbreviations: IRIS, International Renal Interest Society; UP:C, urinary protein:creatinine ratio

prevention of progression and will not result in a cure. Reinfection is likely in endemic areas, particularly without institution of prevention methods.

Prevention

Long-term immunity is not conferred by infection.

Vaccines are no longer available in Brazil; however, a European vaccine is available for use in seronegative dogs. At this time, no vaccines have been endorsed by the World Small Animal Veterinary Association group.

Ectoparasite (sandfly) bite prevention through the use of deltamethrin-containing collars or spot-on repellants (permethrin and imidacloprid) is strongly advised in dogs in endemic areas. Additionally, mesh netting on windows and indoor housing of dogs (especially during peak dusk–dawn sandfly feeding) may reduce risk of bites.

Blood donor screening should be performed for transfusion programs.

Public health and infection control

Leishmania sp. is an important zoonotic disease and culling of seropositive or infected dogs occurs in some regions because of the human infection risk associated with canine reservoirs. Lack of "parasitologic cure" and the frequency of relapse in treated dogs mean that infected dogs remain a reservoir of infection.

LISTERIOSIS
J Scott Weese

Listeria monocytogenes is a rare cause of disease in dogs and cats. Both species are relatively resistant to the bacterium and likely require exposure to very high doses for disease to occur. Young, old and immunosuppressed animals are likely at highest risk of disease.

Clinically, listeriosis is most commonly manifested as septicemia and encephalitis, although other manifestations such as abortion are possible.[202 206] Although it is a relatively ubiquitous saprophyte, there has been increasing concern in recent years about the potential exposure of dogs and cats (and their owners) to *Listeria* sp. in raw pet food, given potentially high contamination rates.[207] Diagnosis is usually based on histology and culture of postmortem specimens. Antemortem, a mononuclear pleocytosis may be evident on CSF cytology. Confirmation can be performed by culture or PCR of CSF. If listeriosis is suspected, amoxicillin, ampicillin, tetracyclines and trimethoprim sulfa are empirical treatment options.

LYME DISEASE (BORRELIOSIS)
Michelle Evason

Definition

Lyme disease (borreliosis) is an infection of dogs caused by the tick vector-borne bacterium *Borrelia burgdorferi*. It is most commonly diagnosed in dogs with a shifting limb lameness that occurs 2–6 months after a bite from an infected *Ixodes* tick (**Figs. 6.60–6.62**). The vast majority of dogs that test positive for *B. burgdorferi* exposure do not show signs of clinical illness (lameness and very rarely kidney disease). Cats do not appear to develop clinical disease, but may become seropositive.[208]

Etiology and pathogenesis

Borrelia burgdorferi sensu lato (and stricto) are spirochetes (**Fig. 6.63**) that are reliant on a host species to survive; therefore, they are transmitted between vertebrate reservoir hosts (small mammals, birds and lizards) and the *Ixodes* spp. tick vector. Deer and moose are most important for adult tick feeding.

Tick attachment for 1–2 days is typically required for transmission of *Borrelia* spirochetes to the host via tick saliva. The outer surface lipoproteins (Osp) of *Borrelia* spp. are responsible for its pathogenicity, in that they allow both survival and persistence of

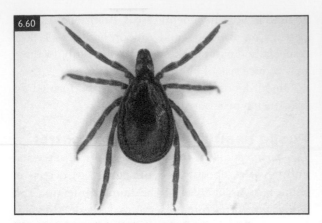

Fig. 6.60 Unfed adult female *Ixodes scapularis* (black-legged or deer tick) (approximately 3 mm in length). (Courtesy of Dr Katie Clow)

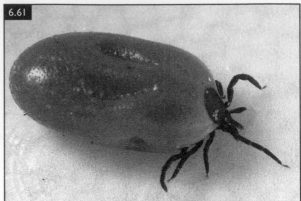

Fig. 6.61 Engorged adult female *Ixodes scapularis* (black-legged or deer tick) (approximately 8 mm in length). (Courtesy of Dr Gary Alpert)

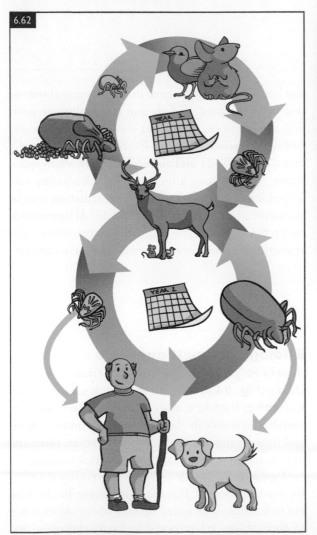

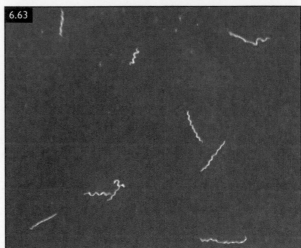

Fig. 6.63 Dark-field microscopy image of *Borrelia* sp. (Courtesy of Adam Replogle)

the spirochete in both the host and the tick vector. OspA has dominant expression and helps *Borrelia* spp. adhere to the tick's mid-gut; during tick feeding on a warm-blooded host OspC is expressed to assist *Borrelia* spp. in moving to the tick's salivary gland/saliva. OspC also enables *Borrelia* spp. to become established in the host, after which levels of variable surface lipoprotein increase and OspC declines.

Fig. 6.62 Lyme disease and *Borrelia burgdorferi* exposure and infection in dogs and humans: life cycle and transmission of *Borrelia burgdorferi* between hosts and the *Ixodes* spp. tick vector.

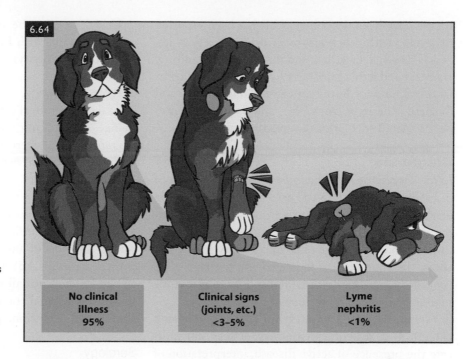

Fig. 6.64 Clinical outcomes and likelihood of clinical disease associated with *Borrelia burgdorferi* exposure and infection in dogs.

| No clinical illness 95% | Clinical signs (joints, etc.) <3–5% | Lyme nephritis <1% |

After an adequate duration of attachment of an infected tick to a dog, the following outcomes can result: (1) no transmission of *Borrelia* sp., (2) transmission of *Borrelia* sp. to the dog, but elimination of the bacterium without it being able to cause disease, or (3) transmission of *Borrelia* sp. to the dog and development of clinical illness (Lyme disease) (**Fig. 6.64**). A minority of the dogs that are exposed to an infected tick develop Lyme disease.

Geography

In North America the deer or black-legged tick, *Ixodes scapularis* (northeastern and upper midwest USA and Canada) and *I. pacificus* and *I. neotomae* (western USA) appear to be involved in infection with *B. burgdorferi* sensu lato. Infected ticks may be spread to new areas via bird migration. In Europe and Asia, the spirochete involved is *Borrelia burgdorferi* sensu stricto, specifically *B. garinii*, *B. afzelii* and *B. burgdorferi*, with the tick vectors *I. ricinus* (Europe) and *I. persulcatus* (Asia).

Incidence and risk factors

The true incidence of clinical disease is unknown. Studies reporting clinical Lyme disease are limited, and estimates range from <3% to 10% of dogs;[209, 210] however, seroprevalence may be much

higher (70–90%)[211] in some endemic areas. Despite the potentially high seroprevalence, very few dogs appear to develop clinical disease that may (or may not) be attributed to *Borrelia* spp.

Risk factors for seropositivity in the northern midwestern USA include tick exposure and factors associated with it, such as time spent outside, living in aforested or urban wooded area, or sandy fertile soil.[211]

Clinical signs

In experimentally infected dogs, clinical disease occurred 2–6 months after tick bite/attachment and seemed to correlate with a rise in antibody titer.[212] In these dogs, acute fever, polyarthropathy (shifting limb lameness), non-specific signs (lethargy, decrease in appetite) and lymphadenopathy were noted and appeared responsive to antibiotics.

Polyarthropathy may correlate with a rise in body temperature and can begin in a single limb and persist for a few days; it may then shift to lameness in another limb, and/or resolve.

Lyme nephritis is a rare but serious form of protein-losing nephropathy (PLN) that may be linked to Lyme disease.[213, 214] Severe and rapidly progressive azotemia, polyuria and polydipsia, uremia, proteinuria, thromboembolic complications, effusions and edema have been described. This has been reported to develop within 24 hours to 8 weeks after a tick bite, and is associated with a sudden onset of vomiting, anorexia and lethargy.[214–216] PLN may be more common in Labrador Retrievers, Golden Retrievers and Bernese Mountain Dogs,[213, 217] and may (or may not) be associated with prior (or concurrent) lameness.

Diagnosis

Lyme disease poses a diagnostic challenge. Signs of disease are often vague and non-specific, and testing methods may be unable to assist with differentiating exposure (i.e. seropositivity) from true clinical illness. There is considerable uncertainty and debate about the approach to dogs who test positive using typical diagnostic tests involving detection of antibodies against the bacterium.

Given that diagnostic testing currently relies on detection of antibodies that may or may not indicate the presence of active disease, interpretation of results and determining whether treatment is needed can be challenging. Further, because testing for these antibodies is commonly performed in apparently healthy dogs as part of screening for other diseases (e.g. heartworm), it is difficult to determine a true beneficial outcome to detection of seropositivity beyond providing support for improvement in tick prevention and increased Lyme disease awareness, and consideration of urinalysis to screen for proteinuria.

Lyme disease diagnosis is based on the potential for exposure (being in, or having been in, an endemic area, ideally with a history of tick exposure), consistent clinical signs (e.g. polyarthropathy, fever), exclusion of other differentials, seropositivity and rapid response to doxycycline therapy.

Although Lyme nephritis is rare, screening urinalysis for proteinuria should be performed in all dogs that are seropositive.

Lab abnormalities

The CBC is usually unremarkable. Non-specific inflammation (such as decreased albumin, hypocalcemia and increased globulins) may be demonstrated by a biochemical profile, as may changes seen with vomiting, diarrhea, dehydration and PLN (azotemia, hypoalbuminemia and electrolyte changes).

Urinalysis may be normal, show inflammation or be consistent with PLN (proteinuria ± decreased urine specific gravity).

Diagnostic imaging

Pleural or peritoneal effusion and non-specific renal changes (thickening and increased echogenicity of the renal cortex, decreased definition of the corticomedullary junction) may be noted with PLN.

Cytology

Joint (synovial) fluid may be normal or consistent with suppurative inflammation, with increased cell counts (5,000–100,000 cells/μL) and predominantly neutrophils (95%).[218] Multiple joints should be tapped because not all may be affected. CSF analysis can be normal, or consistent with subacute to chronic inflammation.

Serology

Antibodies against *Borrelia* spp. are produced in response to a successfully prevented infection as well as disease. These antibodies persist in the body and are the basis of current testing methods. Given that diagnostic testing currently relies on detection of antibodies that may be present in dogs with disease or dogs that have successfully eliminated the bacterium, interpretation of results and determining whether treatment for true clinical disease is needed can be very challenging. This is particularly true in endemic areas, where many dogs may be seropositive, yet few are clinically ill.

Adding to this confusion is the plethora of available diagnostics that have been developed to identify *Borrelia* spp. -infected dogs. Some of these are specifically marketed to try to determine whether clinical infection has occurred (vs. Lyme vaccination), and in some cases what stage of infection is occurring. Some of these tests are also utilized to follow treated dogs for clinical disease resolution, and ongoing monitoring for risk of development of Lyme nephritis, although the effectiveness of this is unknown.

Unfortunately, differentiation of naturally infected vs. vaccinated dogs, and of early vs. later infection, may be difficult. Vaccinated dogs typically have antibodies to OspA (the basis of most vaccines), and OspC antibodies (typically found in unvaccinated dogs) may appear in either vaccinated or unvaccinated dogs. Also, information about early vs. late infection may not be clinically useful.

PCR testing has also been used and is considered insensitive; however, PCR on joint fluid may be of higher yield.[218]

Therapy

It is common practice to proactively and empirically treat seropositive dogs with consistent clinical signs. Improvement is noted within 24–48 hours after antimicrobial therapy. Caution is urged with attributing "response to therapy" entirely to antimicrobials (without pursuit of confirmatory diagnostics) owing to the intermittent nature of lameness, and the chondroprotective effects of doxycycline.[216] Dogs with mild fever and/or polyarthropathy typically recover with minimal therapy.

Treatment is typically advised for 30 days.[216] Doxycycline (5 mg/kg q12h or 10 mg/kg q24h) is considered the drug of choice, in part owing to its efficacy against possible co-infecting pathogens. Amoxicillin is also effective but is most often used in young dogs and dogs that do not tolerate doxycycline.

It is important to note that most dogs will remain seropositive (for months to years) despite antimicrobial therapy and resolution of clinical signs. Therefore, seropositive status should not be used to guide further (or ongoing) therapy.

Controversy and debate surround the topic of empiric therapy of clinically normal seropositive dogs, and centers around the concern over PLN. Clients should be counseled about the rare risk of later-onset progressive and irreversible renal disease, which can occur up to 8 weeks after apparent recovery.[216]

Prognosis/complications

Prognosis and treatment duration are based on severity of presenting clinical signs (fever and lameness vs. PLN) and ability of clients to commit to supportive care and cost. Many dogs with Lyme disease-associated polyarthopathy have mild illness, and the prognosis is excellent in these cases. Dogs with severely progressive PLN have a dismal prognosis, and euthanasia may be warranted, particularly in patients that appear unresponsive to therapy.[214]

Prevention

There are many available and effective vaccine types for prevention of Lyme disease. It is important to remember that vaccination does not provide absolute protection from *Borrelia* spp., and that tick vector control is strongly advised. Vaccination of already infected dogs does not "clear infection" or prevent clinical illness from developing, and it is unknown whether there is any clear benefit to vaccination of seropositive dogs.

Tick prevention is the mainstay of Lyme disease prevention. Application of DEET (diethyltoluamide) to cats and dogs is not advised because of its toxicity.

NEORICKETTSIA HELMINTHOECA (SALMON POISONING)
Michelle Evason

Definition

Salmon poisoning is an acute bacterial infection most common in dogs living in endemic regions, such as the northwestern coast of the USA and Canada. Disease occurs after ingestion of infected, uncooked, freshwater fish, usually salmon. Clinical signs range from mild to severe, and typically manifest as fever, inappetence, lethargy, vomiting and diarrhea.

Etiology and pathogenesis

Neorickettsia helminthoeca is a gram-negative intracellular bacterium with a complex three-host life cycle involving a fluke vector (*Nanophyteus salmincola*), aquatic snail (*Oxytrema silicula*) and freshwater fish (typically salmonids).[219] Typically, dogs are infected after consuming the encysted fluke vector (metacercaria) contained within uncooked fish. Once within the dog, the fluke matures (5–6 days) and transmits the bacterium while feeding deeply on the dog's intestinal mucosa. The incubation period may range from 2 days to 14 days, or up to 1 month. Infected fluke ova are shed in the dog's feces for 60–250 days; once in the environment these develop, hatch and then infect snails. Within the snail, further maturation occurs (to cercariae), and these are ingested or infect fish, which are then eaten by dogs.

Clinical signs are related to the dog's inflammatory response to bacterial replication within macrophages and circulation in the bloodstream, and the resultant local granulomatous response associated with the fluke feeding on the mucosa of the stomach and intestine. Death can occur 18 days after ingestion of infected fish.

Geography

Northwestern coast of North America, with occasional cases in southern Brazil.[219]

Incidence and risk factors

The incidence of clinical disease is unknown. Risk factors for dogs include access to uncooked fish. Dogs that do not live in endemic areas are at risk if ingesting imported fish or consuming store-bought salmon.[220] Less information is available for cats.

Clinical signs
Dogs

Clinical signs typically occur at 5–7 days post-infection and are usually non-specific, including peripheral lymphadenopathy (74%), dehydration (65%), fever (73%) and abdominal pain (28%). Mild-to-severe gastrointestinal (GI) signs such as vomiting (80%) and diarrhea (>70%), may be noted.[219, 220] Severely ill dogs may have respiratory compromise, peripheral edema and tachycardia.[220] Less commonly (<20%), neurologic signs can occur.[220]

Duration can range from peracute (e.g. disseminated intravascular coagulation [DIC], death) to acute with intestinal signs, weight loss or polyuria and polydipsia.

Diagnosis

Diagnosis is based on clinical history (i.e. fish ingestion), together with suggestive clinical signs, CBC changes (thrombocytopenia, anemia) and fecal float with sedimentation to improve sensitivity.[219, 220] Bacterial identification on cytologic or histologic samples (lymph node or splenic aspirates) can confirm the diagnosis. Co-infections with other pathogens, e.g. *Dipyldium caninum* and *Trichuris vulpis*, have been reported.[220]

Therapy

Therapy consists of supportive care for GI signs, along with prompt and appropriate antimicrobial administration. Effective antimicrobials include doxycycline (5 mg/kg PO q12h for 7–14 days), or oxytetracycline, tetracycline and enrofloxacin given for 7 days. Praziquantel (10–30 mg/kg PO q24h for 1–2 days) is advised to reduce fluke infestation.[219]

Monitoring

Clinical improvement typically occurs in 24–72 h, with most dogs responding completely within 1–4 days.[220]

Ongoing monitoring of CBC (e.g. platelet counts) and electrolytes along with supportive care should occur until all changes have resolved, and clinical status is regarded as stable.

Prognosis/complications

The prognosis in dogs with early therapy is excellent; however, those who present with severe complications (e.g. DIC, cardiac or respiratory compromise) have a guarded prognosis. The disease can be fatal, and lack of therapy can result in death within 5–10 days.[219, 220]

Prevention and infection control

Prevention is dependent on proper cooking and freezing of fish. In endemic regions, pet owners should be educated about risks and dogs who swim should be monitored for disease development.

PLAGUE/*YERSINIA PESTIS*
Dennis Spann

Definition
Plague is a multisystemic disease caused by infection with the gram-negative coccobacillus *Yersinia pestis*. It may present as: bubonic plague, affecting the lymph nodes; pneumonic plague, causing severe pneumonia; or septicemic plague, causing multiple organ dysfunction syndrome (MODS). Cats are the most commonly affected domestic animals, but most species are susceptible.

Etiology and pathogenesis
Yersinia pestis is maintained in small mammalian hosts. Cats and dogs become infected primarily through exposure to fleas or tissue from infected small mammals via hunting or scavenging.[221] *Xenopsylla cheopis* is the classic flea to transmit plague (**Fig. 6.65**), but 31 other species have been shown to be competent vectors. *Ctenocephalides felis* is a competent but inefficient vector.[222]

After entering the host via a fleabite, a bite or ingestion of infected tissues, the organism colonizes the local lymph node before spreading in the bloodstream to other lymph nodes and organs. Infection of the lungs results in pneumonic plague (**Fig. 6.66**). Aerosol spread from individuals with pneumonic plague is of concern.

Clinical signs begin 2–6 days after infection. Fever and lymphadenopathy are common early signs. Death often occurs within 10 days of infection. Approximately 75% and 90% of infected cats become bacteremic or have bacteria in their saliva, respectively.

Geography
Plague is present on most continents but is restricted to certain regions. Areas with grasslands and rodents and moderately warm moist climates are more likely to be locations of enzootics. Plague foci are present in the western United States and more frequently reported in states such as New Mexico, Colorado, California, Arizona, Nevada, Oregon, Utah and Wyoming.

Incidence and risk factors
The incidence of plague is low. Free-roaming cats are most commonly affected.[221, 223] Risk factors include exposure to wildlife and hunting in areas where rodents have enzootic plague.

Clinical signs
Clinical signs include fever, ocular discharge, lymphadenopathy, poor thrift and coughing. Fever usually

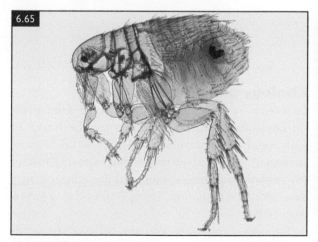

Fig. 6.65 Female *Xenopsylla cheopis*, an important vector of *Yersinia pestis* (approximately 2.5 mm in length). (Courtesy of Ken Gage)

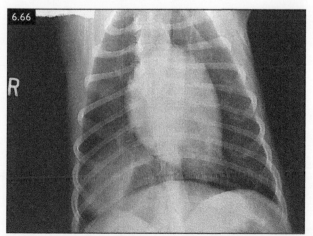

Fig. 6.66 Radiograph of a dog with pneumonic plague. (Courtesy of Dr Jennifer Casebeer and Janine Runfola)

occurs 1–4 days after infection. Submandibular lymph nodes are commonly affected, although others may also be involved. Abscesses can occur on the head or extremities. Lingual ulcers are often found. Cutaneous abscesses can also be noted. Cough and abnormal lung sounds can be seen with secondary pneumonic plague. Death may occur 4–14 days after infection. Pathologic lesions include necrotizing lymphadenitis. Extensive petechiation is seen throughout the tissues examined. Disseminated intravascular coagulation may lead to bleeding from the mouth or nose.

Diagnosis

Diagnosis is often made via culture, which must be done in specialized laboratories. Fluorescent staining of tissue, identification of seroconversion and PCR can also be diagnostic.

Therapy

Streptomycin is the treatment of choice, but other antimicrobials are sometimes used (*Table 6.36*).

Prognosis/complications

With early aggressive antibiotic and supportive care, the prognosis is fair to good. However, disease is often not identified until animals have pneumonic or septicemic plague, in which case the prognosis is very poor.

Table 6.36 **Antimicrobial treatment options for plague**	
ANTIMICROBIAL	**DOSE**
Streptomycin	5 mg/kg IM q12h
Gentamicin	6–8 mg/kg IV/IM/SC q24h
Doxycycline	5–10 mg/kg PO q12h
Chloramphenicol	50 mg/kg PO q8h (dogs) 10–20 mg/kg PO q12h (cats)

Prevention

Keeping cats indoors and effective flea control are the main preventive measures.

Public health and infection control

Zoonotic infections in people caring for infected animals, particularly cats, have been reported.[221, 224–227] Animals suspected of having plague should be treated with appropriate antibiotics, isolated, and appropriate personnel protective equipment (gloves, masks and eyewear) used while handling. They should remain in the hospital for the first 3–5 days while receiving antibiotics, to limit exposure to owners. Appropriate diagnostic testing should be pursued promptly to identify plague and lab personnel should be warned about samples that might present a risk.

PROTOTHECA SPP. (PROTOTHECOSIS)
Michelle Evason

Definition

Protothecosis is an uncommon cause of disseminated disease in dogs, primarily affecting the gastrointestinal (GI) (colitis), ocular or neurologic systems. Prognosis is generally poor. Dermatologic lesions have also been reported in both cats and dogs. It is considered an opportunistic pathogen and can be an environmental contaminant.

Prototheca zopfii is the main pathogen in dogs. It is considered the most aggressive and likely to cause disseminated disease. *P. wickerhamii* is more often associated with the cutaneous form in dogs and cats.

Etiology and pathogenesis

Prototheca spp. are saprophytic algae that grow on environmental debris. They can be found in soil, water and transiently within the GI tract of mammals. These algae prefer decomposing matter for growth (e.g. tree slime), and are consequently associated with manure, sewage and other wet raw materials.

Exposure and infection are believed to occur through trauma or contamination of existing wounds, or possibly through ingestion of algal sporangium. The incubation period is unknown.

Immune compromise has been theorized as playing a role in disease development. However, disease can occur in the absence of immunocompromise or concurrent disease.[228]

Once within the dog, dissemination to ocular and neurologic tissue, the GI tract (colon), kidneys and bones appears most frequent. Cats and occasionally dogs may have localized cutaneous disease.

Geography

Worldwide, but most commonly in warm, wet and swamp or marshy locations in the southern USA, Europe and northeastern Australia.[228, 229]

Incidence and risk factors

Dogs

The incidence of disease may be highest in Collies and Boxers.[228] Young adult, female, middle-sized or large breed dogs may be inherently predisposed or simply at increased risk of environmental exposure, such as through hunting. Concurrent immune compromise may predispose to infection.[230]

Cats

Disseminated disease has not been reported, and the affected cats in the few limited reports have not been immunocompromised by feline leukemia virus or feline immunodeficiency virus.

Clinical signs

In dogs, refractory colitis is the most commonly recognized presentation, and may be present for months (or episodic) before disseminated disease. Systemic disease may be associated with inappetence and weight loss, GI signs (vomiting, diarrhea/colitis), lameness (osteomyelitis), neurologic signs (e.g. seizures, ataxia, deafness) and polyuria/polydipsia.[228–231] Ocular signs may include conjunctivitis, uveitis, hyphema and retinitis with detachment.[229] Rectal exam may reveal melena, hematochezia and mucus. Cutaneous lesions may be nodular and ulcerated. Less commonly, dogs may have localized dermatologic signs with or without disseminated disease.

In cats, single or multiple dermatologic lesions are most frequent and can be present as a single nodule or masses. Typically, these are on the feet, distal limbs and tail base.

Diagnosis

A positive culture and cytologic evidence, together with clinical presentation, are highly suggestive of diagnosis in endemic geographic locations.

Laboratory abnormalities

The CBC, serum chemistry and urinalysis may be normal or reveal changes consistent with inflammation or infection, such as non-regenerative anemia, neutrophilia and eosinophilia. Severe intestinal protein loss may lead to reductions in albumin, globulins and cholesterol. Azotemia and associated urinalysis changes may be present with renal disease. Urinalysis may reveal fungal hyphae in disseminated disease.

Algae may be readily noted on cytology of CSF or ocular fluid, aspirates of lymph node, bone or cutaneous nodules and rectal scrapings (**Fig. 6.67**).[228, 229] The algae are ovoid with a thick cell wall (which does not stain) and may be mistaken for other fungi such as *Blastomyces* or *Candida* spp.[230] Owing to dissemination of disease, finding algae on cytologic exam is quite likely; however, lack of observation does not rule out infection.

The CSF may be normal or reveal inflammation, e.g. elevated cell counts and increased protein. Eosinophilia or organisms may be noted.

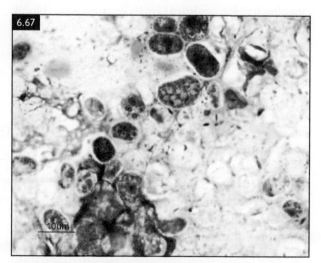

Fig. 6.67 *Prototheca* sp.: ovoid-shaped algae with a thick cell wall are noted on cytology from a rectal scraping. (Courtesy of Dr Theresa Rizzi)

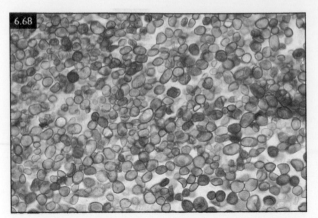

Fig. 6.68 Histopathology of *Prototheca zopfii* infection in a dog. (Courtesy of Dr William Kaplan and Mr Sudman)

Histopathology (biopsy) usually reveals algal sporangia (**Fig. 6.68**). Differentiation from other fungi typically requires culture.

Imaging
Radiographically, osteolytic lesions may be evident in long bones.[228] Abdominal ultrasound may show changes associated with the organ affected, e.g. colonic thickening and abdominal lymphadenopathy, renal changes. MRI or CT of the brain may show changes associated with disseminated disease.

Culture
Specimens for culture include aspirates, blood, urine, CSF or biopsies. The algae are easily grown on standard media within 3–7 days. Organism differentiation requires additional analyses, and susceptibility testing is rarely performed.

Other
Colonoscopy may reveal ulcerated, hyperemic and friable mucosa, but this is non-specific.

Therapy
Surgery may be effective for localized dermatologic disease. Optimal medical therapy for disseminated disease is unknown. Systemic antifungals have included amphotericin B (AMB) and azoles (e.g. itraconazole or fluconazole), or a combination of AMB with an azole. Remission has been documented with AMB; however, relapse is typical. Successful therapy with AMB and itraconazole has occurred in a few cases.

Prognosis/complications
The prognosis is considered guarded to poor with disseminated disease, particularly because clinical signs are advanced by the time of diagnosis. Many dogs do not respond to treatment, relapse or are euthanized.[228, 231] Therapy with AMB or itraconazole may slow progression.

The prognosis with localized dermatologic disease in cats and dogs can be excellent.[228] Cure has been obtained with surgical removal.

Prevention
Avoidance of exposure to warm standing water in endemic regions should be attempted, when possible.

Infection control
Prototheca sp. is an environmental contaminant. Routine disinfection procedures and removal of gross debris are indicated, but this organism poses little infection risk in clinics.

ROCKY MOUNTAIN SPOTTED FEVER/*RICKETTSIA RICKETTSII*
Michelle Evason

Definition
Rocky Mountain spotted fever (RMSF) is caused by the tick-borne bacterium *Rickettsia rickettsii*. In dogs, infection and subsequent vasculitis typically result in acute (and vague) multisystem clinical signs (**Fig. 6.69**). Prompt treatment with doxycycline is warranted when there is a suspicion of RMSF.

Etiology and pathogenesis
Rickettsia rickettsii is an intracellular, gram-negative bacterium reliant on a host tick for transmission. Tick vectors include *Rhipicephalus sanguineus* (**Fig. 6.70**), *Dermacentor variabilis* and *D. andersoni*.

Ticks are infected when they feed on incidental hosts (e.g. dogs or humans) and reservoir hosts (e.g. voles, rodents, small mammals) during each stage

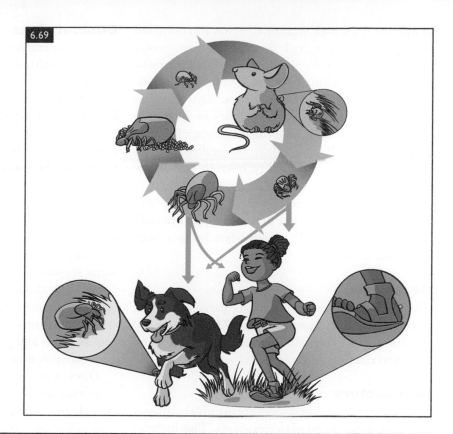

Fig. 6.69 Rocky Mountain spotted fever: tick life cycle and tick vector transmission of *Rickettsia rickettsii* to dog or human incidental host.

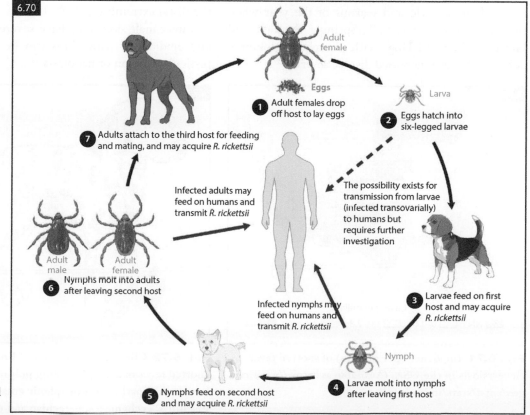

Fig. 6.70 Life cycles of the brown dog tick (*Rhipicephalus sanguineus*) and *Rickettsia rickettsii*. (Courtesy of Centers for Disease Control and Prevention)

of molting. However, transmission has also occurred through exposure to tick fluids.[232] In dogs, transmission is believed to require 5–20 hours of attachment.[232] Once within the dog's endothelial cells, rapid infection, multiplication and dissemination through the vasculature (lymphatics or blood) to other parts of the body (and further damage to endothelial cells) result in vasculitis. Generalized edema, increased vascular permeability, microthrombus formation and necrosis cause clinical signs of disease.

Infection and clinical disease are acute and rapid, with an incubation period of approximately 2–14 days.[232] A chronic disease state has not been described in dogs.

Geography

RMSF can be found in various parts of North, Central and South America (**Fig. 6.71**). The regional incidence varies depending on tick distributions and infection rates of reservoir hosts.

Risk factors

Risk factors for clinical disease are mainly those associated with likelihood of tick exposure. This includes an outdoor lifestyle and seasons of the year when ticks are most active.[232, 233] Springer Spaniels and German Shepherd Dogs with phosphofructokinase deficiencies have increased disease severity.[233]

Clinical signs

Acute fever and non-specific systemic signs, such as lethargy, shifting limb lameness, weakness, vomiting, diarrhea and decrease in appetite, predominate (**Fig. 6.72**). Lymphadenopathy, splenomegaly and hepatomegaly are usually present. Upper respiratory tract signs, ocular discharge or gangrene can occur. Petechiae and ecchymoses are usually found on the mucous membranes, and edema is typically found at the distal limbs or peripheries (e.g. ear tips).

Ocular signs due to vasculitis, bleeding tendencies or thromboembolism (e.g. uveitis, subretinal bleeding, hyphema) may be noted. Neuromuscular signs secondary to bleeding or meningitis may be focal or widespread, including seizures, ataxia, stupor, tremors or additional CNS signs, such as vestibular disease. Polyarthritis and joint swelling, stiffness and generalized muscle or abdominal pains are common.

Dogs with higher antibody titers or delayed diagnoses may have more advanced and severe neurologic signs, edema and vasculitis lesions (e.g. petechiae, ecchymoses) as well as gangrene of the distal extremities.[232, 233]

Intact male dogs may have severe scrotal edema and epididymal pain. This can be confused with testicular torsion or neoplasia.[234]

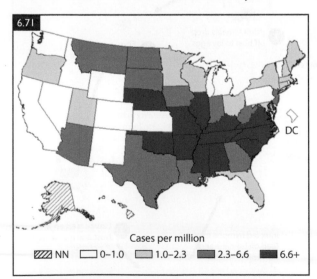

Fig. 6.71 Incidence (per million) of spotted fever rickettsiosis in the USA. (Available at https://www.cdc.gov/rmsf/stats/index.html)

Cases per million
NN   0–1.0   1.0–2.3   2.3–6.6   6.6+

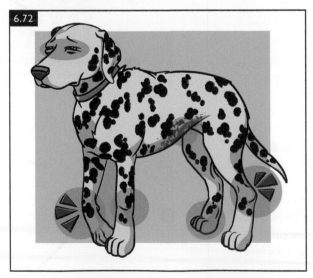

Fig. 6.72 Clinical presentation of Rocky Mountain spotted fever in a dog, including polyarthopathy, lymphadenopathy, liver or splenic enlargement, vasculitis, ecchymoses, petechiae and uveitis.

Diagnosis

Patient history (e.g. tick vector endemic area), taken together with compatible (often mild and non-specific) clinical signs, serology or PCR is needed for diagnosis. Few dogs (approximately 20%) have a history of known tick exposure.[232, 233]

Laboratory abnormalities

Moderate-to-severe thrombocytopenia occurs in most (but not all) clinically affected dogs.[233] Mild non-regenerative anemia and leukopenia or leukocytosis with toxic change may be noted.

Non-specific changes in serum biochemistry associated with vasculitis and inflammation may be present, such as decreased albumin, hypocalcemia and increased globulins. Elevated alkaline phosphatase and bilirubin, and hyponatremia, may also occur. Urinalysis may be normal, indicate inflammation or be consistent with protein-losing nephropathy.[233]

Cytology of lymph node aspirates, joint taps and CSF may be normal or consistent with inflammation. Histopathology of skin or organ biopsy with immunofluorescent assay can show vasculitis, inflammation and bacteria.[232] This may be very sensitive in acute disease, particularly when petechiae or ecchymosis lesions are sampled. False negatives and lack of organism differentiation can occur. Culture is not routinely used because of the low yield and enhanced laboratory biosafety practices that are required.

A variety of assays is available for RMSF testing (Table 6.37).

Therapy

Rapid clinical improvement (within 24–48 hours of antimicrobials) is typical and supports the diagnosis. Treatment consists of supportive care and antimicrobial therapy for 7 days. Doxycycline (5 mg/kg PO q12h) is the drug of choice, but chloramphenicol, tetracycline and enrofloxacin may also be effective.[235, 236] Delay in antimicrobial therapy will increase morbidity and mortality, and treatment should be promptly initiated in all suspect cases.[232]

Co-infections are common, and this should be investigated if response to antimicrobial therapy is slow or incomplete.

Prognosis/complications

Dogs that are treated promptly with appropriate therapy usually respond completely and rapidly, and have an excellent prognosis.[233] Advanced neurologic signs or tissue necrosis (gangrene) can worsen prognosis. Neurologic signs may persist in severely affected dogs despite appropriate treatment.[232]

Prevention

Prevention is dependent on effective tick control. Ideally, a product that prevents tick attachment or kills ticks shortly after attachment should be used. Tick control is particularly important in kennels, boarding facilities, during canine group events or on importation, especially with *R. sanguineus* infected dogs. Recovery from infection is thought to confer long-lasting immunity.[232] Dogs can be sentinels of human exposure because both humans and their pets may be exposed to infected ticks in the same environments.

Table 6.37 Laboratory assays for RMSF

DIAGNOSTIC	SAMPLE	TARGET	OUTCOME/UTILITY
Indirect microimmunofluorescence assay	Serum	IgM and IgG antibodies	A fourfold rise between acute and convalescent titers (taken 2–3 weeks apart) is required for diagnosis. A single high titer (≥1:1,024) within a week of consistent clinical signs can be diagnostic. Limitations: initial (early or acute) results can be negative owing to lack of antibody development or use of antimicrobials. Positive results may represent prior exposure vs. true clinical disease. Extensive cross-reaction with other pathogens (e.g. *Bartonella* spp.) can occur
PCR or real-time PCR	Whole blood, skin or tissue biopsy	DNA	Confirms active infection in acute disease. Limitations: false negatives can occur in acute disease owing to low numbers of bacteria or antimicrobial therapy. Lab variability and availability can be concerns

SURGICAL SITE INFECTIONS
Ameet Singh

Definition
Surgical site infections (SSIs) develop at surgical sites or in relation to a surgical procedure; the outcome can range from minor to life threatening.

Etiology and pathogenesis
Following creation of a surgical incision, the skin barrier is compromised, and bacterial contamination will occur during and/or after the procedure. However, the majority of surgically created wounds will not develop SSIs because the host's own defenses are able to prevent contamination from resulting in an infection. This is dependent on several factors, which include patient health, type of surgical procedure and the dose/virulence of contaminating organism(s).

The sources of most pathogens recovered from SSIs are the patient, medical caregivers and the environment. The most common bacteria include *Staphylococcus pseudintermedius*, *S. aureus*, Enterobacteriaceae, *Enterococcus* spp. and *Pseudomonas* spp. Commensal opportunistic pathogens are likely the most common cause, with staphylococci of greatest concern. *S. pseudintermedius* is a commensal organism of most dogs and cats and is also the leading cause of SSIs in these species.

Incidence and risk factors
Various epidemiologic studies have provided SSI rates of 0.8–18%, depending on surgery type.[237–241]

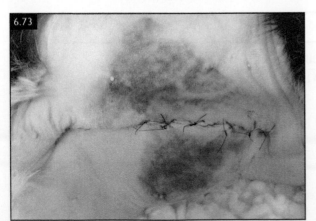

Fig. 6.73 Marked inflammation of the skin associated with surgical site preparation.

Discussion of various risk factors is beyond the scope of this text, but factors that compromise the patient (e.g. endocrinopathy, hypotension) or the surgical site (e.g. traumatic skin preparation [**Fig. 6.73**]) complicate or delay surgery, result in more contamination of the surgical site (e.g. open fracture, dirty procedures) or facilitate colonization of contaminating bacteria (e.g presence of a surgical implant) can increase risk.

Clinical signs
A broad range of clinical signs can be encountered. Most SSIs are superficial and exhibit a mucopurulent or serosanguineous discharge, pain upon palpation, redness, swelling or even complete incisional dehiscence. SSIs must be differentiated from non-infectious inflammation, although this can be challenging in some instances. This differentiation is of particular importance because most post-surgical wounds exhibit varying degrees of inflammation that do not have an infectious cause. Sometimes, however, the skin incision may appear normal despite the presence of a severe deep infection (**Figs. 6.74, 6.75**).

Diagnosis
Prompt diagnosis is essential to allow appropriate SSI therapy. Client education regarding signs of infection (pain, lameness, swelling, redness) is critical because this may prompt them to seek veterinary attention. Diagnosis of an SSI is primarily based on clinical examination, with adjunctive measures such as cytologic evaluation, culture, hematology and diagnostic imaging used to characterize the infection and determine the optimal treatment. Bacterial culture and susceptibility testing of all wounds should be performed where an SSI is suspected, and are particularly important when a deep or organ/space SSI is present (or suspected).

Therapy
SSI treatment depends on the location and severity. Conservative therapy, consisting of removal of skin sutures and/or topical biocidal treatment, may be useful in superficial SSIs. The presence of local cellulitis, systemic evidence of disease or potential

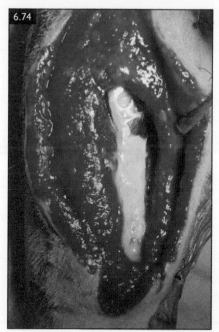

Fig. 6.74 Surgical site infection after tibial plateau levelling osteotomy. Note the inflamed tissue and purulent debris over the surgical implant.

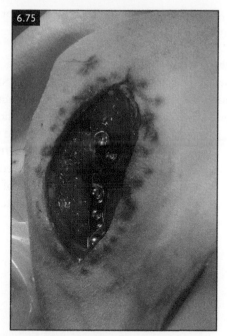

Fig. 6.75 Surgical site infection after tibial plateau levelling osteotomy, following lavage and debridement.

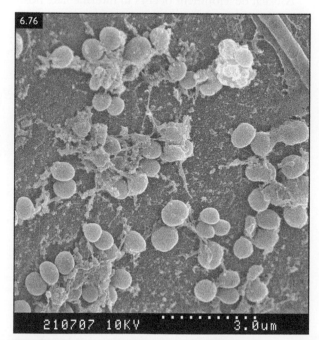

Fig. 6.76 Electron micrograph of *Staphylococcus pseudintermedius* colonization of a surgical implant. Note the adherent cocci and presence of the associated biofilm.

deep/organ/space infection indicates the need for systemic antimicrobials. Empiric antimicrobial therapy based on expected pathogens can be justified while awaiting the results of culture and susceptibility testing. Drugs with efficacy against staphylococci are good choices empirically in most cases, such as amoxicillin/clavulanic acid or cephalexin. However, multidrug-resistant pathogens (e.g. meticillin-resistant *S. pseudintermedius*) are increasingly involved.[241, 242]

Surgical intervention to debride necrotic tissue and perform wound lavage may be indicated in selected cases.

Implant-associated SSIs are extremely challenging to treat because implants can become colonized with a bacterial biofilm that protects the pathogens from antimicrobials and the host immune response (**Fig. 6.76**). Generally, implant removal is the only method of resolving an implant-associated SSI; however, this can only occur following fracture consolidation or when the implants are no longer required. Antimicrobial therapy may need to be administered in a palliative manner until implant removal can be performed.

Prevention

Because of the tremendous impact that SSIs can have, both on patients and on pet owners, practitioners should focus on preventive strategies. These are based on reducing the risk and improving the ability of the patient to eliminate bacterial contamination. The strategies discussed have been adopted from human surgical practice because many of these measures have not yet been validated in veterinary medicine (*Table 6.38*).

Table 6.38 **Surgical site infection prevention strategies**	
TYPE	**STRATEGY**
Preoperative	Managing patient risk factors
	Surgical site preparation
	Surgeon preparation
	Surgical planning
	Perioperative antimicrobials (when indicated)
Operative	Proper operating environment
	Sterilization of instruments
	Proper surgical attire
	Surgical efficiency
	Surgical technique (use of Halsted's principles)
	Atraumatic tissue handling
	Prevention of tissue dessication
	Intraoperative antimicrobial redosing, when indicated
Postoperative	Clean recovery and housing environments
	Proper wound care and monitoring

TOXOPLASMA GONDII (TOXOPLAMOSIS)
Craig Datz and Michelle Evason

Definition

Toxoplasmosis is a protozoal disease found in animals and humans worldwide. Common clinical signs include anorexia, lethargy, fever, respiratory distress and neurologic disorders.

Etiology and pathogenesis

Toxoplasma gondii is a coccidian parasite that can infect almost all animals. Cats and other Felidae serve as definitive hosts. The life cycle in cats starts with ingestion of bradyzoite tissue cysts from animal tissues, often small prey such as rodents (**Figs. 6.77, 6.78**). Ingestion of oocysts from the environment is less common. In the stomach and intestine, bradyzoites are released from the cysts and penetrate epithelial cells in the intestinal lining to develop into merozoites. Fertilization occurs (sexual reproduction) and new oocysts are passed in the feces within 3–10 days of ingestion in an unsporulated (uninfective) form. Oocysts sporulate 1–5 days after shedding. These oocysts containing infective sporozoites can survive for months to years in the environment and serve as a reservoir for transmission.

Asexual development occurs in intermediate hosts as well as in Felidae. After oocyst ingestion, sporozoites penetrate intestinal epithelial cells and divide into tachyzoites. These can infect other cells in the body, multiply, form bradyzoites, and encyst in muscles, visceral organs and the CNS, although clinical effects are uncommon. Congenital (transplacental) infection may occur, and other routes of transmission such as lactation, transfusion and transplantation have been reported.

Geography

Toxoplasmosis is found worldwide, more commonly in warm and tropical climates and less commonly in dry and cold areas.

Incidence and risk factors

Reports of seroprevalence in cats range from 13% to 44%,[175, 243–245] although active oocyst shedding is rare in adult cats. Seroprevalence is highest in older cats, especially those that are kept outdoors or found in shelters.

The major risk factor in cats is hunting behavior and ingestion of prey. Exposure to raw or

Fig. 6.77
Toxoplasma gondii life cycle. (Courtesy of Dr Alexander J da Silva and Melanie Moser)

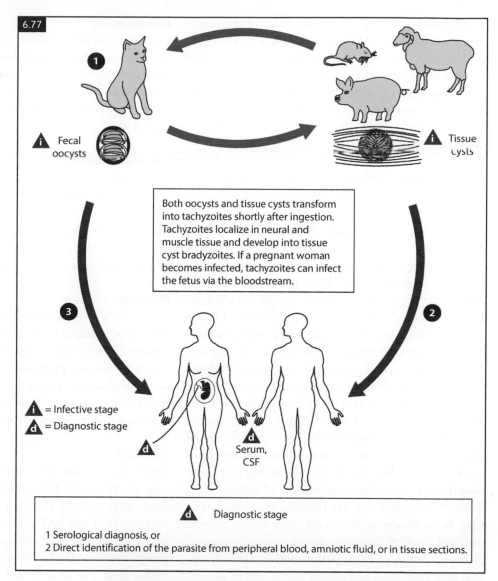

Both oocysts and tissue cysts transform into tachyzoites shortly after ingestion. Tachyzoites localize in neural and muscle tissue and develop into tissue cyst bradyzoites. If a pregnant woman becomes infected, tachyzoites can infect the fetus via the bloodstream.

i Fecal oocysts

i Tissue cysts

i = Infective stage
d = Diagnostic stage

Serum, CSF

d Diagnostic stage

1 Serological diagnosis, or
2 Direct identification of the parasite from peripheral blood, amniotic fluid, or in tissue sections.

Fig. 6.78 Toxoplasmosis life cycle with feline definitive host: a cat consumes a mouse infected with *Toxoplasma gondii* bradyzoite tissue cysts. After ingestion, bradyzoites penetrate the cat's intestinal cells and develop into merozoites. Oocysts are passed in feces, sporulation occurs and oocysts containing infective sporozoites act as a reservoir for transmission.

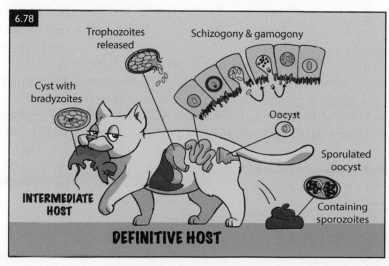

Trophozoites released

Schizogony & gamogony

Cyst with bradyzoites

Oocyst

Sporulated oocyst

INTERMEDIATE HOST

Containing sporozoites

DEFINITIVE HOST

undercooked meat is a common route of transmission to dogs and other animals. Similarly, although exposure to cats and especially litterboxes is thought to be a significant risk to humans, studies indicate that ingestion of undercooked meat is the main source of *T. gondii* exposure.[246, 247]

Clinical signs

Cats

Initial intestinal infection in cats is usually subclinical or results in mild, self-limiting diarrhea.[248] If tachyzoites spread to other tissues, signs can be more severe, as determined by the affected organ system. For example, pneumonia leads to anorexia, lethargy, coughing and/or respiratory distress. Involvement of the liver, pancreas and other abdominal organs may result in weight loss, vomiting, abdominal discomfort and icterus. Ocular lesions include anterior or posterior uveitis and/or chorioretinitis. Neurologic signs from CNS infection include ataxia, circling, paralysis, seizures, blindness and behavioral changes. Non-specific signs such as intermittent or persistent fever, lymphadenopathy or joint pain may occur. Cats that have feline leukemia virus- or feline immunodeficiency virus-associated disease or are receiving immunomodulating drugs such as ciclosporin may have more severe or rapidly progressing signs from activation of latent infections.[248] Neonates that are infected transplacentally may be stillborn or die soon after birth. Kittens exposed through lactation often have severe disease. Lethargy, depression, hypothermia, excessive sleeping, or vocalization and ascites may occur in kittens, as may "fading" syndrome.

Dogs

In puppies less than 1 year of age, generalized infection causes non-specific signs such as fever, vomiting and diarrhea. Pneumonia and liver disease (icterus) may occur. In older dogs, the neuromuscular system is often affected, with seizures, cranial nerve deficits, ataxia, paresis, paralysis and myositis. Canine toxoplasmosis is often confused with *Neospora caninum* infection, although ocular and dermatologic signs are less common.

Diagnosis

Confirmation of toxoplasmosis as the cause of clinical signs can be difficult because evidence of the organism can be found in healthy as well as affected animals. Diagnostic tests can either detect *T. gondii* directly or provide evidence of exposure (immune response).

Laboratory tests

In affected cats, hematology is non-specific but may show anemia, leukocytosis or leukopenia. Serum biochemistry results may indicate liver, pancreas or muscle involvement, for example increased alanine aminotransferase, aspartate transaminase, bilirubin, amylase, lipase or creatine kinase.

Imaging

In cats with lung involvement, thoracic radiography may show a patchy or diffuse alveolar or interstitial pattern and/or evidence of pleural effusion. Nodular (discrete masses) pulmonary patterns can also be seen. Abdominal radiography and/or ultrasonography may show mass lesions in the intestines, organs or mesenteric lymph nodes with or without effusion.

Serology

Antibody titers are often used to rule in or out exposure to *T. gondii*. Enzyme-linked immunosorbent assay and indirect fluorescent antibody tests can measure IgM and IgG antibodies. Reference ranges may vary among laboratories, but a common interpretation is that the test is positive if the IgM titer is higher than 1:64 or if the IgG titer increases at least fourfold over 2–3 weeks. However, antibody tests only indicate exposure and single titers cannot be used to confirm toxoplasmosis.

Fecal analysis

Fecal flotation may reveal *T. gondii* oocysts, which are approximately 10 µm in size, or one-fourth the size of *Cystoisospora* oocysts. They are indistinguishable from *Hammondia* or *Besnoitia* spp., which are rarely pathogenic. There are no clinical signs associated with the oocyst shedding phase.

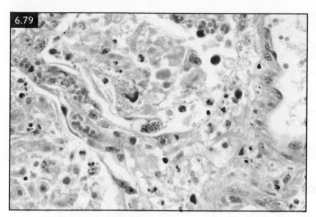

Fig. 6.79 Bronchointerstitial pneumonia due to pulmonary toxoplasmosis in a cat. (Courtesy of Dr Ryan Jennings)

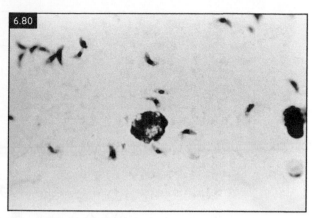

Fig. 6.80 Free-swimming, crescent-shaped *Toxoplasma gondii* tachyzoites in peritoneal effusion from a mouse (1,125× magnification). (Courtesy of Centers for Disease Control and Prevention)

Tissue analysis

Cytology or histopathology of affected tissues may identify tachyzoites or bradyzoites (**Figs. 6.79, 6.80**). PCR testing of whole blood, bronchoalveolar lavage fluid, CSF or aqueous humor is available. However, PCR cannot distinguish between acute and latent (tissue cyst) infection.[248, 249]

Therapy

Clindamycin (at least 10 mg/kg PO q12h for 4 weeks) is often used to treat disseminated toxoplasmosis.[248, 249] Clinical improvement, such as resolution of fever and increased appetite, is usually seen within 24–48 hours. Respiratory, ophthalmic and neurologic complications take longer to resolve. If clindamycin is not tolerated, alternative treatments include trimethoprim sulfa (combined 15 mg/kg PO q12h for 4 weeks) or pyrimethamine (0.5 mg/kg PO q12h for 4 weeks) combined with a sulfa drug.[248, 249]

Prognosis/complications

The prognosis for most animals exposed to *T. gondii* is very good because the majority will seroconvert without signs of disease. Cats with pulmonary, hepatic or CNS involvement, or immunosuppression, have a fair to guarded prognosis depending on the severity.

Prevention

Keeping cats indoors so that they do not hunt and ingest prey should prevent most cases. Dogs, cats and other animals should not be fed raw or undercooked meat.[248, 249] Experimental vaccines have been developed but none are currently available. The increased use of immunosuppressive medications such as ciclosporin may lead to a higher risk of acute or reactivated toxoplasmosis.[248]

Public health and infection control

Toxoplasmosis is zoonotic and a serious disease that can affect human fetuses (stillbirth, CNS disease) and immunocompromised people.[247, 249] In healthy humans, infection may lead to transient fever and lymphadenopathy. The main risk factor is consumption of raw or undercooked meat or other animal products such as raw goat's milk (**Fig. 6.81**). Cat ownership does not appear to increase the risk of exposure or clinical toxoplasmosis.[246, 248, 249] Exposure to sandboxes or soil is also a risk factor.

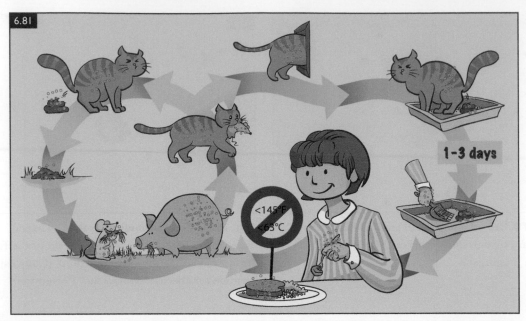

Fig. 6.81 Toxoplasmosis transmission to humans: the main human risk factors are consumption of uncooked meat or other animal products and exposure to infective oocysts in sandboxes or soil.

TRYPANOSOMIASIS
Michelle Evason

Definitions

Trypanosomiasis results from infection with *Trypanosoma cruzi* (Chagas' disease, American trypanosomiasis), *T. brucei* and *T. congolense* (African trypanosomiasis) (**Figs. 6.82, 6.83**). In North America, transmission of *T. cruzi* occurs following a bite from (or ingestion of) an infected "kissing" or "assassin" bug (triatomine or reduviid insect). The tsetse fly is the vector of *T. brucei* and *T. congolense* in Africa. Dogs and cats can be clinically infected and act as reservoirs in endemic areas.

American trypanosomiasis can manifest in young dogs (<6 months) as inappetence, lethargy, pallor, lymphadenopathy and sudden death due to

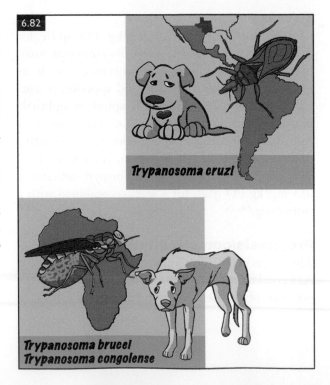

Fig. 6.82 Top: Chagas' disease (*Trypanosoma cruzi* infection): transmitted by a "kissing bug" vector and occurring in the southern USA (Texas). Bottom: African trypanosomiasis (*Trypanosoma brucei* and *T. congolense* infection): transmitted by the tsetse fly and occurring throughout Africa.

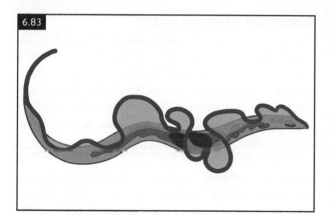

Fig. 6.83 A spindle-shaped *Trypanosoma* sp. trypomastigote found in an infected dog.

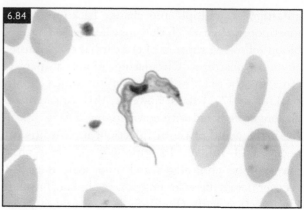

Fig. 6.84 *Trypanosoma* sp. trypomastigote. (Courtesy of Dr Blaine Mathison)

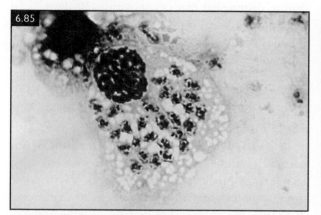

Fig. 6.85 Intracellular development of *Trypanosoma cruzi*. (Courtesy of Dr AJ Sulzer)

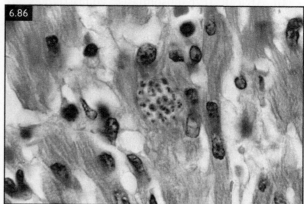

Fig. 6.86 Trypomastigotes within myocardiocytes in a dog with trypanosomiasis. (Courtesy of LL Moore Jr)

heart disease. Chronically infected adult dogs may have heart murmurs, arrhythmias, lethargy, congestive heart failure (typically right-sided) or sudden death. Signs of canine African trypanosomiasis may include fever, weight loss, lymphadenopathy, ocular or neurologic signs, ascites or peripheral edema.

Species affected

Dogs, humans, and multiple wild and domestic mammals can be affected. Cats may act as a reservoir host, along with various rodents, skunks, raccoons, opossums, guinea pigs and armadillos.

Etiology and pathogenesis

Trypanosoma spp. are protozoal parasites that exist in three forms: (1) the spindle-shaped trypomastigote that circulates in the host's blood (**Fig. 6.84**), (2) the intracellular spherical amastigote (**Fig. 6.85**) and (3) the flagellated epimastigote form which is found within the blood-feeding insect vector.

In the Americas, the kissing bug vector is infected after ingestion of trypomastigotes from infected animals or humans. Animals are most commonly infected after trypomastigote-infected insect vector feces contaminate the bite site, with transfer to the mucous membranes, or after ingestion of the insect and parasite release into the mouth.[250] Transmission may also occur through blood transfusion or transplacentally.[250]

After infection, trypomastigotes circulate within the blood, or enter macrophages, change into amastigotes and multiply by binary fission. Trypomastigotes may infect myocardiocytes (**Fig. 6.86**), convert to amastigotes, multiply and change back into trypo-mastigotes, after which they may be released into the blood following rupture of the cardiac cells, causing acute myocarditis. Circulating protozoa (parasitemia) may be noted at 3 days post-infection, typically peaking at 17–21 days; however, this parasitemia is no longer detected with cytology by 30 days.

In the acute phase of infection, myocarditis can occur at 14–30 days. In some dogs the acute phase may not be clinically noted, and some dogs will recover (latent phase) or progress to chronic infection. Co-infection with *Dirofilaria immitis* or *Leishmania* spp. may occur,[251] and can complicate presentation, diagnosis and the affected animal's immune response.

In African trypanosomiasis, epimastigotes are transmitted in the tsetse fly saliva during feeding on animals. There is no amastigote form, and the protozoa disseminate throughout the host via the circulation (blood and lymph) over a prolonged time frame (weeks to months). Dogs may become parasitemic in 2–3 days. This leads to vascular permeability changes and phagocyte proliferation, and in some cases neurologic signs related to meningoencephalitis.

Geography

Trypanosoma cruzi is found in South and Central America, Mexico and in the southern USA (Texas).[250, 252] *T. brucei* and *T. congolense* are found throughout Africa.

Incidence and risk factors

The incidence of clinical disease is unknown. This is believed to be an emerging disease in some regions, likely due to expansion of vector endemic ranges globally and importation. The seroprevalence of American trypanosomiasis in dogs or cats ranges from less than 10% to greater than 60%, depending on the region, study and animal type (e.g. client owned vs. stray, roaming ability, presence of vector control).[250, 253–256]

Risk factors for seropositivity in dogs and cats include age (<1 year or >9 years), outdoor lifestyle, stray, rural area, use for hunting (dogs), sleeping indoors, living with a dog (cats) and living in an area lacking sustained vector control.[250, 252] Clusters of disease can occur within local geographic areas (e.g. village), households or kennels.

Common clinical signs

Trypanosomiasis is a multisystem disease in dogs. In American trypanosomiasis, cardiac disease is most common and may present as acute or chronic myocarditis, arrhythmias or sudden death. Neurologic disease can also occur. Other dogs may be subclinically infected for life and may (or may not) progress to overt clinical signs.

In the acute phase, fever, non-specific systemic signs (e.g. lethargy, weakness, decreased appetite), lymphadenopathy, pallor, diarrhea, and splenic or hepatic enlargement can be noted, particularly with puppies. Sudden death (usually cardiac disease) and neurologic signs (which may be confused with canine distemper) can occur within 30 days.[257] In older dogs, clinical signs are usually less severe.

Dogs that progress to chronic infection are typically subclinical (latent phase) for a time. Some dogs develop chronic myocarditis within 8–36 months, and ultimately display signs consistent with heart failure (first right-sided and then progressing to left-sided), similar to dilated cardiomyopathy.

In dogs with African trypanosomiasis, fever, edema and ascites can occur together with lethargy, inappetence, pallor and weight loss. Neurologic signs, lymphadenopathy, ocular signs or oculonasal discharge, bloody vomit or diarrhea may be noted.

Clinical disease has not been reported in cats, despite high seroprevalence in some areas.

Diagnosis

American trypanosomiasis should be considered in any dog with cardiac disease and a history of living in or travelling to an endemic area. African trypanosomiasis should be considered in persistently febrile dogs, especially with signs of edema or ascites, that live in endemic regions.

American trypanosomiasis

The CBC may be normal in the latent or chronic state. In the acute phase anemia, neutrophilia, lymphocytosis, eosinophilia and monocytosis can be noted.[257] In acute disease, trypanomastigotes may be observed. Visualization of the pathogen can be improved using buffy coat evaluation, together with Wright or Giemsa stains, and further improved by pelleting (intense centrifugation) technique and examination. In addition to blood smears, the parasite (amastigote or more likely trypanomastigote) may be identified in lymph nodes and effusions in acute infections. In chronic infection, cytology may be of low yield.

Serum biochemistry may be non-specific for inflammation and acute mycocarditis, such as increased alanine aminotransferase, aspartate transaminase, creatinine and urea. Urinalyses may be normal.

Electrocardiography may reveal tachycardia, ventricular arrhythmias and/or conduction abnormalities, e.g. atrioventricular or bundle-branch block.

Radiology/imaging may show evidence of cardiomegaly, congestive heart failure (effusion or edema) and organ (liver or spleen) enlargement. Echocardiography may show changes consistent with dilated cardiomyopathy.

Serology (immunofluorescent assay, enzyme-linked immunosorbent assay) is typically used for diagnosis, particularly during the latent and chronic stages of infection. Antibodies may be detected 15–30 days post-infection. Cross-reaction may occur with *Leishmania* (exposure or vaccination) and confuse diagnosis.[258] In these cases (and when the history is not helpful) two different testing methods are advised for clarification. All results must be interpreted in light of the clinical signs.

PCR (whole blood, plasma, pelleted sample, lymph node aspirate, heart sample or ascites) is considered the optimal and most sensitive route of diagnosis.[250, 254, 259] However, sensitivity may vary with level of parasitemia, co-pathogens or laboratory.

Xenodiagnosis (testing of parasite feces for the pathogen) may be used as a complement to serology and can identify canine feeding.

African trypanosomiasis

The most common CBC changes include anemia, thrombocytopenia, and lowered or raised white cell counts. Serum biochemistry may show azotemia, elevated liver enzymes and hyperglobulinemia with hypoalbuminemia.

Protozoal identification with cytology is typically used for diagnosis. Samples may be obtained from blood smears, fluid (ascites or edema) and aspirates (e.g. lymph node). PCR has been used to identify *Trypanosoma* spp.

Therapy
American trypanosomiasis
The acute phase of disease is rarely noted; however, treatment with benznidazole (5–10 mg/kg PO q24h for 2 months) and a glucocorticoid has been used to reduce arrhythmias and cardiac fibrosis. In chronic disease, specific anti-protozoal therapy is rarely beneficial, and treatment is directed at alleviation of clinical signs related to heart failure and reduction of arrhythmias.

African trypanosomiasis
Treatment with diminazene aceturate has been used for *T. brucei*; however, this may be difficult to obtain and relapses with drug resistance commonly occur. Isometamidium chloride has also been used with reported success as chemoprophylaxis.[260]

Prognosis/complications
Prognosis is based on severity of presenting clinical signs; however, it is typically poor because of the lack of curative therapy and treatment options, and rapidly progressive disease. Older dogs with American trypanosomiasis (mean 9 years) usually survive longer than younger dogs.

Public health
American trypanosomiasis is a zoonotic concern, particularly in rural areas with low standards of housing and hygiene, the presence of domestic animals (e.g. chickens, goats, pigs) and a lack of vector control programs. In these areas dogs and cats can serve as reservoirs for human infection and should be kept outside, as increased risk has been associated with increased numbers of household dogs. Dogs and cats may also serve as sentinels for human disease risk.

Veterinarians and clinic staff should take precautions in suspected cases, and lab workers should be notified when handling samples. Any potential exposure (e.g. needle stick) should be immediately reported to public health authorities.

Canine African trypanosomiasis species rarely infect humans. However, care should be taken by personnel such as lab workers and veterinary staff, who have the potential for needlestick injury or other high-risk blood exposures.

TULAREMIA (*FRANCISELLA TULARENSIS*)
Dennis Spann

Definition

Francisella tularensis is an aerobic, gram-negative, non-spore-forming, non-motile coccobacillus (**Fig. 6.87**). Tularemia is a highly infectious multisystemic disease that develops when *F. tularensis* infects an animal via ingestion, animal or insect bites, contact with infected tissues, contaminated water, soil or inhalation. Subspecies include: *F. tularensis tularensis, holartica, mediasiatica* and *novicida*. *F. tularensis* creates a febrile glandulo-ulcerative disease with high morbidity. Cats are more commonly affected than dogs. Chronically infected rodents and rabbits likely serve as a reservoir for zoonotic outbreaks. Cats most frequently contract tularemia by preying on infected rabbits, as well as voles or other rodent hosts.

Etiology and pathogenesis

Tularemia is predominately an acute febrile illness that occurs after ingestion (e.g. consumption of infected tissues, food or water), inhalation (e.g. after aerosolization from close contact with infected animals or animal tissues aerosolized by lawnmowers or other equipment), arthropod transfer (various biting insects, including biting flies, mosquitoes, and *Ixodes, Dermacentor* and *Amblyomma* ticks) (**Fig. 6.88**), or direct contact between mucous membranes or broken skin and the bacterium. The incubation period is 1–10 days.

Only a few organisms (10–50 bacteria) are required to create an infection. The organism can survive in the environment for extended periods in water, soil, food and carcasses, and is highly resistant to freezing. An ulcer often develops at the site of infection. Bacteria are phagocytized by macrophages, where they evade reactive oxygen species and replicate in the cytoplasm before being released to infect other cells. Bacteria initially spread to local lymph nodes before spreading systemically.

Geography

Francisella tularensis has worldwide distribution but is found focally within endemic countries. Occurrence is predominately in the northern hemisphere, in North America and Eurasia, although a case has been reported in Australia. In North America, tularemia is caused by infection with either *F. tularensis* subspecies *tularensis* (type A) or *F. tularensis* subspecies *holarctica* (type B); however, in Eurasia type A is not observed and the primary subspecies is type B.

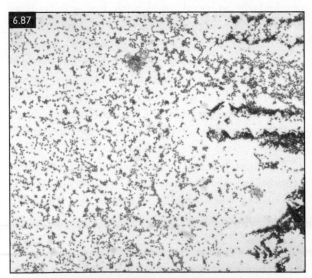

Fig. 6.87 Gram stain of *Francisella tularensis*. (Courtesy of PHIL CDC/Larry Stauffer, Oregon State Public Health Laboratory)

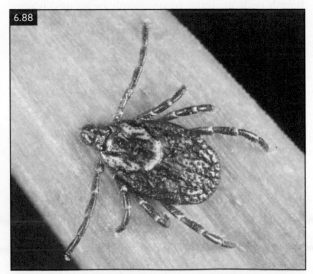

Fig. 6.88 *Dermacentor variabilis* is one of several biting insects that is competent to transmit *Francisella tularensis*. (Courtesy of CDC Public Health Image Library)

Incidence and risk factors

Tularemia is a rare disease worldwide. It is associated with lagomorphs, beavers, squirrels, voles and musk-rats. Hunting rodents and lagomorphs, tick and deer fly exposure are risk factors for infection. Biting flies are a greater risk factor in the western United States, whereas, from the Rocky Mountains east, ticks are more commonly a risk. Hot summer weather may be associated with increased outbreaks of tularemia due to intensified biting insect activity. There appears to be a bimodal distribution of cases in cats, in the spring and fall.[261] Serologic studies in the Midwest have identified that 8% of cats have antibodies to *F. tularensis.*[261, 262]

Clinical signs

Disease is usually acute, but chronic infections can occur, particularly in dogs and humans. Systemic disease can be ulcerative, ulceroglandular, typhoidal and/or pneumonic. Septicemia is often reported in susceptible animals, but subclinical infections may also be common, especially in more resistant species such as dogs and cattle.

Disease affecting the liver, spleen and lymphoreticular organs is common. The pathologic lesion is necrosis. Animals can develop disseminated intravascular coagulation, systemic inflammatory response syndrome and multiple organ dysfunction syndrome (**Fig. 6.89**).

In cats, anorexia, dehydration, lethargy, icterus, draining abscesses, orolingual ulceration, white patches, tachypnea, lymphadenomegaly, hepatomegaly and splenomegaly are common. In dogs, more subtle signs such as fever, lethargy, lymphadeno-megaly and ocular discharge may develop.

Diagnosis

A presumptive clinical diagnosis is made from appropriate clinical signs in endemic regions where there is a history of exposure to rabbits and rodents, or areas that could be frequented by them or contaminated with their carcasses. Hematologic changes are non-specific, and may include elevated alanine aminotransferase, alkaline phosphatase and bilirubin. Marked neutrophilia is common, although neutropenia and thrombocytopenia can also occur. Bilirubinuria and hemoglobinuria may be present.

Definitive diagnosis is based on bacterial culture, direct immunofluorescence (**Fig. 6.90**), serology, enzyme-linked immunosorbent assay or PCR. Culture should be performed only by specialized facilities. PCR technologies promise to be the most rapid, sensitive, specific and safe techniques for diagnosis.

Therapy

Supportive care is essential, along with prompt antimicrobial therapy. Infection control practices should include the use of protective outerwear (gowns, gloves, mask and eye protection) and isolation. Streptomycin, gentamicin, doxycycline and ciprofloxacin are all used for humans. Streptomycin is the drug of choice in humans, but is not readily available. Consequently, gentamicin is usually considered the most suitable alternative (*Table 6.39*).

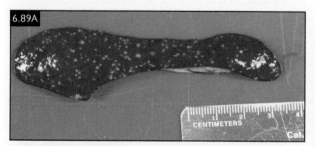

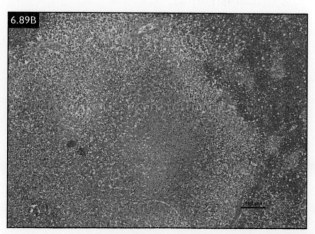

Fig. 6.89 (A) Spleen of a cat with multiple organ dysfunction syndrome caused by tularemia. The white spots are areas of intense inflammation and necrosis. (B) Histology of splenic lesions. (Courtesy of Dr Jerome Nietfeld)

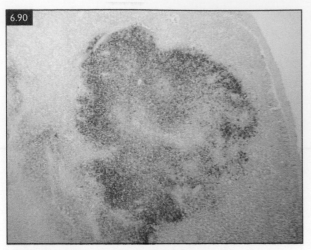

Fig. 6.90 Immunohistochemical stain of
F. tularensis. (Courtesy of Dr Jerome Nietfeld)

Table 6.39 **Treatment options for tularemia**

DRUG	SPECIES	DOSE
Gentamicin	Cat	5–8 mg/kg IM/IV/SC q24h for 14 days
	Dog	9–12 mg/kg IM/IV/SC q24h for 14 days
Marbofloxacin	Cats	2.75–5.5 mg/kg PO q24h for 14–21 days
Enrofloxacin	Dogs	10 mg/kg PO q24h for 14–21 days
Doxycycline	Dogs and cats	5 mg/kg PO q12h for 14–21 days

Prognosis/complications

Prognosis is fair to good with treatment. Fatalities still occur.

Prevention

Prevention of cats from hunting, and tick and fly control decrease transmission of *F. tularensis* and other vector-borne pathogens. Avoidance of feeding raw rabbit meat, mowing over carcasses in long grass, and wearing masks and safety glasses while mowing tall grass or dressing rabbit carcasses is advised for prevention.

Public health and infection control

Animals suspected of having tularemia should be isolated and handled with contact precautions, including dedicated outerwear, gloves, and respiratory and eye protection (e.g. mask and goggles or face shield). The bacterium is susceptible to routine disinfectants, if they are used properly.

REFERENCES

1 McHugh, KE *et al.* (2017) The cytopathology of *Actinomyces*, *Nocardia*, and their mimickers. *Diagn Cytopathol* **45**:1105–15.

2 Sykes, J (2014) Anaerobic bacterial infections. In *Canine and Feline Infectious Diseases*. J Sykes, ed. Elsevier, St. Louis, MO, pp.364–71.

3 Greene, CE *et al.* (2012) Anaerobic infections. In *Infectious Diseases of the Dog and Cat*. CE Greene, ed. Elsevier, St. Louis, MO, pp.411–16.

4 Jang, SS *et al.* (1997) Organisms isolated from dogs and cats with anaerobic infections and susceptibility to selected antimicrobial agents. *J Am Vet Med Assoc* **210**:1610–14.

5 Barenfanger, J *et al.* (2002) Outcomes of improved anaerobic techniques in clinical microbiology. *Clin Infect Dis* **35**:S78–83.

6 Lawhon, SD *et al.* (2013) Frequency of resistance in obligate anaerobic bacteria isolated from dogs, cats, and horses to antimicrobial agents. *J Clin Microbiol* **51**:3804–10.

7 Greiner, M *et al.* (2007) Bacteraemia in 66 cats and antimicrobial susceptibility of the isolates (1995–2004). *J Feline Med Surg* **9**:404–10.

8 Greiner, M *et al.* (2007) Bacteraemia and antimicrobial susceptibility in dogs. *Vet Rec* **160**:529–30.

9 Conboy, G (2004) Natural infections of *Crenosoma vulpis* and *Angiostrongylus vasorum* in dogs in Atlantic Canada and their treatment with milbemycin oxime. *Vet Rec* **155**:16–18.

10 Morgan, ER *et al.* (2008) *Angiostrongylus vasorum* and *Eucoleus aerophilus* in foxes (*Vulpes vulpes*) in Great Britain. *Vet Parasitol* **154**:48–57.

11 Koch, J *et al.* (2009) Canine pulmonary angiostrongylosis: an update. *Vet J* **179**:348–59.

12 Willesen, JL *et al.* (2009) Haematological and biochemical changes in dogs naturally infected with

Angiostrongylus vasorum before and after treatment. *Vet J* **180**:106–11.

13 Chapman, PS *et al.* (2004) *Angiostrongylus vasorum* infection in 23 dogs (1999–2002). *J Small Anim Pract* **45**:435–40.

14 Birkenhauer, A (2014) Babesiosis. In *Canine and Feline Infectious Diseases*. J Sykes, ed. Elsevier, St. Louis, MO, pp.727–38.

15 Birkenheuer, AJ *et al.* (2005) Geographic distribution of babesiosis among dogs in the United States and association with dog bites: 150 cases (2000–2003). *J Am Vet Med Assoc* **227**: 942–7.

16 Stegeman, JR *et al.* (2003) Transfusion-associated *Babesia gibsoni* infection in a dog. *J Am Vet Med Assoc* **222**:959–63, 952.

17 Böhm, M *et al.* (2006) Capillary and venous *Babesia canis rossi* parasitaemias and their association with outcome of infection and circulatory compromise. *Vet Parasitol* **141**:18–29.

18 Eichenberger, RM *et al.* (2016) Prognostic markers in acute *Babesia canis* infections. *J Vet Intern Med* **30**: 174–82.

19 Penzhorn, BL *et al.* (2004) Feline babesiosis in South Africa – A review. *Ann N Y Acad Sci* **1026**:183–6.

20 Schoeman, T *et al.* (2001) Feline babesiosis: signalment, clinical pathology and co-infections. *J South Afr Vet Assoc* **72**:4–11.

21 Macintire, DK *et al.* (2002) *Babesia gibsoni* infection among dogs in the southeastern United States. *J Am Vet Med Assoc* **220**:325–9.

22 Tuttle, AD *et al.* (2003) Concurrent bartonellosis and babesiosis in a dog with persistent thrombocytopenia. *J Am Vet Med Assoc* **223**:1306–10.

23 Movilla, R *et al.* (2017) Molecular detection of vector-borne pathogens in blood and splenic samples from dogs with splenic disease. *Parasit Vectors* **10**:131.

24 Breitschwerdt, EB (2008) Feline bartonellosis and cat scratch disease. *Vet Immunol Immunopathol* **123**:167–71.

25 Lappin, MR *et al.* (2009) Presence of *Bartonella* species and *Rickettsia* species DNA in the blood, oral cavity, skin and claw beds of cats in the United States. *Vet Dermatol* **20**:509–14.

26 Hegarty, BC *et al.* (2014) Analysis of seroreactivity against cell culture-derived *Bartonella* spp. antigens in dogs. *J Vet Intern Med* **28**: 38–41.

27 Guptill, L (2010) Feline bartonellosis. *Vet Clin North Am Small Anim Pract* **40**:1073–90.

28 Guptill, L *et al.* (1997) Experimental infection of young specific pathogen-free cats with *Bartonella henselae*. *J Infect Dis* **176**: 206–16.

29 Breitschwerdt, EB (2014) Bartonellosis: One Health perspectives for an emerging infectious disease. *Inst Lab Anim Res J* **55**:46–58.

30 Guptill, L *et al.* (2004) Prevalence, risk factors, and genetic diversity of *Bartonella henselae* infections in pet cats in four regions of the United States. *J Clin Microbiol* **42**:652–9.

31 Stutzer, B *et al.* (2012) Chronic bartonellosis in cats: what are the potential implications? *J Feline Med Surg* **14**:612–21.

32 Chomel, BB *et al.* (2009) *Bartonella* endocarditis: a pathology shared by animal reservoirsand patients. *Ann N Y Acad Sci* **1166**:120–6.

33 Cockwill, KR *et al.* (2007) *Bartonella vinsonii* subsp. *berkhoffii* endocarditis in a dog from Saskatchewan. *Can Vet J* **48**:839–44.

34 Sykes, JE *et al.* (2006) Evaluation of the relationship between causative organisms and clinical characteristics of infective endocarditis in dogs: 71 cases (1992–2005). *J Am Vet Med Assoc* **228**:1723–34.

35 Sykes, J (2014) Bartonellosis. In *Canine and Feline Infectious Diseases*. J Sykes, ed. Elsevier, St. Louis, MO, pp.498–511.

36 Breitschwerdt, E *et al.* (2006) Canine bartonellosis. In *Infectious Diseases of the Dog and Cat*. CE Greene, ed. Saunders Elsevier, Philadephia, PA, pp.518–24.

37 Wardrop, KJ *et al.* (2005) Canine and feline blood donor screening for infectious disease. *J Vet Intern Med* **19**:135–42.

38 Greene, RT (2012) Coccidioidomycosis and paracoccidioidomycosis. In *Infectious Diseases of the Dog and Cat*, 4th ed. CE Greene, ed. Elsevier, St. Louis, MO, pp.634–45.

39 Sykes, J (2014) Coccidioidomycosis. In *Canine and Feline Infectious Diseases*, J. Sykes, ed. Elsevier, St. Louis, MO, pp.613–23.

40 Graupmann-Kuzma, A *et al.* (2008) Coccidioidomycosis in dogs and cats: a review. *J Am Vet Med Assoc* **44**:226–35.

41 Simões, DM *et al.* (2016) Retrospective analysis of cutaneous lesions in 23 canine and 17 feline cases of coccidiodomycosis seen in Arizona, USA (2009–2015). *Vet Dermatol* **27**:346–e87.

42 Davidson, AP *et al.* (1994) Canine coccidioidomycosis: 1970 to 1993. *5th International Conference on Coccidioidomycosis*, Stanford University, CA, pp.155–62.

43 Butkiewicz, CD *et al.* (2005) Risk factors associated with *Coccidioides* infection in dogs. *J Am Vet Med Assoc* **226**:1851–4.

44 Shubitz, LE *et al.* (2005) Incidence of *Coccidioides* infection among dogs residing in a region in which the organism is endemic. *J Am Vet Med Assoc* **226**:1846–50.

45 Mehrkens, LR *et al.* (2016) Clinicopathologic and histopathologic renal abnormalities in dogs with coccidioidomycosis. *J Vet Int Med* **30**:1667–71.

46 Ajithdoss, DK *et al.* (2011) Coccidioidomycosis presenting as a heart base mass in two dogs. *J Comp Pathol* **145**:132–7.

47 Ramírez-Romero, R *et al.* (2016) Coccidioidomycosis in biopsies with presumptive diagnosis of malignancy in dogs: report of three cases and comparative discussion of published reports. *Mycopathologia* **181**: 151–7.

48 Gaidici, A *et al.* (2009) Transmission of coccidioidomycosis to a human via a cat bite. *J Clin Microbiol* **47**:505–6.

49 Kohn, GJ *et al.* (1992) Acquisition of coccidioidomycosis at necropsy by inhalation of coccidioidal endospores. *Diagn Microbiol Infect Dis* **15**:527–30.

50 Angelakis, E *et al.* (2010) Q fever. *Vet Microbiol* **140**:297–309.

51 Shapiro, AJ *et al.* (2015) Seroprevalence of *Coxiella burnetii* in domesticated and feral cats in eastern Australia. *Vet Microbiol* **177**:154–61.

52 Komiya, T *et al.* (2003) Seroprevalence of *Coxiella burnetii* infections among cats in different living environments. *J Vet Med Sci* **65**:1047–8.

53 Buhariwalla, F *et al.* (1996) A dog-related outbreak of Q fever. *Clin Infect Dis* **23**:753–5.

54 Langley, JM *et al.* (1988) Poker players' pneumonia. An urban outbreak of Q fever following exposure to a parturient cat. *N Engl J Med* **319**:354–6.

55 La Scola, B *et al.* (1996) Serological cross-reactions between *Bartonella quintana*, *Bartonella henselae*, and *Coxiella burnetii*. *J Clin Microbiol* **34**: 2270–4.

56 Egberink, H *et al.* (2013) Coxiellosis/Q fever in cats: ABCD guidelines on prevention and management. *J Feline Med Surg* **15**:573–5.

57 Kopecny, L *et al.* (2013) Investigating *Coxiella burnetii* infection in a breeding cattery at the centre of a Q fever outbreak. *J Feline Med Surg* **15**:1037–45.

58 D'Amato, F *et al.* (2014) Draft genome sequence of *Coxiella burnetii* Dog Utad, a strain isolated from a dog-related outbreak of Q fever. *New Microbes New Infect* **2**:136–7.

59 Pennisi, MG *et al.* (2013) Cryptococcosis in cats: ABCD guidelines on prevention and management. *J Feline Med Surg* **15**:611–18.

60 Vorathavorn, VI *et al.* (2013) Cryptococcosis as an emerging systemic mycosis in dogs. *J Vet Emerg Crit Care* **23**:489–97.

61 Lester, SJ *et al.* (2011) Cryptococcosis: update and emergence of *Cryptococcus gattii*. *Vet Clin Pathol* **40**:4–17.

62 Trivedi, SR *et al.* (2011) Clinical features and epidemiology of cryptococcosis in cats and dogs in California: 93 cases (1988–2010). *J Am Vet Med Assoc* **239**:357–69.

63 Danesi, P *et al.* (2014) Molecular identity and prevalence of *Cryptococcus* spp. nasal carriage in asymptomatic feral cats in Italy. *Med Mycol* **52**:667–73.

64 Trivedi, SR *et al.* (2011) Feline cryptococcosis: impact of current research on clinical management. *J Feline Med Surg* **13**:163–72.

65 Duncan, CG *et al.* (2006) Evaluation of risk factors for *Cryptococcus gattii* infection in dogs and cats. *J Am Vet Med Assoc* **228**:377–82.

66 Lester, SJ *et al.* (2004) Clinicopathologic features of an unusual outbreak of cryptococcosis in dogs, cats, ferrets, and a bird: 38 cases (January to July 2003). *J Am Vet Med Assoc* **225**:1716–22.

67 Sykes, JE *et al.* (2010) Clinical signs, imaging features, neuropathology, and outcome in cats and dogs with central nervous system cryptococcosis from California. *J Vet Intern Med* **24**:1427–38.

68 Sherrill, MK *et al.* (2015) Cytauxzoonosis: diagnosis and treatment of an emerging disease. *J Feline Med Surg* **17**:940–8.

69 Thomas, JE *et al.* (2018) Minimum transmission time of *Cytauxzoon felis* by *Amblyomma americanum* to domestic cats in relation to duration of infestation, and investigation of ingestion of infected ticks as a potential route of transmission. *J Feline Med Surg* **20**:67–72.

70 Diaz-Reganon, D *et al.* (2017) Molecular detection of *Hepatozoon* spp. and *Cytauxzoon* sp. in domestic and stray cats from Madrid, Spain. *Parasit Vectors* **10**:112.

71 Rizzi, TE *et al.* (2015) Prevalence of *Cytauxzoon felis* infection in healthy cats from enzootic areas in Arkansas, Missouri, and Oklahoma. *Parasit Vectors* **8**:13.

72 Cohn, LA *et al.* (2011) Efficacy of atovaquone and azithromycin or imidocarb dipropionate in cats with acute cytauxzoonosis. *J Vet Intern Med* **25**:55–60.

73 Venco, L *et al.* (2015) Feline heartworm disease: a 'Rubik's-cube-like' diagnostic and therapeutic challenge. *J Vet Cardiol* **17**(Suppl 1):S190–201.

74 Little, SE *et al.* (2014) Canine infection with *Dirofilaria immitis*, *Borrelia burgdorferi*, *Anaplasma* spp., and *Ehrlichia* spp. in the United States, 2010–2012. *Parasit Vectors* **7**:257.

75 Bowman, DD *et al.* (2009) Heartworm biology, treatment, and control. *Vet Clin North Am Small Anim Pract* **39**:1127–58, vii.

76 Lorentzen, L *et al.* (2008) Incidence of positive heartworm antibody and antigen tests at IDEXX Laboratories: trends and potential impact on feline heartworm awareness and prevention. *Vet Parasitol* **158**:183–90.

77 Bové, CM *et al.* (2010) Outcome of minimally invasive surgical treatment of heartworm caval syndrome in dogs: 42 cases (1999–2007). *J Am Vet Med Assoc* **236**:187–92.

78 Neer, TM *et al.* (2002) Consensus statement on ehrlichial disease of small animals from the infectious disease study group of the ACVIM. *J Vet Intern Med* **16**: 309–15.

79 Savidge, C *et al.* (2016) *Anaplasma phagocytophilum* infection of domestic cats: 16 cases from the northeastern USA. *J Feline Med Surg* **18**:85–91.

80 Lappin, MR *et al.* (2015) Evidence of *Anaplasma phagocytophilum* and *Borrelia burgdorferi* infection in cats after exposure to wild-caught adult *Ixodes scapularis*. *J Vet Diagn Invest* **27**:522–5.

81 Harrus, S *et al.* (1997) Canine monocytic ehrlichiosis: a retrospective study of 100 cases, and an epidemiological investigation of prognostic indicators for the disease. *Vet Rec* **141**:360–3.

82 Harrus, S *et al.* (2011) Diagnosis of canine monocytotropic ehrlichiosis (*Ehrlichia canis*): an overview. *Vet J* **187**:292–6.

83 Carrade, DD *et al.* (2009) Canine granulocytic anaplasmosis: a review. *J Vet Intern Med* **23**:1129–41.

84 Gaunt, S *et al.* (2010) Experimental infection and co-infection of dogs with *Anaplasma platys* and *Ehrlichia canis:* hematologic, serologic and molecular findings. *Parasit Vectors* **3**:33.

85 Little, SE *et al.* (2010) *Ehrlichia ewingii* infection and exposure rates in dogs from the southcentral United States. *Vet Parasitol* **172**:355–60.

86 Shipov, A *et al.* (2008) Prognostic indicators for canine monocytic ehrlichiosis. *Vet Parasitol* **153**:131–8.

87 Komnenou, AA *et al.* (2007) Ocular manifestations of natural canine monocytic ehrlichiosis (*Ehrlichia canis*): a retrospective study of 90 cases. *Vet Ophthalmol* **10**: 137–42.

88 Neer, TM *et al.* (2006) Canine monocytotropic ehrlichiosis and neorickettsiosis. In *Infectious Diseases of the Dog and Cat*. CE Greene, ed. Saunders Elsevier, Philadelphia, PA, pp.203–16.

89 Gremiao, I *et al.* (2011) Treatment of refractory feline sporotrichosis with a combination of intralesional amphotericin B and oral itraconazole. *Aust Vet J* **89**:346–51.

90 Talbot, JJ *et al.* (2014) What causes canine sino-nasal aspergillosis? A molecular approach to species identification. *Vet J* **200**:17–21.

91 Barrs, VR *et al.* (2014) Feline aspergillosis. *Vet Clin North Am Small Anim Pract* **44**:51–73.

92 Barrs, VR *et al.* (2013) *Aspergillus felis* sp. nov., an emerging agent of invasive aspergillosis in humans, cats, and dogs. *PLoS ONE* **8**:e64871.

93 Schultz, RM *et al.* (2008) Clinicopathologic and diagnostic imaging characteristics of systemic aspergillosis in 30 dogs. *J Vet Intern Med* **22**:851–9.

94 Barrs, VR *et al.* (2012) Sinonasal and sino-orbital aspergillosis in 23 cats: aetiology, clinicopathological features and treatment outcomes. *Vet J* **191**:58–64.

95 Sykes, J (2014) Aspergillosis. In *Canine and Feline Infectious Diseases*. J Sykes, ed. Elsevier, St. Louis, MO, pp.633–48.

96 De Lorenzi, D *et al.* (2006) Diagnosis of canine nasal aspergillosis by cytological examination: a comparison of four different collection techniques. *J Small Anim Pract* **47**:316–19.

97 Saunders, JH *et al.* (2004) Radiographic, magnetic resonance imaging, computed tomographic, and rhinoscopic features of nasal aspergillosis in dogs. *J Am Vet Med Assoc* **225**:1703–12.

98 Pomrantz, JS *et al.* (2007) Comparison of serologic evaluation via agar gel immunodiffusion and fungal culture of tissue for diagnosis of nasal aspergillosis in dogs. *J Am Vet Med Assoc* **230**:1319–23.

99 Whitney, J *et al.* (2013) Evaluation of serum galactomannan detection for diagnosis of feline upper respiratory tract aspergillosis. *Vet Microbiol* **162**:180–5.

100 Billen, F *et al.* (2009) Comparison of the value of measurement of serum galactomannan and *Aspergillus*-specific antibodies in the diagnosis of canine sino-nasal aspergillosis. *Vet Microbiol* **133**:358–65.

101 Barrs, VR *et al.* (2015) Detection of *Aspergillus*-specific antibodies by agar gel double immunodiffusion and IgG ELISA in feline upper respiratory tract aspergillosis. *Vet J* **203**:285–9.

102 Garcia, RS *et al.* (2012) Sensitivity and specificity of a blood and urine galactomannan antigen assay for diagnosis of systemic aspergillosis in dogs. *J Vet Intern Med* **26**:911–19.

103 Peeters, D *et al.* (2008) Whole blood and tissue fungal DNA quantification in the diagnosis of canine sino-nasal aspergillosis. *Vet Microbiol* **128**:194–203.

104 Sharman, MJ *et al.* (2012) Sinonasal aspergillosis in dogs: a review. *J Small Anim Pract* **53**:434–44.

105 Corrigan, VK *et al.* (2016) Treatment of disseminated aspergillosis with posaconazole in 10 dogs. *J Vet Intern Med* **30**:167–73.

106 Greene, CE (2012) Aspergillosis and penicilliosis. In *Infectious Diseases of the Dog and Cat*, 4th ed. CE Greene, ed. Elsevier, St. Louis, MO, pp.651–66.

107 Meason-Smith, C *et al.* (2016) Characterization of the cutaneous mycobiota in healthy and allergic cats using next generation sequencing. *Vet Dermatol* **28**:71–e17.

108 Dye, C *et al.* (2009) *Alternaria* species infection in nine domestic cats. *J Feline Med Surg* **11**:332–6.

109 Evans, N *et al.* (2011) Focal pulmonary granuloma caused by *Cladophialophora bantiana* in a domestic short haired cat. *Med Mycol* **49**:194–7.

110 Singh, K *et al.* (2006) Fatal systemic phaeohyphomycosis caused by *Ochroconis gallopavum* in a dog (*Canis familaris*). *Vet Pathol* **43**:988–92.

111 Bentley, RT *et al.* (2011) Successful management of an intracranial phaeohyphomycotic fungal granuloma in a dog. *J Am Vet Med Assoc* **239**:480–5.

112 Tennant, K *et al.* (2004) Nasal mycosis in two cats caused by *Alternaria* species. *Vet Rec* **155**:368–70.

113 Chakrabarti, A *et al.* (2016) Brain abscess due to *Cladophialophora bantiana*: a review of 124 cases. *Med Mycol* **54**:111–19.

114 Booth, TM *et al.* (2000) Stifle abscess in a pony associated with *Mycobacterium smegmatis*. *Vet Rec* **147**:452–4.

115 Gleich, SE *et al.* (2009) Prevalence of feline immunodeficiency virus and feline leukaemia virus among client-owned cats and risk factors for infection in Germany. *J Feline Med Surg* **11**:985–92.

116 Levy, JK *et al.* (2007) Seroprevalence of *Dirofilaria immitis*, feline leukemia virus, and feline immunodeficiency virus infection among dogs and cats exported from the 2005 Gulf Coast hurricane disaster area. *J Am Vet Med Assoc* **231**:218–25.

117 Matteucci, D *et al.* (1993) Detection of feline immunodeficiency virus in saliva and plasma by cultivation and polymerase chain reaction. *J Clin Microbiol* **31**:494–501.

118 Allison, RW *et al.* (2003) Covert vertical transmission of feline immunodeficiency virus. *AIDS Res Hum Retroviruses* **19**:421–34.

119 Jordan, HL *et al.* (1998) Feline immunodeficiency virus is shed in semen from experimentally and naturally infected cats. *AIDS Res Hum Retroviruses* **14**:1087–92.

120 Ueland, K *et al.* (1992) No evidence of vertical transmission of naturally acquired feline immunodeficiency virus infection. *Vet Immunol Immunopathol* **33**:301–8.

121 Jordan, HL *et al.* (1998) Horizontal transmission of feline immunodeficiency virus with semen from seropositive cats. *J Reprod Immunol* **41**:341–57.

122 Burling, AN *et al.* (2017) Seroprevalences of feline leukemia virus and feline immunodeficiency virus infection in cats in the United States and Canada and risk factors for seropositivity. *J Am Vet Med Assoc* **251**:187–94.

123 Cohen, ND *et al.* (1990) Epizootiologic association between feline immunodeficiency virus infection and feline leukemia virus seropositivity. *J Am Vet Med Assoc* **197**:220–5.

124 Little, S *et al.* (2009) Seroprevalence of feline leukemia virus and feline immunodeficiency virus infection among cats in Canada. *Can Vet J* **50**:644–8.

125 Levy, J *et al.* (2008) 2008 American Association of Feline Practitioners' feline retrovirus management guidelines. *J Feline Med Surg* **10**:300–16.

126 Little, S *et al.* (2011) Feline leukemia virus and feline immunodeficiency virus in Canada: recommendations for testing and management. *Can Vet J* **52**:849–55.

127 Hartmann, K *et al.* (2007) Quality of different in-clinic test systems for feline immunodeficiency virus and feline leukaemia virus infection. *J Feline Med Surg* **9**:439–45.

128 Hosie, MJ *et al.* (2009) Feline immunodeficiency. ABCD guidelines on prevention and management. *J Feline Med Surg* **11**:575–84.

129 Little, S (2011) A review of feline leukemia virus and feline immunodeficiency virus seroprevalence in cats in Canada. *Vet Immunol Immunopathol* **143**:243–5.

130 Domenech, A *et al.* (2011) Use of recombinant interferon omega in feline retrovirosis: from theory to practice. *Vet Immunol Immunopathol* **143**:301–6.

131 Williams, BH *et al.* (2000) Coronavirus-associated epizootic catarrhal enteritis in ferrets. *J Am Vet Med Assoc* **217**:526–30.

132 Addie, D *et al.* (2009) Feline infectious peritonitis. ABCD guidelines on prevention and management. *J Feline Med Surg* **11**:594–604.

133 Kipar, A *et al.* (2010) Sites of feline coronavirus persistence in healthy cats. *J Gen Virol* **91**:1698–1707.

134 Chang, HW *et al.* (2010) Feline infectious peritonitis: insights into feline coronavirus pathobiogenesis and epidemiology based on genetic analysis of the viral 3c gene. *J Gen Virol* **91**:415–20.

135 Brown, MA *et al.* (2009) Genetics and pathogenesis of feline infectious peritonitis virus. *Emerg Infect Dis* **15**:1445–52.

136 Takano, T *et al.* (2011) Mutation of neutralizing/antibody-dependent enhancing epitope on spike protein and 7b gene of feline infectious peritonitis virus: influences of viral replication in monocytes/macrophages and virulence in cats. *Virus Res* **156**:72–80.

137 Rohrbach, BW *et al.* (2001) Epidemiology of feline infectious peritonitis among cats examined at veterinary medical teaching hospitals. *J Am Vet Med Assoc* **218**:1111–15.

138 Pesteanu-Somogyi, LD *et al.* (2006) Prevalence of feline infectious peritonitis in specific cat breeds. *J Feline Med Surg* **8**:1–5.

139 Worthing, KA *et al.* (2012) Risk factors for feline infectious peritonitis in Australian cats. *J Feline Med Surg* **14**:405–12.

140 Foley, JE *et al.* (1997) Risk factors for feline infectious peritonitis among cats in multiple-cat environments with endemic feline enteric coronavirus. *J Am Vet Med Assoc* **210**:1313–18.

141 Norris, JM *et al.* (2005) Clinicopathological findings associated with feline infectious peritonitis in Sydney, Australia: 42 cases (1990–2002). *Aust Vet J* **83**:666–73.

142 Addie, DD *et al.* (1995) Risk of feline infectious peritonitis in cats naturally infected with feline coronavirus. *Am J Vet Res* **56**:429–34.

143 Hartmann, K (2005) Feline infectious peritonitis. *Vet Clin North Am Small Anim Pract* **35**:39–79, vi.

144 Ishida, T *et al.* (2004) Use of recombinant feline interferon and glucocorticoid in the treatment of feline infectious peritonitis. *J Feline Med Surg* **6**:107–9.

145 Legendre, AM *et al.* (2009) Effect of polyprenyl immunostimulant on the survival times of three cats with the dry form of feline infectious peritonitis. *J Feline Med Surg* **11**:624–6.

146 Ritz, S *et al.* (2007) Effect of feline interferon-omega on the survival time and quality of life of cats with feline infectious peritonitis. *J Vet Intern Med* **21**:1193–7.

147 Pedersen, NC *et al.* (2018) Efficacy of a 3C-like protease inhibitor in treating various forms of acquired feline infectious peritonitis. *J Feline Med Surg* **20**:378–92.

148 Scherk, MA *et al.* (2013) 2013 AAFP Feline Vaccination Advisory Panel Report. *J Feline Med Surg* **15**:785–808.

149 Lauring, AS *et al.* (2001) Specificity in receptor usage by T-cell-tropic feline leukemia viruses: implications for the in vivo tropism of immunodeficiency-inducing variants. *J Virol* **75**:8888–98.

150 Nakata, R *et al.* (2003) Reevaluation of host ranges of feline leukemia virus subgroups. *Microbes Infect* **5**:947–50.

151 Stewart, MA *et al.* (1986) Nucleotide sequences of a feline leukemia virus subgroup A envelope gene and long terminal repeat and evidence for the recombinational origin of subgroup B viruses. *J Virol* **58**:825–34.

152 Gomes-Keller, MA *et al.* (2009) Fecal shedding of infectious feline leukemia virus and its nucleic acids: a transmission potential. *Vet Microbiol* **134**:208–17.

153 Pacitti, AM *et al.* (1986) Transmission of feline leukaemia virus in the milk of a non-viraemic cat. *Vet Rec* **118**:381–4.

154 Vobis, M *et al.* (2003) Evidence of horizontal transmission of feline leukemia virus by the cat flea (*Ctenocephalides felis*). *Parasitol Res* **91**:467–70.

155 Hofmann-Lehmann, R *et al.* (1998) Feline immunodeficiency virus (FIV) infection leads to increased incidence of feline odontoclastic resorptive lesions (FORL). *Vet Immunol Immunopathol* **65**:299–308.

156 Major, A *et al.* (2010) Exposure of cats to low doses of FeLV: seroconversion as the sole parameter of infection. *Vet Res* **41**:17.

157 O'Connor, TP, Jr *et al.* (1991) Report of the National FeLV/FIV Awareness Project. *J Am Vet Med Assoc* **199**:1348–53.

158 Gleich, S *et al.* (2009) Hematology and serum biochemistry of feline immunodeficiency virus-infected and feline leukemia virus-infected cats. *J Vet Intern Med* **23**:552–8.

159 de Mari, K *et al.* (2004) Therapeutic effects of recombinant feline interferon-omega on feline leukemia virus (FeLV)-infected and FeLV/feline immunodeficiency virus (FIV)-coinfected symptomatic cats. *J Vet Intern Med* **18**:477–82.

160 Hartmann, K *et al.* (1992) Use of two virustatica (AZT, PMEA) in the treatment of FIV and of FeLV seropositive cats with clinical symptoms. *Vet Immunol Immunopathol* **35**:167–75.

161 Nelson, P *et al.* (1995) Therapeutic effects of diethylcarbamazine and 3'-azido-3'-deoxythymidine on feline leukemia virus lymphoma formation. *Vet Immunol Immunopathol* **46**:181–94.

162 Addie, DD *et al.* (2000) Long-term impact on a closed household of pet cats of natural infection with feline coronavirus, feline leukaemia virus and feline immunodeficiency virus. *Vet Rec* **146**:419–24.

163 Vail, DM *et al.* (1998) Feline lymphoma (145 cases): proliferation indices, cluster of differentiation 3 immunoreactivity, and their association with prognosis in 90 cats. *J Vet Intern Med* **12**:349–54.

164 Lutz, H *et al.* (2009) Feline leukaemia. ABCD guidelines on prevention and management. *J Feline Med Surg* **11**:565–74.

165 Tasker, S *et al.* (2009) Description of outcomes of experimental infection with feline haemoplasmas: copy numbers, haematology, Coombs' testing and blood glucose concentrations. *Vet Microbiol* **139**:323–32.

166 Baumann, J *et al.* (2013) Establishment and characterization of a low-dose *Mycoplasma haemofelis* infection model. *Vet Microbiol* **167**:410–16.

167 Compton, SM *et al.* (2012) *Candidatus Mycoplasma haematoparvum* and *Mycoplasma haemocanis* infections in dogs from the United States. *Comp Immunol Microbiol Infect Dis* **35**:557–62.

168 do Nascimento, NC *et al.* (2012) *Mycoplasma haemocanis* – the canine hemoplasma and its feline counterpart in the genomic era. *Vet Res* **43**:66.

169 Hulme-Moir, KL *et al.* (2010) Use of real-time quantitative polymerase chain reaction to monitor antibiotic therapy in a dog with naturally acquired *Mycoplasma haemocanis* infection. *J Vet Diagn Invest* **22**: 582–7.

170 Aquino, LC *et al.* (2016) Analysis of risk factors and prevalence of haemoplasma infection in dogs. *Vet Parasitol* **221**:111–17.

171 Soto, F *et al.* (2017) Occurrence of canine hemotropic mycoplasmas in domestic dogs from urban and rural areas of the Valdivia Province, southern Chile. *Comp Immunol Microbiol Infect Dis* **50**:70–7.

172 Seneviratna, P *et al.* (1973) Transmission of *Haemobartonella canis* by the dog tick, *Rhipicephalus sanguineus*. *Res Vet Sci* **14**:112–14.

173 Ishak, AM *et al.* (2007) Prevalence of *Mycoplasma haemofelis*, "Candidatus *Mycoplasma haemominutum*", *Bartonella* species, *Ehrlichia* species, and *Anaplasma phagocytophilum* DNA in the blood of cats with anemia. *J Feline Med Surg* **9**:1–7.

174 Kamrani, A *et al.* (2008) The prevalence of *Bartonella*, hemoplasma, and *Rickettsia felis* infections in domestic cats and in cat fleas in Ontario. *Can J Vet Res* **72**:411–19.

175 Levy, JK *et al.* (2011) Prevalence of infectious diseases in cats and dogs rescued following Hurricane Katrina. *J Am Vet Med Assoc* **238**:311–17.

176 Novacco, M *et al.* (2010) Prevalence and geographical distribution of canine hemotropic mycoplasma infections in Mediterranean countries and analysis of risk factors for infection. *Vet Microbiol* **142**:276–84.

177 Tasker, S *et al.* (2003) Use of a PCR assay to assess the prevalence and risk factors for *Mycoplasma haemofelis* and "Candidatus *Mycoplasma haemominutum*" in cats in the United Kingdom. *Vet Rec* **152**:193–8.

178 Dowers, KL *et al.* (2009) Use of pradofloxacin to treat experimentally induced *Mycoplasma hemofelis* infection in cats. *Am J Vet Res* **70**:105–11.

179 Ishak, AM *et al.* (2008) Marbofloxacin for the treatment of experimentally induced *Mycoplasma haemofelis* infection in cats. *J Vet Intern Med* **22**:288–92.

180 Novacco, M *et al.* (2018) Consecutive antibiotic treatment with doxycycline and marbofloxacin clears bacteremia in *Mycoplasma haemofelis*-infected cats. *Vet Microbiol* **217**:112–20.

181 Dowers, KL *et al.* (2002) Use of enrofloxacin for treatment of large-form *Haemobartonella felis* in experimentally infected cats. *J Am Vet Med Assoc* **221**:250–3.

182 Wardrop, KJ *et al.* (2016) Update on canine and feline blood donor screening for blood-borne pathogens. *J Vet Intern Med* **30**:15–35.

183 Vincent-Johnson, NA (2003) American canine hepatozoonosis. *Vet Clin North Am Small Anim Pract* **33**:905–20.

184 Li, Y *et al.* (2008) Diagnosis of canine *Hepatozoon* spp. infection by quantitative PCR. *Vet Parasitol* **157**:50–8.

185 Panciera, RJ *et al.* (2000) Skeletal lesions of canine hepatozoonosis caused by *Hepatozoon americanum*. *Vet Pathol* **37**:225–30.

186 Sasanelli, M *et al.* (2010) Failure of imidocarb dipropionate to eliminate *Hepatozoon canis* in naturally infected dogs based on parasitological and molecular evaluation methods. *Vet Parasitol* **171**:194–9.

187 Macintire, DK *et al.* (2001) Treatment of dogs infected with *Hepatozoon americanum*: 53 cases (1989–1998). *J Am Vet Med Assoc* **218**:77–82.

188 Schumacher, LL *et al.* (2013) Canine intestinal histoplasmosis containing hyphal forms. *J Vet Diagn Invest* **25**:304–7.

189 Cunningham, L *et al.* (2015) Sensitivity and specificity of histoplasma antigen detection by enzyme immunoassay. *J Am Anim Hosp Assoc* **51**:306–10.

190 Wilson, AG *et al.* (2018) Clinical signs, treatment, and prognostic factors for dogs with histoplasmosis. *J Am Vet Med Assoc* **252**:201–9.

191 Schulman, RL *et al.* 1999. Use of corticosteroids for treating dogs with airway obstruction secondary to hilar lymphadenopathy caused by chronic histoplasmosis: 16 cases (1979–1997). *J Am Vet Med Assoc* **214**:1345–8.

192 Aulakh, HK *et al.* (2012) Feline histoplasmosis: a retrospective study of 22 cases (1986–2009). *J Am Anim Hosp Assoc* **48**:182–7.

193 Hodges, RD *et al.* (1994) Itraconazole for the treatment of histoplasmosis in cats. *J Vet Intern Med* **8**:409–13.

194 Reinhart, JM *et al.* (2012) Feline histoplasmosis: fluconazole therapy and identification of potential sources of *Histoplasma* species exposure. *J Feline Med Surg* **14**:841–8.

195 Vides, JP *et al.* (2011) *Leishmania chagasi* infection in cats with dermatologic lesions from an endemic area of visceral leishmaniosis in Brazil. *Vet Parasitol* **178**:22–8.

196 Vida, B *et al.* (2016) Immunologic progression of canine leishmaniosis following vertical transmission in United States dogs. *Vet Immunol Immunopathol* **169**:34–8.

197 Schantz, PM *et al.* (2005) Autochthonous visceral leishmaniasis in dogs in North America. *J Am Vet Med Assoc* **226**:1316–22.

198 Solano-Gallego, L *et al.* (2009) Directions for the diagnosis, clinical staging, treatment and prevention of canine leishmaniosis. *Vet Parasitol* **165**:1–18.

199 Cortes, S *et al.* (2012) Risk factors for canine leishmaniasis in an endemic Mediterranean region. *Vet Parasitol* **189**:189–96.

200 Paltrinieri, S *et al.* (2010) Guidelines for diagnosis and clinical classification of leishmaniasis in dogs. *J Am Vet Med Assoc* **236**:1184–91.

201 Torres, M *et al.* (2016) Adverse urinary effects of allopurinol in dogs with leishmaniasis. *J Small Anim Pract* **57**:299–304.

202 Decker, RA *et al.* (1976) Listeriosis in a young cat. *J Am Vet Med Assoc* **168**:1025.

203 Pritchard, JC *et al.* (2016) *Listeria monocytogenes* septicemia in an immunocompromised dog. *Vet Clin Pathol* **45**:254–9.

204 Raith, K *et al.* (2010) Encephalomyelitis resembling human and ruminant rhombencephalitis caused by *Listeria monocytogenes* in a feline leukemia virus-infected cat. *J Vet Intern Med* **24**:983–5.

205 Schroeder, H *et al.* (1993) Generalised *Listeria monocytogenes* infection in a dog. *J S Afr Vet Med Assoc* **64**:133–6.

206 Sturgess, CP (1989) Listerial abortion in the bitch. *Vet Rec* **124**:177.

207 Nemser, SM *et al.* (2014) Investigation of *Listeria*, *Salmonella*, and toxigenic *Escherichia coli* in various pet foods. *Foodborne Pathog Dis* **11**:706–9.

208 Burgess, EC (1992) Experimentally induced infection of cats with *Borrelia burgdorferi*. *Am J Vet Res* **53**:1507–11.

209 Levy, S *et al.* (2002) Utility of an in-office C6 ELISA test kit for determination of infection status of dogs naturally exposed to *Borrelia burgdorferi*. *Vet Ther* **3**:308–15.

210 Levy, SA *et al.* (2008) Quantitative measurement of C6 antibody following antibiotic treatment of *Borrelia burgdorferi* antibody-positive nonclinical dogs. *Clin Vaccine Immunol* **15**:115–19.

211 Magnarelli, LA *et al.* (2001) Reactivity of dog sera to whole-cell or recombinant antigens of *Borrelia burgdorferi* by ELISA and immunoblot analysis. *J Med Microbiol* **50**:889–95.

212 Summers, BA *et al.* (2005) Histopathological studies of experimental Lyme disease in the dog. *J Comp Pathol* **133**:1–13.

213 Dambach, DM *et al.* (1997) Morphologic, immunohistochemical, and ultrastructural characterization of a distinctive renal lesion in dogs putatively associated with *Borrelia burgdorferi* infection: 49 cases (1987–1992). *Vet Pathol* **34**:85–96.

214 Littman, MP (2013) Lyme nephritis. *J Vet Emerg Crit Care (San Antonio)* **23**:163–73.

215 Littman, MP *et al.* (2018) ACVIM consensus update on Lyme borreliosis in dogs and cats. *J Vet Intern Med* **32**:887–903.

216 Littman, MP *et al.* (2006) ACVIM small animal consensus statement on Lyme disease in dogs: diagnosis, treatment, and prevention. *J Vet Intern Med* **20**:422–34.

217 Gerber, B *et al.* (2007) Increased prevalence of *Borrelia burgdorferi* infections in Bernese Mountain Dogs: a possible breed predisposition. *BMC Vet Res* **3**:15.

218 Susta, L *et al.* (2012) Synovial lesions in experimental canine Lyme borreliosis. *Vet Pathol* **49**:453–61.

219 Headley, SA *et al.* (2011) *Neorickettsia helminthoeca* and salmon poisoning disease: a review. *Vet J* **187**:165–73.

220 Sykes, JE *et al.* (2010) Salmon poisoning disease in dogs: 29 cases. *J Vet Intern Med* **24**:504–13.

221 Gage, KL *et al.* (2000) Cases of cat-associated human plague in the Western US, 1977–1998. *Clin Infect Dis* **30**:893–900.

222 Eisen, RJ *et al.* (2008) Early-phase transmission of *Yersinia pestis* by cat fleas (*Ctenocephalides felis*) and their potential role as vectors in a plague-endemic region of Uganda. *Am J Trop Med Hyg* **78**:949–56.

223 Eidson, M *et al.* (1991) Clinical, clinicopathologic, and pathologic features of plague in cats: 119 cases (1977–1988). *J Am Vet Med Assoc* **199**:1191–7.

224 Doll, JM *et al.* (1994) Cat-transmitted fatal pneumonic plague in a person who traveled from Colorado to Arizona. *Am J Trop Med Hyg* **51**:109–14.

225 Gould, LH *et al.* (2008) Dog-associated risk factors for human plague. *Zoonoses Publ Hlth* **55**:448–54.

226 Thornton, DJ *et al.* (1975) Cat bite transmission of *Yersinia pestis* infection to man. *J S Afr Vet Med Assoc* **46**:165–9.

227 Weniger, BG *et al.* (1984) Human bubonic plague transmitted by a domestic cat scratch. *JAMA* **251**:927–8.

228 Stenner, VJ *et al.* (2007) Prototothecosis in 17 Australian dogs and a review of the canine literature. *Med Mycol* **45**:249–66.

229 Shank, AM *et al.* (2015) Canine ocular prototothecosis: a review of 14 cases. *Vet Ophthalmol* **18**:437–42.

230 Manino, PM *et al.* (2014) Disseminated prototothecosis associated with diskospondylitis in a dog. *J Am Anim Hosp Assoc* **50**:429–35.

231 Font, C *et al.* (2014) Paraparesis as initial manifestation of a *Prototheca zopfii* infection in a dog. *J Small Anim Pract* **55**:283–6.

232 Warner, RD *et al.* (2002) Rocky Mountain spotted fever. *J Am Vet Med Assoc* **221**:1413–17.

233 Gasser, AM *et al.* (2001) Canine Rocky Mountain Spotted fever: a retrospective study of 30 cases. *J Am Anim Hosp Assoc* **37**:41–8.

234 Ober, CP *et al.* (2004) Orchitis in two dogs with Rocky Mountain spotted fever. *Vet Radiol Ultrasound* **45**:458–65.

235 Breitschwerdt, EB *et al.* (1991) Efficacy of chloramphenicol, enrofloxacin, and tetracycline for treatment of experimental Rocky Mountain spotted fever in dogs. *Antimicrob Agents Chemother* **35**:2375–81.

236 Breitschwerdt, EB *et al.* (1999) Efficacy of doxycycline, azithromycin, or trovafloxacin for treatment of experimental Rocky Mountain spotted fever in dogs. *Antimicrob Agents Chemother* **43**:813–21.

237 Brown, DC *et al.* (1997) Epidemiologic evaluation of postoperative wound infections in dogs and cats. *J Am Vet Med Assoc* **210**:1302–6.

238 Eugster, S *et al.* (2004) A prospective study of postoperative surgical site infections in dogs and cats. *Vet Surg* **33**:542–50.

239 Frey, TN *et al.* (2010) Risk factors for surgical site infection-inflammation in dogs undergoing surgery for rupture of the cranial cruciate ligament: 902 cases (2005–2006). *J Am Vet Med Assoc* **236**:88–94.

240 Nicholson, M *et al.* (2002) Epidemiologic evaluation of postoperative wound infection in clean-contaminated wounds: a retrospective study of 239 dogs and cats. *Vet Surg* **31**:577–81.

241 Turk, R *et al.* (2011) Post-hospital discharge procedure-specific surgical site infection surveillance in small animal patients. *2nd ASM/ESCMID Conference on methicillin-resistant staphylococci in animals*, September 8–11, 2011, Washington, DC.

242 Nicoll, C *et al.* (2014) Economic impact of tibial plateau leveling osteotomy surgical site infection in dogs. *Vet Surg* **43**:899–902.

243 Jones, JL *et al.* (2014) *Toxoplasma gondii* seroprevalence in the United States 2009–2010 and comparison with the past two decades. *Am J Trop Med Hyg* **90**:1135–9.

244 Lykins, J *et al.* (2016) Understanding toxoplasmosis in the United States through "large data" analyses. *Clin Infect Dis* **63**:468–75.

245 Vollaire, MR *et al.* (2005) Seroprevalence of *Toxoplasma gondii* antibodies in clinically ill cats in the United States. *Am J Vet Res* **66**:874–77.

246 Cook, AJ *et al.* (2000) Sources of *Toxoplasma* infection in pregnant women: European multicentre case–control study. European Research Network on Congenital Toxoplasmosis. *BMJ* **321**:142–7.

247 Jones, JL *et al.* (2014) Neglected parasitic infections in the United States: toxoplasmosis. *Am J Trop Med Hyg* **90**:794–9.

248 Foster, S (2016) Dealing with toxoplasmosis: clinical presentation, diagnosis, treatment, and prevention. In *August Consultations in Feline Internal Medicine*, SE Little, ed. Elsevier, St. Louis, MO, pp.73–83.

249 Dubey, JP *et al.* (2012) Toxoplasmosis and neosporosis. In *Infectious Diseases of the Dog and Cat*, 4th ed. CE Greene, ed. Elsevier Saunders, St. Louis, MO, pp.807–21.

250 Curtis-Robles, R *et al.* (2017) Epidemiology and molecular typing of *Trypanosoma cruzi* in naturally-infected hound dogs and associated triatomine vectors in Texas, USA. *PLoS Negl Trop Dis* **11**:e0005298.

251 Cruz-Chan, JV *et al.* (2010) *Dirofilaria immitis* and *Trypanosoma cruzi* natural co-infection in dogs. *Vet J* **186**:399–401.

252 Cardinal, MV *et al.* (2007) Impact of community-based vector control on house infestation and *Trypanosoma cruzi* infection in *Triatoma infestans*, dogs and cats in the Argentine Chaco. *Acta Trop* **103**:201–11.

253 Cardinal, MV *et al.* (2006) A prospective study of the effects of sustained vector surveillance following community-wide insecticide application on *Trypanosoma cruzi* infection of dogs and cats in rural Northwestern Argentina. *Am J Trop Med Hyg* **75**:753–61.

254 Ramirez, JD *et al.* (2013) Understanding the role of dogs (*Canis lupus familiaris*) in the transmission dynamics of *Trypanosoma cruzi* genotypes in Colombia. *Vet Parasitol* **196**:216–19.

255 Rosypal, AC *et al.* (2007) Serological survey of *Leishmania infantum* and *Trypanosoma cruzi* in dogs from urban areas of Brazil and Colombia. *Vet Parasitol* **149**:172–7.

256 Rosypal, AC *et al.* (2007) Prevalence of antibodies to *Leishmania infantum* and *Trypanosoma cruzi* in wild canids from South Carolina. *J Parasitol* **93**:955–7.

257 Quijano-Hernandez, IA *et al.* (2013) Preventive and therapeutic DNA vaccination partially protect dogs against an infectious challenge with *Trypanosoma cruzi*. *Vaccine* **31**:2246–52.

258 Troncarelli, MZ *et al.* (2009) *Leishmania* spp. and/or *Trypanosoma cruzi* diagnosis in dogs from endemic and nonendemic areas for canine visceral leishmaniasis. *Vet Parasitol* **164**:118–23.

259 Enriquez, GF *et al.* (2013) Detection of *Trypanosoma cruzi* infection in naturally infected dogs and cats using serological, parasitological and molecular methods. *Acta Trop* **126**:211–17.

260 Watier-Grillot, S *et al.* (2013) Chemoprophylaxis and treatment of African canine trypanosomosis in French military working dogs: a retrospective study. *Vet Parasitol* **194**:1–8.

261 Mani, RJ *et al.* (2016) Ecology of tularemia in central US endemic region. *Curr Trop Med Rep* **3**:75–9.

262 Larson, MA *et al.* (2014) *Francisella tularensis* bacteria associated with feline tularemia in the United States. *Emerg Infect Dis* **20**:2068–71.

Note: Page numbers in *italic* refer to content of tables

Printed and bound by CPI Group (UK) Ltd, Croydon, CR0 4YY

17/10/2024

01775663-0011